Handbook of
Systemic Autoimmune Diseases

Volume 4

Reproductive and Hormonal Aspects of Systemic Autoimmune Diseases

Edited by:

Michael Lockshin
Hospital of Special Surgery
Barbara Volcker Centre, New York, USA

and

D. Ware Branch
Department of Obstetrics and Synecology
University of Utah, Salt Lake City, USA

Series Editor

Ronald A. Asherson

ELSEVIER

Amsterdam – Boston – Heidelberg – London – New York – Oxford
Paris – San Diego – San Francisco – Singapore – Sydney – Tokyo

ELSEVIER B.V.

P.O. Box 211, 1000 AE
Amsterdam. The Netherlands

ELSEVIER Inc.
525 B Street
Suite 1900. San Diego
CA 92101-4495, USA

ELSEVIER Ltd.
The Boulevard
Langford Lane, Kidlington,
Oxford OX5 1GB, UK

ELSEVIER Ltd.
84 Theobalds Road
London WC1X 8RR
UK

First edition 2006

Library of Congress Cataloging in Publication Data
A catalog record is available from the Library of Congress.

British Library Cataloguing in Publication Data
A catalogue record is available from the British Library.

ISBN-13: 978-0-444-51801-9
ISBN-10: 0-444-51801-0
ISSN: 1571-5078 (Series)

Transferred to digital printing 2008

Series Editor

Ronald A. Asherson

Dr Ronald A Asherson, MD, FACP, MD (Hon), FRCP (London), FCP (SA), FACR, is Honorary Consultant Physician at the Rheumatic Disease Unit, Department of Medicine, University of Cape Town Health Sciences Centre in Cape Town, as well as being Consultant Rheumatologist at the Rosebank Clinic in Johannesburg, South Africa. He is also a Visiting Professor at the Systemic Autoimmune Diseases Unit at the Hospital Clinic, Barcelona, Spain where he regularly visits and coordinates research projects.

From 1976 to 1981 he was Assistant Clinical Professor of Medicine at the New York Hospital – Cornell Medical Center in New York under the late Professor Henry Heineman. From 1981 to 1986 he was associated with the Rheumatology Department at the Royal Postgraduate Medical School of London where he developed his interests in connective tissue diseases and antiphospholipid antibodies.

In 1986 he moved to the Rayne Institute and St Thomas' Hospital in London, where he was appointed Honorary Consultant Physician and Senior Research Fellow and remained there until 1991.

In 1998 he was elected as Fellow of the American College of Physicians (FACP) as well as a Founding Fellow of the American College of Rheumatology (FACR). From 1988 to 1991 he served on the Council of the Royal Society of Medicine in London. In 1992 he was co-winner of the European League Against Rheumatism (EULAR) Prize and in 1993 was the co-recipient of the International League Against Rheumatism (ILAR) Prize, both for his research on antiphospholipid antibodies. In 1994 he was elected as a Fellow of the Royal College of Physicians (FRCP) of London. In 2002 he was awarded an Honorary Doctorate in Medicine from the University of Pleven in Bulgaria.

Dr Asherson has been an invited speaker at many universities and on the Scientific Committees of many international conferences both in the USA and Europe. He is the author of more than 280 papers on connective tissue diseases and has contributed to more than 30 textbooks of medicine, rheumatology and surgery as well as having co-edited "*Problems in the Rheumatic Diseases*", the "*Phospholipid Binding Antibodies*", two editions of "*The Antiphospholipid Syndrome*" and "*Vascular Manifestations of the Systemic Autoimmune Diseases*" He is on the Editorial Boards of many international and Internet Rheumatology journals. He is currently engaged in research on connective tissue diseases, particularly on the antiphospholipid syndrome. In 1999, he was the co-recipient of the Juan Vivancos Prize in Spain and in 2003 was the co-recipient of the Abbott Prize, awarded at the European League Against Rheumatism (EULAR) International Meeting, held in Lisbon, Portugal. In September 2003 was Co-Chairman of the First Latin American Congress on Autoimmunity, held in the Galapagos Islands, Ecuador. In 2005, he was honored by the South African Rheumatism and Arthritis Association and made a Life Member.

His original description of the "Catastrophic Antiphospholipid Syndrome" and the publishing of more than 40 papers on this new disease was rewarded by the attachment of the eponym "Asherson's Syndrome" to this condition at the November 2002 International Phospholipid Conference held in Sicily.

He is currently Series Editor of 12 volumes entitled "The Handbook of Systemic Autoimmune Disease" (Elsevier, Holland).

Volume Editors

Michael D. Lockshin

Dr. Lockshin received his bachelor's and medical degrees from Harvard University, the latter in 1963, and his clinical training in New York. He joined the Hospital for Special Surgery and Cornell University Medical College in 1970, rising to the position of Professor of Medicine and Attending Physician. In 1989 he moved to the National Institutes of Health where he was Extramural Director, then Acting Director of the National Institute of Arthritis and Musculoskeletal and Skin Diseases, National Institutes of Health, before returning to the Hospital for Special Surgery in 1997 as Director of the Barbara Volcker Center for Women and Rheumatic Diseases, Co-Director of the Mary Kirkland Center for Lupus Research, and Professor of Medicine and Obstetrics-Gynecology.

Dr. Lockshin's research interests have focused on systemic lupus erythematosus, antiphospholipid antibody syndrome, especially pregnancy and lupus and antiphospholipid antibody syndrome. His most recent interests have been on sex distribution of disease. He is the author of more than 230 scientific papers and textbook chapters and a book on health policy, *Guarded Prognosis.* He was a member of the Institute of Medicine Committee on Understanding the Biology of Sex and Gender Differences. He is now Editor-in-Chief, *Arthritis & Rheumatism.*

List of Contributors

Kjersti M. Aagaard-Tillery
Division of Maternal-Fetal Medicine, Department of Obstetrics and Gynecology, University of Utah Health Sciences Center, Salt Lake City, UT, USA

D.W. Branch
Department of Obstetrics and Gynecology, Division of Maternal Fetal Medicine, University of Utah Health Sciences Center, Salt Lake City, UT, USA

Chiara Briani
Department of Neurosciences, University of Padova, Italy

Antonio Brucato
Department of Internal Medicine, Niguarda Hospital, Milano, Italy

Jill P. Buyon
Division of Rheumatology, Hospital for Joint Diseases, New York University School of Medicine, New York, NY, USA

Rolando Cimaz
Istituti Clinici di Perfezionamento, Milano, Italy

Megan E.B. Clowse
Division of Rheumatology, Johns Hopkins School of Medicine, Baltimore, MD, USA

Andrea Doria
Division of Rheumatology, Department of Clinical and Experimental Sciences, University of Padova, Italy

David Faden
Department of Obstetrics and Gynecology, General Hospital and University of Brescia, Brescia, Italy

Micol Frassi
Rheumatology and Clinical Immunology, General Hospital and University of Brescia, Brescia, Italy

Pier Franca Gambari
Division of Rheumatology, Department of Clinical and Experimental Sciences, University of Padova, Italy

Anna Ghirardello
Division of Rheumatology, Department of Clinical and Experimental Sciences, University of Padova, Italy

Shawn Gurtcheff
General Division of Obstetrics and Gynecology, Department of Obstetrics and Gynecology, University of Utah Health Sciences Center, Salt Lake City, UT, USA

Harry Hatasaka
Division of Reproductive Endocrinology, Department of Obstetrics and Gynecology, University of Utah Health Sciences Center, Salt Lake City, UT, USA

Calla M. Holmgren
Division of Maternal-Fetal Medicine, Department of Obstetrics and Gynecology, University of Utah Health Sciences Center, Salt Lake City, UT, USA

Luca Iaccarino
Division of Rheumatology, Department of Clinical and Experimental Sciences, University of Padova, Italy

Nathalie C. Lambert
Laboratoire d'Immuno-Rhumatologie, INSERM U639, Marseille Cedex France

Roger A. Levy
Disciplina de Reumatologia, Faculdade de Ciências Médicas, Universidade do Estado do Rio de Janeiro, RJ, Brasil

M. Lockshin
Department of Rheumatology, Hospital for Special Surgery, New York City, NY, USA

Michael D. Lockshin
Joan and Sanford Weill Medical College of Cornell University, Hospital for Special Surgery, New York, NY, USA

Andrea Lojacono
Department of Obstetrics and Gynecology, General Hospital and University of Brescia, Brescia, Italy

Pierluigi Meroni
IRCCS Ist. Auxologico University of Milan, Milano, Italy

Mario Motta
Neonatal Intensive Care Unit, General Hospital and University of Brescia, Brescia, Italy

Michelle Petri
Division of Rheumatology, Johns Hopkins School of Medicine, Baltimore, MD, USA

Chiara Biasini Rebaioli
Rheumatology and Clinical Immunology, General Hospital and University of Brescia, Brescia, Italy

Ann M. Reed
Department of Medicine and Pediatrics, Mayo Clinic, Rochester, MN, USA

Lisa R. Sammaritano
Department of Medicine, Weill Medical College of Cornell University, Hospital for Special Surgery, New York, NY, USA

James R. Scott
Division of General Obstetrics and Gynecology, Department of Obstetrics and Gynecology, University of Utah Health Sciences Center, Salt Lake City, UT, USA

Felicia Tenedios
Hospital for Special Surgery, Weill Medical College of Cornell University, New York, NY, USA

Angela Tincani
Rheumatology and Clinical Immunology, General Hospital and University of Brescia, Brescia, Italy

Sandra Zampieri
Division of Rheumatology, Department of Clinical and Experimental Sciences, University of Padova, Italy

Sonia Zatti
Department of Obstetrics and Gynecology, General Hospital and University of Brescia, Brescia, Italy

Contents

Series Editor v
Volume Editors vii
List of Contributors ix

Introduction 1
D. Ware Branch

Sex Differences in Autoimmune Disease 3
Michael D. Lockshin

Maternal–Fetal Aspects of Autoimmune Disease 11
Nathalie C. Lambert, Ann M. Reed

Fertility and Autoimmune Disease 29
Shawn Gurtcheff, Harry Hatasaka

Pregnancy and Systemic Lupus Erythematosus 43
Megan E.B. Clowse, Michelle Petri

Antiphospholipid Syndrome 59
D.W. Branch, M. Lockshin

Pregnancy in Rheumatoid Arthritis, Sjögren Syndrome and Other Rare Autoimmune Rheumatic Diseases 77
Andrea Doria, Luca Iaccarino, Anna Ghirardello, Chiara Briani, Sandra Zampieri, Angela Tincani, Pier Franca Gambari

A Bedside Perspective of Neonatal Lupus 95
Jill P. Buyon

Use of Anti-Rheumatic Drugs in Pregnancy 101
Roger A. Levy

Offspring of Women with Systemic Autoimmune Diseases: Fetal and Neonatal Complications and Inheritance of Autoimmune Diseases 111
Chiara Biasini Rebaioli, Mario Motta, Micol Frassi, Antonio Brucato, Rolando Cimaz, Pierluigi Meroni, Andrea Doria, Andrea Lojacono, Sonia Zatti, David Faden, Angela Tincani

Contraception in Women with Autoimmune Diseases 123
Lisa R. Sammaritano

Gynecologic Problems in Women with Autoimmune Diseases 141
Kjersti M. Aagaard-Tillery, Calla M. Holmgren, James R. Scott

The Climacteric and Osteoporosis in Women with Autoimmune Diseases 161
Felicia Tenedios

Index 181

Handbook of Systemic Autoimmune Diseases, Volume 4
Reproductive and Hormonal Aspects of Systemic Autoimmune Diseases
Michael Lockshin and D. Ware Branch, editors

CHAPTER 1

Introduction

D. Ware Branch, M.D.

March 2005

This volume of the series entitled Handbook of Systemic Autoimmune Diseases represents a medical collaboration focusing primarily on female aspects of rheumatic diseases. This collaboration recognizes the need to understand and optimally manage the care of women with autoimmune conditions that may affect their reproduction and hormonal status in a variety of ways. Thus, the authors who contributed to this volume, including rheumatologists, immunologists, obstetrician-gynecologists, perinatologists and reproductive endocrinologists, all share an academic interest in the unique relationship between being a woman and having an autoimmune disease.

This handbook will doubtlessly prove useful to clinicians as well as curious researchers. It covers very practical points, ranging from which anti-rheumatic medications are safe in pregnancy to how to counsel women with scleroderma contemplating pregnancy. It also touches on numerous controversial topics, such as the mechanism of antiphospholipid-related fetal loss and whether or not non-steroidal anti-inflammatory agents should be used in pregnancy. Finally, we have included critical and balanced reviews of the controversial association between autoimmune disease and female infertility, as well as the infrequently addressed spectrum of gynecologic problems, including sexual dysfunction, in female rheumatologic patients.

As one who has been involved in the reproductive aspects of women with autoimmune diseases for over 20 years, I am proud of our collaborative effort for several reasons. Perhaps most importantly for the readers, this handbook represents a useful, state-of the-art compilation by expert clinicians and scientists. Beyond this, our collaboration also has begun to unmask the complexity of medicine in ways that ignore traditional medical specialty boundaries to the benefit of our patients. Finally, we have become friends and colleagues in the vision of improving the whole-person care of our patients. As mentioned by Dr. Lockshin, a key component in the genesis of this volume was the Fourth International Congress on Sex Hormones, Pregnancy, and Rheumatic Disease, in Stresa, Italy September 2004. The co-chairs, Bianca Canesi and Maurizio Montecucco, and the scientific program directors, Antonio Brucato, Roberto Caporali, and Angela Tincani, have done much to nurture both friendship and intellect.

DOI: 10.1016/S1571-5078(05)04001-8

Handbook of Systemic Autoimmune Diseases, Volume 4
Reproductive and Hormonal Aspects of Systemic Autoimmune Diseases
Michael Lockshin and D. Ware Branch, editors

CHAPTER 2

Sex Differences in Autoimmune Disease

Michael D. Lockshin*

Joan and Sanford Weill Medical College of Cornell University, Hospital for Special Surgery, New York, NY, USA

1. Introduction

Some autoimmune rheumatic diseases mainly affect women. The reasons for sex predominance are unclear. Sex predominance is an epidemiological construct indicating female:male (F/M) incidence ratios; it is not a clinical construct that denotes disease severity. Authors often cite high F/M ratios of autoimmune diseases to support the hypothesis that estrogen, by modulating the process of immune response controls an illness. However, basic facts regarding F/M ratios are contested and less reliable than assumed; uncited illnesses in which males predominate contradict claims of estrogen control.

To argue that estrogen drives autoimmunity, authors selectively cite illnesses that are demonstrably female predominant (Shoenfeld and Cervera, 1999; Feltkamp, 1999; Janeway et al., 1999): thyroid diseases (Hashimoto, Graves), rheumatic diseases (lupus, rheumatoid arthritis, scleroderma, Sjögren), and hepatic diseases (autoimmune hepatitis, primary biliary cirrhosis), while failing to account for ankylosing spondylitis, vasculitis, Goodpasture disease, juvenile onset diabetes, and inflammatory bowel disease, diseases that are sex neutral or male predominant. Selective citation is possible in part because definitions for autoimmunity differ. Some clinical definitions include high F/M ratios as a relevant characteristic; definitions that focus on the autoimmune process largely ignore the relevance of sex, except insofar as estrogen controls quantitative (usually) in vitro response.

2. Prevalence and epidemiology

Reported F/M ratios are imprecise and vary with age. In authoritative texts, F/M ratios vary 10-fold (from 10 to 50) for Hashimoto disease, sevenfold (from 1.5 to 10) for multiple sclerosis, five-fold (from 0.2 to 1) for Goodpasture disease, four-fold (from 3 to 12) for scleroderma, and threefold (from 7 to 20) for lupus (AARDA, 2000; Rose and Mackay, 1998; Beeson, 1994) (Fig. 1; see Table 1).

3. Etiology/pathogenesis

High F/M ratios do not by themselves imply greater disease severity in women; indeed, most sex discrepant *human* illnesses are equally severe in both sexes (Weyand et al., 1998). In contrast, in *animal* models of autoimmune disease, female predominance usually describes predominance of *both* severity *and* incidence, raising serious questions about the validity of imputations from animals.

Arguments that estrogen drives differences in sex incidence usually focus on estrogen's effects on in vitro immunity, on in vivo amelioration of

*Corresponding author.
Joan and Sanford Weill Medical College of Cornell University, Hospital for Special Surgery, 535 E 70th Street, New York, NY 10021, USA.
E-mail address: LockshinM@HSS.edu (M.D. Lockshin).

DOI: 10.1016/S1571-5078(05)04002-X

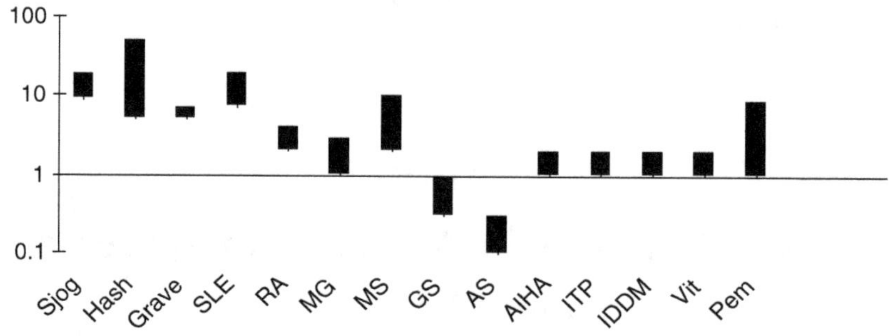

Figure 1. Maximum (top of bar) and minimum (bottom of bar) F/M ratios reported for various autoimmune diseases. Sjog, Sjögren; Hash, Hashimoto; Grave, Graves; SLE, systemic lupus erythematosus; MG, myasthenia gravis; MS, multiple sclerosis; GS, Goodpasture syndrome; AS, ankylosing spondylitis; AIHA, autoimmune hemolytic anemia; ITP, idiopathic thrombocytopenic purpura; IDDM, insulin-dependent diabetes mellitus; vit, vitiligo; pem, pemphigus foliaceus.

Table 1
Female/Male ratios cited by various authors and the American Autoimmune and Related Diseases Association (AARDA)

Disease	Beeson	Rose	Janeway	AARDA
Sjögren	19	15	—	9
Hashimoto thyroiditis	6	18	5	50
Graves hyperthyroidism	6	7	5	7
Lupus erythematosus	7	9	20	9
Rheumatoid arthritis	2	3	3	4
Scleroderma	4	12	—	3
Myasthenia gravis	1	3	1	2
Multiple sclerosis	1.5	2	10	—
Goodpasture	0.2	—	1	—

experimental disease by female castration or worsening by male castration/estrogen supplement, or on human case reports in which castration or pharmacologic intervention has altered the severity of a clinical course. A relevant test of the hypothesis that females have intrinsically different immune systems than men (possibly because of estrogen) might look at sex differences of responses to vaccination, infection, and immunomodulation, since the same immunologic processes that are aberrant in autoimmunity are called into play with these natural and available challenges. If immune response is inherently different between men and women, responses to these tests should differ between the sexes.

Those few studies that look at sex differences after vaccination sometimes show higher antibody titers in females but most such studies show no sex differences. Sex differences in clinical protection by, or adverse reactions to, vaccination have rarely been noted. Most studies find male and female responses identical; however, arthritic reactions to rubella may be more common in women, a point not pursued in depth. Viral and bacterial infections affect men and women equally. In chronic Lyme disease—a possible infection model for rheumatoid arthritis—male and female severity are similar. Sex-specific attack rates of most mycobacterial, fungal, and parasitic diseases are equal, except when exposure to the infecting agent differs by sex (see below). Therapeutically administered cytokines sometimes induce autoimmune rheumatic symptoms; they do so equally in both men and women (Ioannou and Isenberg, 2000), but more women than men receiving the anti-TNFα agent infliximab for Crohn's disease develop antinuclear antibodies (Vermeire et al., 2003). Thus, although antibody titers tend to be higher in women, intrinsic male–female differences in clinically important immune response, displayed by response to vaccination and infection, do not appear to be quantitatively great enough to account for the high F/M ratios of rheumatic disease.

Other possible explanations for high F/M ratios include environmental causes, non-immunologic effects of hormones, genetic explanations, and explanations that focus on a whole body or life event differences between the sexes.

In many 'experiments of nature' environmental agents cause autoimmune or autoimmune-like disease. When they do, F/M ratios vary with exposure ratios rather than with specific diseases.

More men than women take drugs that induce lupus, and, unlike idiopathic lupus, drug-induced lupus is male predominant (Yung et al., 1997); more men are exposed to silica inducers of scleroderma-like disease, also male predominant; more women were exposed to the contaminated cooking oil that caused a scleroderma-like illness in Spain, which was female predominant (Abaitua Borda et al., 1998). More women than men took contaminated L-tryptophan, a putatively 'natural' antidepressant; the resulting epidemic of eosinophilia-myalgia syndrome was female predominant (Shulman, 1990). When infection induces arthritis, for instance chronic Lyme disease, there is no sex discrepancy, although boys are more often affected by acute Lyme disease because of their greater exposure in outdoor play to infected ticks (Carlson et al., 2000).

Autoimmune diseases such as lupus likely begin decades before the first symptoms appear (Reichlin et al., 1992; Arbuckle et al., 2003). If an environmental factor such as infection causes this illness, sex discrepant exposure to that factor will have to be sought decades, rather than months, before occurrence of the first symptoms. Sex differences for environmental causes of autoimmune disease are easy to postulate: different exposures due to sociologically different experiences (young boys playing in wooded areas); differences in processing infecting organisms due to different routes of exposure (hormonally variable mucosal susceptibility; menstruation and intercourse render women susceptible to infection in ways that men are not); vulnerable periods (the high attack rate of malaria in the *post partum* period is an example) (Diagne et al., 2000); or threshold differences in immune responses (see below).

Hormonal differences clearly distinguish men from women. Case reports of amelioration of autoimmune disease after castration or worsening after estrogen treatment suggest that gonadal hormones modulate disease severity in individuals (Lahita, 1999b) do not constitute compelling evidence for differences of incidence. Population studies on effects of hormone therapy show either no or very small increases of incidence of rheumatoid arthritis and lupus in patients taking these drugs. Estrogen replacement therapy, oral contraceptives, and ovulation induction probably do not worsen lupus (Guballa et al., 2000; Petri et al., 2004). Although synoviocyte estrogen receptors may be target organs in rheumatoid arthritis (Castagnetta et al., 1999), a disease that is modestly female predominant, these receptors are presumably present in synovium of patients with chronic Lyme disease and ankylosing spondylitis, which are not female predominant. Androgens have no apparent role in the male predominance of ankylosing spondylitis (Giltay et al., 1999).

Although studies often attribute pregnancy-associated remission or flare to the effect of pregnancy-associated hormones, clinical course in pregnancy differs among autoimmune diseases. Rheumatoid arthritis and multiple sclerosis remit during pregnancy (Nelson et al., 1993). Lupus does not or only slightly worsens during pregnancy (Lockshin, 1993). Ankylosing spondylitis worsens. If there were a consistent change during pregnancy, it could be due to other pregnancy characteristics than direct hormone effect, for instance increased circulation, increased fluid volume, metabolic rate, hemodilution, and other factors.

A threshold mechanism, i.e., a requirement for a specific level of estrogen at a vulnerable time, could explain a hormone-associated increase in disease incidence without a corresponding increase in severity. An animal model suggests this possibility: estrogen may permissively allow survival of forbidden autoimmune clones (Bynoe et al., 2000).

Hormones might influence F/M ratios by affecting cells not normally considered as a part of the immune system. Vascular pathology is prominent in the systemic autoimmune diseases. Hypothetically, hormone effects on endothelium might be critical for disease initiation. An unknown sex difference related to ovulation or menstruation cytokines, to vascular rheology, or to a biological clock might be responsible for different disease experiences of the two sexes. In some mouse strains, healing of injuries is sexually dimorphic, the dimorphism being under estrogen control (Heber-Katz et al., 2004). At the level of single-cell behavior in cell culture, male and female cells are strikingly different independent of estrogen (Zakeri, Z. personal communication, December 2004; Huard, J. personal communication, December 2004).

Abundant evidence confirms genetic control of autoimmunity: family and twin studies demonstrating high family incidence of disease, HLA associations of specific illnesses, disease susceptibility or resistance genes, and transgene experiments (Seldin et al., 1999; Taurog et al., 1999) rendering animals susceptible to illness through genetic manipulation. Evidence of this type is particularly strong for spondyloarthropathy, rheumatoid arthritis, and lupus. HLA genes by themselves do not explain sex dimorphism, but sex-discrepant HLA-associated effects are possible (Lambert et al., 2000). The X and Y genes are not the likely causes of sex discrepancy: ankylosing spondylitis, the only sex discrepant human rheumatic disease studied for X-chromosome markers to date, has no X-chromosome susceptibility locus (Hoyle et al., 2000). Except for CD40 ligand, few putative autoimmune markers are on the X or Y chromosome. However, in the male-predominant BXSB mouse model of lupus, susceptibility resides on the Y chromosome (Schrott et al., 1993). Regarding other sexually dimorphic genetic mechanisms, no evidence for imprinting or differential X-inactivation differences exists for autoimmune diseases, but differences in these mechanisms have been rarely sought in autoimmunity (Stewart, 1998; Trejo et al., 1994). Skewed X-inactivation in the thymus may lead to inadequate thymic deletion and hence loss of T-cell tolerance (Chitnis et al., 2000). In a mouse model of diabetes, mutation of a tissue/developmental stage-specific proteasome product is sex discrepant. Sex dimorphism of T-cell trafficking may be due to sex-determined cell surface markers (Vermeire et al., 2003). Thus, specific chromosomal differences between males and females are possible, largely unexplored, reasons for the sex discrepancy of autoimmune disease.

Immunization, in-breeding, transgenic and gene knockout animal models of autoimmune disease give mixed messages about causes of sex discrepancy. In strains of mice and rats that are susceptible to experimental thyroiditis, estrogen increases anti-thyroid antibody titer but not histologic thyroiditis. In contrast, the severity of induced mouse thyroiditis varies with iodide content of diet and with types of chow. Genetic and extrinsic factors, therefore, influence experimental thyroiditis incidence more than hormones do.

While the $(NZB \times NZW)F_1$ mouse model of lupus shows high female incidence and severity, the MRL *lpr/lpr* model is sex neutral and the BXSB model is male predominant (Lahita, 1999a). Castration/replacement experiments in $(NZB \times NZW)F_1$ mice demonstrate estrogen enhancement and testosterone suppression of spontaneous disease severity and incidence. Genetic susceptibility is linked to MHC and other immune-relevant genes, such as those controlling complement and apoptosis. Like its human counterpart, lupus in mice develops in young adulthood, implying that incubation, maturation, or cumulative damage is required for disease expression. At maturation, but not before, susceptible mouse strains have more numerous and more avid estrogen receptors on lymphoid and uterine tissue than do non-susceptible strains, a possible explanation for strain susceptibility differences but not necessarily for sex differences (Dhaher et al., 2000).

Male and female mice in germ-free environments are equally affected by lupus, but germ-free females develop higher autoantibody levels. Germ-free, antigen-free animals have less frequent disease than do germ-free or conventionally raised animals, indicating environmental contribution to illness, and leaving open the possibility that differential exposure causes sex discrepancy in humans (Maldonado et al., 1999). Both the p21 knockout and the DNAse 1 knockout mouse lupus models show slightly higher autoantibody levels in females. Inexplicably, glomerulonephritis is much worse in female p21 knockouts but equals that of males in DNAse 1 knockouts (Balomenos et al., 2000; Napirei et al., 2000). The human HLA B27 gene transgenically expressed in rats induces a phenotype with features of psoriasis and ankylosing spondylitis. In a germ-free environment, the spondylitis does not occur. Introduction of specific gastrointestinal pathogens to the germ-free animal induces spondylitis (Taurog et al., 1999). Male predominance is true of this model, as it is of the human disease, but the reasons are unknown. In these animal models of autoimmune disease, genetic, hormone, life stage, and environmental factors are all relevant to disease causation. No consistent cause for sex discrepancy appears.

Men and women differ in whole body ways that are not easily explained by hormones, chromosomes, or specific genes. Body size is the most apparent manifestation of this effect. A monthly (chronobiologic) cycle in women is another. Most female predominant diseases cluster in the young-adult years, while autoimmune diseases that affect younger or older patients are more evenly divided between the sexes. Whole body characteristics of young adulthood that may explain female predominance include mode of sexual intercourse, pregnancy, chronobiology, non-hormonal effects of menstrual cycles, vascular responses, and as yet unknown other variables. The large quantity and long duration of circulating fetal cells in scleroderma and other autoimmune disease patients (Evans et al., 1999) and the finding of chimerism in sites of autoimmune disease (Clancy, personal communication, September 2004; Khosrotehrani et al., 2004) suggests a profound new biological difference between men and women, the implications of which are unknown.

Table 2
Non-immunologic mechanisms by which males and females differ in disease incidence, according to biological levels of study

Level of study	Mechanism	Example
In utero	In utero nutrition, hormone exposure determine adult phenotype	Sexual behavior, prostate size, adult onset diabetes can be influenced by prenatal exposures in animals; girls with prenatal growth restriction have insulin resistance, ovarian hyporesponsiveness later in life
Imprinted gene	Maternal or paternal origin of a gene influences phenotype differently in males and females	Turner syndrome patients whose X chromosome is of paternal origin are more aggressive than are those whose X chromosome is of maternal origin
X-inactivation	Because of incomplete inactivation, XX cells may produce higher levels of an X-chromosome gene product than do XY cells	Gastrin-releasing peptide receptor is higher in women, causing increased risk of lung cancer in women smokers compared to men
X-chromosome mosaicism	In the presence of a mutated X-chromosome gene, XX individuals have one healthy allele, but an XY or XO individual does not	Females survive incontinentia pigmenti because unaffected X chromosomes exist in mosaic with affected; males have only affected X chromosomes and die
Hormone	Estrogen affects non-hormone cell receptors	Women have a longer QTc interval than men. Cardiac ion channel sensitivity renders women more susceptible to drug-induced arrhythmia.
Organ difference	Organ function differs between the sexes	Men and women use different parts of the brain in language; gastrointestinal transit times differ in men and women
Exposure	Sexes encounter exogenous substances at different rates	Toxic-oil scleroderma affects women; procainamide-induced lupus affects men
Exogenous chemical processing	Exogenous substances are handled differently by the sexes	Kappa opioid drugs are more effective in young adult women than men
Life event	Effects of pregnancy	Fetal cells circulate longer and at higher quantity in scleroderma patients than controls; rheumatoid arthritis remits during pregnancy, related to HLA mismatch between mother and fetus
Behavior	Social activities have different effects in the sexes	Athleticism, diet lead to amenorrhea and osteoporosis in women but not men

4. Explanations for sex discrepancy

Table 2 shows mechanisms that account at various biological levels for sex differences in non-autoimmune human illnesses. The most striking differences of incidence occur when exposures to infectious agents or toxins differ between the sexes. If (unidentified) infections or toxins induce autoimmune rheumatic disease, differences in exposure (perhaps decades before onset of clinical illness) remain as plausible explanations for the sex differences. If gonadal hormones play a role they likely do so through a threshold or permissive mechanism rather than through quantitative immunomodulation. Differences related to X-inactivation, imprinting, X-or Y-chromosome genetic modulators, and intrauterine influences remain as alternate, theoretical, explanations for sex differences of incidence. The epidemiology of some autoimmune diseases—young, female—suggests that an explanation for female predominance lies in exposure, vulnerable periods, or thresholds, rather than in the immune response itself. These topics remain to be explored.

Key points

- Some autoimmune diseases are female predominant, but many are not. Among autoimmune diseases, female/male ratios prevalence range from 10:1 to 1:3.
- For most human autoimmune diseases, severity is similar in both sexes; in mouse models, severity is often but not always greater in females.
- Immunological responses of humans to infection and immunization are similar in the two sexes.
- Estrogen influences in vitro immune function, but its role as an explanation for sex prevalence differences in human disease is unproven.
- Environmental exposure and estrogen-independent cellular, chromosomal, and genetic differences between the sexes are testable hypotheses to explain female predominant disease.

References

AARDA Home page, November 17, 2000, http://www.aarda.org/.

Abaitua Borda, I., Philen, R.M., Posada de la Paz, M., Gomez de la Camara, A., Diez Ruiz-Navarro, M., Gimenez Ribota, O., Alvargonzalez Soldevilla, J., Terracini, B., Severiano Pena, S., Fuentes Leal, C., Kilbourne, E.M. 1998. Toxic oil syndrome mortality: the first 13 years. Int. J. Epidemiol. 27, 1057–1063.

Arbuckle, M.R., McClain, M.T., Rubertone, M.V., Scofield, R.H., Dennis, G.J., James, J.A., Harley, J.B. 2003. Development of autoantibodies before the clinical onset of systemic lupus erythematosus. N. Engl. J. Med. 349 (16), 1526–1533.

Balomenos, D., Martin-Caballero, J., Garcia, M.I., Prieto, I., Flores, J.M., Serrano, M., Martinez-, A.C. 2000. The cell cycle inhibitor p21 controls T-cell proliferation and sex-linked lupus development. Nat. Med. 6, 171–176.

This is one of several highlighted papers that offer estrogen-independent explanations for sex differences of disease prevalence. Sex differences of disease severity are irrelevant to this model.

Beeson, P. 1994. Age and sex association of 40 autoimmune diseases. Am. J. Med. 96, 457–462.

Bynoe, M.S., Grimaldi, C.M., Diamond, B. 2000. Estrogen up-regulates Bcl-2 and blocks tolerance induction of naïve B cells. Proc. Natl. Acad. Sci. USA 97 (6), 2703–2708.

Carlson, D., Hernandez, J., Bloom, B.J., Coburn, J., Aversa, J.M., Steere, A.C. 2000. Lack of Borrelia Burgdorferi DNA in synovial samples from patients with antibiotic treatment-resistant Lyme arthritis. Arthritis Rheum. 42, 2705–2709.

Castagnetta, L., Cutolo, M., Granata, O.M., Di Falco, M., Bellavia, V., Carruba, G. 1999. Endocrine end-points in rheumatoid arthritis. Ann. NY Acad. Sci. 876, 180–191.

Chitnis, S., Monteiro, J., Glass, D., Apatoff, B., Salmon, J., Concannon, P., Gregersen, P.K. 2000. The role of X-chromosome inactivation in female predisposition to autoimmunity. Arthritis Res. 2 (5), 399–406.

This is one of several highlighted papers that offer estrogen-independent explanations for sex differences of disease prevalence. Sex differences of disease severity are irrelevant to this model.

Dhaher, Y.Y., Greenstein, B., de Fougerolles Nunn, E., Khamashta, M., Hughes, G. 2000. Strain differences in binding properties of estrogen receptors in immature and adult BALB/c and MRL-lpr/lpr mice, a model of systemic lupus erythematosus. Int. J. Immunopharmacol. 22, 247–254.

Diagne, N., Rogier, C., Sokhna, C.S., Tall, A., Fontenille, D., Roussilhon, C., Spiegel, A., Trape, J.-F. 2000. Increased susceptibility to malaria during the early postpartum period. New Engl. J. Med. 343, 598–603.

Evans, P.C., Lambert, N., Maloney, S., Furst, D.E., Moore, J.M., Nelson, J.L. 1999. Long-term fetal microchimerism in peripheral blood mononuclear cell subsets in healthy women and women with scleroderma. Blood 93, 2033–2037.

Microchimerism (fetal cells circulating in maternal blood long after conclusion of a pregnancy) is an extraordinarily new and bizarre observation that has great, though unknown, implications for sex differences in human disease and physiology.

Feltkamp, T.E.W. 1999. The mystery of autoimmune diseases. In: Y. Shoenfeld (Ed.), The Decade of Autoimmunity. Elsevier, Amsterdam, pp. 1–5.

Giltay, E.J., van Schaardenburg, D., Gooren, L.J. 1999. Androgens and ankylosing spondylitis: a role in the pathogenesis?. Ann. NY Acad. Sci. 876, 340–364.

Guballa, N., Sammaritano, L., Schwartzman, S., Buyon, J., Lockshin, M. 2000. Ovulation induction and in vitro fertilization in systemic lupus erythematosus and antiphospholipid syndrome. Arthritis Rheum. 43, 550–556.

Heber-Katz, E., Chen, P., Clark, L., Zhang, X.M., Troutman, S., Blankenhorn, E.P. 2004. Regeneration in MRL mice: further genetic loci controlling the ear hole closure trait using MRL and M.m. Castaneus mice Wound Repair Regen. 12 (3), 384–392.
This is an interesting new observation that highlights some of the unexpected ways in which females and males differ. Implications for other differences that modulate disease expression are great.

Hoyle, E., Laval, S.H., Calin, A., Wordsworth, B.P., Brown, M.A. 2000. The X-chromosome and susceptibility to ankylosing spondylitis. Arthritis Rheum. 43, 1353–1355.

Ioannou, Y., Isenberg, D.A. 2000. Current evidence for the induction of autoimmune rheumatic manifestations by cytokine therapy. Arthritis Rheum. 43, 1431–1442.

Janeway, C.A., Travers, P., Walport, M., Capra, J.D. (Eds.), 1999. Immunobiology, 4th ed., Chapter 13. Elsevier Science Ltd./Garland Publishing, New York, pp. 489–509.

Khosrotehrani, K., Johnson, K.L., Cha, D.H., Salomon, R.N., Bianchi, D.W. 2004. Transfer of fetal cells with multilineage potential to maternal tissue. JAMA 292 (1), 75–80.
Microchimerism (fetal cells circulating in maternal blood long after conclusion of a pregnancy) is an extraordinarily new and bizarre observation that has great, though unknown, implications for sex differences in human disease and physiology.

Lahita, R.G. 1999a. Gender and age in lupus. In: R.G. Lahita (Ed.), Systemic Lupus Erythematosus, 3rd ed., Academic Press, San Diego, p. 131.

Lahita, R.G. 1999b. The role of sex hormones in systemic lupus erythematosus. Curr. Opin. Rheumatol. 11, 352–356.

Lambert, N.C., Distler, O., Muller-Ladner, U., Tylee, T.S., Furst, D.E., Nelson, J.L. 2000. HLA-DQA1 *0501 is associated with diffuse systemic sclerosis in Caucasian men. Arthritis Rheum. 43, 2005–2010.

Lockshin, M.D. 1993. Does lupus flare during pregnancy?. Lupus 2, 1–2.

Maldonado, M.A., Kakkanaiah, V., MacDonald, G.C., Chen, F., Reap, E.A., Balish, E., Farkas, W.R., Jennette, J.C., Madaio, M.P., Kotzin, B.I., Cohen, P.I., Eisenberg, R.A. 1999. The role of environmental antigens in the spontaneous development of autoimmunity in MRL-lpr mice. J. Immunol. 162, 6322–6330.
This is one of several highlighted papers that offer estrogen-independent explanations for sex differences of disease prevalence. Sex differences of disease severity are irrelevant to this model.

Napirei, M., Karsunky, H., Zevnik, B., Stephan, H., Mannherz, H.G., Moroy, T. 2000. Features of systemic lupus erythematosus in Dnase 1-deficient mice. Nat. Gen. 25, 177–181.

Nelson, J.L., Hughes, K.A., Smith, A.G., Nisperos, B.B., Branchaud, A.M., Hansen, J.A. 1993. Maternal–fetal disparity in HLA class II alloantigens and the pregnancy-induced amelioration of rheumatoid arthritis. New Engl. J. Med. 329, 466–471.

Petri, M., Buyon, J.P., Kim, M., Kalunian, K., Grossman, J., Hahn, B., Sammaritano, L., Lockshin, M., Merrill, J., Belmont, H.M., Askanase, A.D., McCune, W.J., Hearth-Holmes, M., Dooley, M., Von Feldt, J., Friedman, A., Tan, M., Davis, J., Cronin, M., Diamond, B., Mackay, M., Sigler, L., Fillius, M. 2004. Combined oral contraceptives (OC) are not associated with an increased rate of flare in SLE patients in SELENA. Arthritis Rheum. 50, s239. (abst).

Reichlin, M., Harley, J.B., Lockshin, M.D. 1992. Serologic studies of monozygotic twins with systemic lupus erythematosus. Arthritis Rheum. 35, 457–464.

Rose, N.R., Mackay, I.R. 1998. The Autoimmune Diseases. 3rd ed., Academic Press, San Diego, pp, 1–4.

Schrott, L.M., Waters, N.S., Boehm, G.W., Sherman, G.F., Morrison, L., Rosen, G.D., Behan, P.O., Galaburda, A.M., Denenberg, V.H. 1993. Behavior, cortical ectopias, and autoimmunity in BXSB-Yaa and BXSB-Yaa+mice. Brain Behav. Immun. 7 (3), 205–223.

Seldin, M.F., Amos, C.I., Ward, R., Gregersen, P.K. 1999. The genetics revolution and the assault on rheumatoid arthritis. Arthritis Rheum. 42, 1071–1079.

Shoenfeld, Y., Cervera, R. 1999. Innovations in autoimmunity in the last decade. In: Y. Shoenfeld (Ed.), The Decade of Autoimmunity. Elsevier, Amsterdam, pp. 7–18.

Shulman, L.E. 1990. The eosinophilia–myalgia syndrome associated with ingestion of L-tryptophan. Arthritis Rheum. 33, 913–917.

Stewart, J.J. 1998. The female X-inactivation mosaic in systemic lupus erythematosus. Immunol. Today 19, 352–357.
This is one of several highlighted papers that offer estrogen-independent explanations for sex differences of disease prevalence. Sex differences of disease severity are irrelevant to this model.

Taurog, J.D., Maika, S.D., Satumtira, N., Dorris, M.L., McLean, I.L., Yanagisawa, H., Sayad, A., Stagg, A.J., Fox, G.M., Le O'Brien, A., Rehman, M., Zhou, M., Weiner, A.L., Splawski, J.B., Richardson, J.A., Hammer, R.E. 1999. Inflammatory disease in HLA-B27 transgenic rats. Immunol. Rev. 169, 209–223.

Trejo, V., Derom, C., Vlietinck, R., Ollier, W., Silman, A., Ebers, G., Derom, R., Gregersen, P.K. 1994. X chromosome inactivation patterns correlate with fetal–placental anatomy in monozygotic twin pairs: implications for immune relatedness and concordance for autoimmunity. Mole. Med. 1, 62–70.

Vermeire, S., Noman, M., Van Assche, G., Baert, F., Van Steen, K., Esters, N., Joossens, S., Bossuyt, X., Rutgeerts, P. 2003. Autoimmunity associated with anti-tumor necrosis factor alpha treatment in Crohn's disease: a prospective cohort study. J. Gastroenterol. 125 (1), 32–39.

Weyand, C.M., Schmidt, D., Wagner, U., Goronzy, J.J. 1998. The influence of sex on the phenotype of rheumatoid arthritis. Arthritis Rheum. 41, 817–822.

Yung, R., Williams, R., Johnson, K., Phillips, C., Stoolman, L., Chang, S., Richardson, B. 1997. Mechanisms of drug-induced lupus. III. Sex-specific differences in T cell homing may explain increased disease severity in female mice. Arthritis Rheum. 40, 1334–1343.

Handbook of Systemic Autoimmune Diseases, Volume 4
Reproductive and Hormonal Aspects of Systemic Autoimmune Diseases
Michael Lockshin and D. Ware Branch, editors

CHAPTER 3

Maternal–Fetal Aspects of Autoimmune Disease

Nathalie C. Lambert[a], Ann M. Reed[b]

[a]*Laboratoire d'Immuno-Rhumatologie, INSERM U639, Marseille Cedex France*
[b]*Department of Medicine and Pediatrics, Mayo Clinic, Rochester, MN, USA*

In pregnancy, genetically and immunologically semi-foreign tissues and cells survive without rejection. Over the past several decades, concepts have changed regarding the immunology of implantation, maternal–fetal immunology, and autoimmune disease. The maternal–fetal interface, once considered an immunologically privileged site, is now known as a site of recognition of the fetus as foreign and of placental exchange of fetal and maternal cells. In addition, unique human leukocyte antigen (HLA) expression, natural killer (NK) cell markers, and cytokine profile response shifts occur during pregnancy. Maternal–fetal interaction plays a role in autoimmune disease, beginning with the immunology of conception and followed by immune alterations during and after pregnancy. This chapter discusses factors of the maternal–fetal interaction associated with autoimmune disease susceptibility and disease activity in the offspring and in the mother.

1. Immunomodulation during pregnancy

1.1. A role of tolerance in healthy pregnancy

Immunomodulation of peripheral blood lymphocyte subsets occurs during pregnancy. Total T-cell number in the maternal circulation remains stable throughout pregnancy, although some reports claim a decreased CD4/CD8 ratio. The number of cytotoxic T-cell decreases during pregnancy, thought to reflect a need for suppression or downregulation of cytotoxic cell activity (Le Bouteiller, 1994; Pazmany et al., 1996; Poole and Claman, 2004; Wegmann et al., 1993). Downregulation of NK-cell activity at the maternal and fetal interface is crucial. HLA class I and II proteins are not expressed by cells at the maternal–fetal interface, with the exception of HLA-G and low, transient levels of HLA-C (Ober, 1998; Poole and Claman, 2004). HLA-G binds to killer inhibitor receptors (KIR), which are expressed on and lead to inhibition of NK-cells, thus preventing placental cell death. HLA-G also induces a shift to TH2 cytokine profile and downregulates TNFα and IFNγ (Morales et al., 2003; Rajagopalan and Long, 1999; van der Meer et al., 2004).

It is a common belief that a TH2-type cytokine shift in maternal immune response is required to maintain pregnancy and that a TH1 response may be involved in preeclampsia and spontaneous abortions (Jonsson et al., 2004; Wegmann et al., 1993). The proposed cytokine shift is local rather than systemic; it includes interleukin (IL)-10, granulocyte–macrophage colony-stimulating factor (GM-CSF), IL-3, CSF-1, and the TH2 cytokines IL-4 and IL-5 (Borish and Steinke, 2003; Le Bouteiller, 1994; Poole and Claman, 2004).

The number of cytotoxic T $\gamma\delta$ cell decreases during pregnancy; T cells remain stable and are activated and express progesterone receptors (Barakonyi et al., 1999; Rukavina and Gill, 1997). Cytotoxic T $\gamma\delta$ cell excrete IL-10 and progesterone-induced blocking factor (PIBF) which also suppresses NK activity (Check et al., 1997;

DOI: 10.1016/S1571-5078(05)04003-1

Szekeres-Bartho, 2002). This correlates with an increase of serum IL-1 and IL-6. The ratio of IFNγ/IL-4 decreases with the shift toward a TH2 response (Matthiesen et al., 1998). IL-10, GM-CSF, CSF- and IL-3 influence the development of the trophoblast cells. Th2 cytokines (IL-4 and IL-5) in the local milieu protect the fetus (Piccinni et al., 1995; Roberts et al., 2001; Wegmann et al., 1993). However, small amounts of tumor necrosis factor (TNF)α and interferon (IFN)γ occur early in pregnancy and during labor, IFNγ being involved in normal vascular remodeling and decidual (feto–maternal interface) integrity (Ashkar et al., 2000; Vassiliadis et al., 1998).

Th3 cells, producing immunosuppressive cytokines (tumor growth factor (TGFβ) and IL-10) have anti-inflammatory properties and produce antigen-specific tolerance (Borish and Steinke, 2003). CD4+CD25+ regulatory T cells (Treg) are a specialized population of T cells that suppress T-cell responses by the production of IL-10 and TGF in the decidua in early pregnancy (Nagaeva et al., 2002)

1.2. A beneficial or pathogenic role in autoimmune diseases

Pregnancy is a special immunotolerant state that could contribute temporarily to the stabilization, degradation, or amelioration of autoimmune disease. For a long time it was thought that immune responses are depressed during pregnancy and that the placenta is a barrier between fetal and maternal circulation that prevents maternal attack. However, studies of maternal pregnancy immunology are controversial. For example, peripheral blood T-cell levels are said to decline, remain unchanged or increase during pregnancy. Immunomodulation of pregnancy is more complicated; simple immune suppression would not make evolutionary sense. Moreover, the placenta is not an absolute barrier since trafficking of cells occurs in both directions.

For cell-mediated TH1 autoimmune diseases, such as rheumatoid arthritis (RA) (this statement itself an oversimplification), remissions of symptoms could come from changes to a TH2-response. A recent study shows absence of a TH2 type cytokine profile but elevation of circulating levels of anti-inflammatory cytokines in pregnant patients with RA and ankylosing spondylitis (Østensen et al., 2005). Therefore the theory that a Th1/Th2 shift is responsible of remission in Th1 diseases is likely simplistic.

Decreased levels of IL-10 and TGF, thought to be produced by Tregs, in many autoimmune diseases suggest the possibility that Tregs induced during pregnancy create a transient moment of tolerance (Shevach, 2000; Shevach et al., 2001). Recent data validate this theory: pregnancy-induced expansion of Tregs may mediate lessening of multiple sclerosis activity (Sanchez-Ramon et al., 2005).

The effects of tryptophane-catabolizing enzyme indoleamine 2, 3-dioxygenase (IDO), a potential candidate for depleting the essential amino acid tryptophan in the placenta, and thus suppressing T-cell proliferation, are of recent interest. Inhibition of IDO induces rapid T-cell rejection of allogeneic fetuses in pregnant mice, suggesting a role in human pregnancy (Mellor and Munn, 1999; Munn et al., 1998; Schrocksnadel et al., 1996).

Although amelioration, stabilization, or degradation of autoimmune diseases during pregnancy remains to be clearly defined at both the clinical and the cellular level, other factors related to the feto–maternal traffic of cells are suggested by the fact that RA women, pregnant with an HLA class II disparate fetus, are more likely to improve during pregnancy (Nelson et al., 1993).

2. Feto–maternal exchange during pregnancy and subsequent persistent microchimerism

2.1. A normal physiological condition

The placenta is not an immunological barrier. Rather, maternal and fetal cells traffic across the placenta in a state of mutual tolerance that exists between maternal and fetal circulations during normal gestation, a fact known since the 1940s, when it was recognized that erythrocytes cross the placenta and cause complications in both mother and fetus. Prior to 1989, identification of fetal cells in the maternal blood depended on morphologic or cytogenetic characteristics. DNA amplification by polymerase chain reaction (PCR) now allows detection of a small quantity of fetal DNA within a large amount of maternal DNA. Why nucleated fetal cells appear in the maternal circulation is not well understood; one hypothesis is that the fetus influences its mother's immune system by sending cells to her. Fetal cells are detectable primarily by identifying male karyotypes in maternal blood as early as 5–6 weeks of gestation. Passage of maternal cells into the fetal circulation also occurs (Lo et al., 2000), though quantitative-PCR techniques find less mother-to-fetus trafficking than fetus-to-mother. Fetal cells in a mother or maternal cells in a fetus are referred to as chimerism, and low levels as microchimerism (Mc).

In 1996, Bianchi et al., studying women who had previously given birth to males and using PCR amplification of male-specific Y-chromosome sequences, reported that fetal cells persist in the maternal circulation up to 27 years after childbirth (Bianchi et al., 1996). Maternal cells appear in fetal cord blood samples as early as 13 weeks gestation (Lo et al., 1998) and in abnormal tissue of newborns with congenital anomalies (Srivatsa et al., 2003). Persistence of maternal cells, or of DNA of presumably maternal origin, in the offspring has been described in infants with immunodeficiency and in immunocompetent adults (Lambert et al., 2004; Maloney et al., 1999; Pollack et al., 1982). Thus significant maternal-fetal interface trafficking is apparently bi-directional.

2.2. A possible trigger to autoimmunity

Many chimeric cells have long-term survival and might be associated with autoimmune disease (Table 1). Fetal tolerance toward maternal cells is long-lasting, as evidenced by unresponsiveness of adult B cells to non-inherited HLA antigens.

Nelson et al. took observations based on transplant immunology and asked whether microchimerism arising from pregnancy could mimic graft-versus-host disease (cGVHD), a model for autoimmune disease (Nelson, 1996). Patients with cGVHD have symptoms of inflammatory myositis (polymyositis, dermatomyositis, systemic lupus erythematosus (SLE), scleroderma (SSc), primary biliary cirrhosis (PBC), Sjögren's, immune thrombocytopenia, immune pancytopenia, and neutropenia). Over 50 percent of patients with cGVHD have positive ANA or anti-nuclear antibodies and, occasionally, double-stranded DNA antibody.

2.2.1. Scleroderma

The first study to investigate Mc in an autoimmune disease was a prospective blinded study of fetal Mc in women with SSc compared to matched healthy controls (Nelson et al., 1998). Women with SSc and healthy women who had previously given birth to at least one son were recruited. Semi-quantitative PCR assay using Y-chromosome-specific sequences were amplified in the maternal blood looking for the presence of male DNA. Y-chromosome specific DNA was detected in 25% of the control patients and 59% of the SSc patients, and cell number was significantly increased in the SSc patients (Nelson et al., 1998). In another study, Y-chromosome DNA sequences were found in 46% of patient's blood samples versus 4% of controls (Artlett et al., 1998) and 58% of the skin biopsy samples of 19 women with SSc had male DNA, much higher than in control females (Artlett et al., 1998). However, this latter study has been criticized for technical flaws (Nakagome et al., 1990, 1991). In a Japanese study looking at skin biopsies with another Y-chromosome-specific sequence (p49a, used in previous published studies (Nelson et al., 1998)), no difference in rate of positive male DNA occurred between cases and controls, but the number of male cells per 80 ng of tissue DNA was higher in SSc patients compared to healthy controls (Ohtsuka et al., 2001). Johnson et al. (2001b) tested specimens obtained at autopsies of mothers who had had sons who had either SSc or no autoimmune disease. They analysed adrenal gland, heart, intestine, kidney, liver, lung, lymph node, pancreas, parathyroid, skin, and spleen for male cells by fluorescence in situ hybridization. Male cells occurred in at least one site

Table 1
Representative table of known studies of chimerism in autoimmune disease, not meant to be totally comprehensive

Reference	No of cases included	No of controls included	Type of Mc detected	Detection technique	No of + for Mc/ total No cases; controls	Levels of Mc [cases]; [controls][a]	Specimen studied	Difference between controls and cases[b]	Origin of the populations	HLA association	Disease studied[c]
Nelson et al. (1998)	17	16 7 healthy SSc sisters	Male	Semi-Q Y (p49a) PCR	10/17; 4/16 2/7	[11.1/16cc] [0.4/16cc] [1.3/16cc]	Blood	S	North America	ND	SSc
Artlett et al. (1998)	69	25	Male	Nest.Y (DYZ1) PCR	32/69; 1/25	NA	Blood	S	North America	ND	SSc
	19	68	Male	Nest.Y (DYZ1) PCR	11/19; 0/68	NA	Skin biopsies	S			
	3	2	Male	FISH	3/3; 0/2	[0–3/3000] [0]	CD3, CD14, CD45 PBMC	NA			
	7	10	Male	FISH	7/7; 0/10		Skin biopsies	ND			
Evans et al. (1999)	20	35 13 SSc sisters	Male	Nest.Y (SRY) PCR	12/20; 11/35 5/13	NA	PBMC	S	North America	ND	SSc
	10	9	Male		3/9; 3/10		CD3 PBMC	NS			
	8	9	Male		5/8; 4/9		CD56/CD16 PBMC	NS			
	9	11	Male		2/9; 4/11		CD14 PBMC	NS			
	8	11	Male		2/8; 5/11		CD19 PBMC	NS			
Maloney et al. (1999)	9	22	Maternal	HLA PCR	6/9; 11/22	NA	PBMC	NS	North America	ND	SSc
Murata et al. (1999)	13	12	Male	Nest.Y (DYZ1) PCR	8/13; 6/12	NA	PBMC	NS	Japan	ND	SSc
Lambert et al. (2000)	12	19	Male	Nest.Y (SRY) PCR	ND	ND	CD3 PBMC	ND	North America	DQA1*0501	SSc
Artlett et al. (2000a)	63	64 24 disease ctrl	Any Mc	HLA (Cw) PCR	41/63; 18/64 8/24	NA	PBMC	S	North America		SSc
Miyashita et al. (2000)	20	41	Male	Nest Y (DYZ1) PCR	6/20; 8/41	NA	Blood	S	Japan	ND	SSc
Ohtsuka et al. (2001)	49	57 30 CTD	Male	Semi-Q Y (p49a) PCR	14/49; 20/57 6/30 CTD	[4.59 ± 9.63] [1.83 ± 4.96] per 80 ng	Skin tissues	Freq: NS Levels: S	Japan	NA	SSc
Johnson et al. (2001)	5	3	Male	FISH	5/5 0/3	NA	11 different tissues	ND	North America	NA	SSc
Scaletti et al. (2002)	3	3	Male	FISH	NA	NA	T cells		Italy	NA	SSc

Lambert et al. (2002)	39	39	Male	Real time Y (DYS14) PCR	20/39 12/39	[0–12.5] [0–4.4] per 10^6	PBMC	Freq: NS Levels: S	North America	ND	SSc
	19	18			5/19 12/18	[1.6–44.8] [0.3–68.7]	T cells	NS		ND	
	10	13			3/10 4/13	[0.5–13.7] [0.2–50.3]	CD4 T cells	NS		ND	
	8	11			3/8 7/11	[1.1–24.2] [0.6–16.3]	CD8 T cells	NS		ND	
Artlett et al. (2002)	47	22	Male	Real time Y (SRY) PCR	39/47 14/22	median [$19/10^5$] [$5/10^5$]	Pos and neg CD4, CD8 cells	Freq: NS Levels: S	North America	ND	SSc
	47	22			28/47 9/22	median [$1/10^5$] [$0/10^5$]	CD4 T cells	Freq: NS Levels: S			
	47	22			23/47 8/22	median [$0/10^5$] [$0/10^5$]	CD8 T cells	Freq: NS Levels: NS			
Artlett et al. (2003)	47	27	Male and Any Mc	Real time-Y (SRY) PCR, HLA (Cw) PCR	33/47 13/27		PBMC	NS	North America	Recipient HLA: no association	SSc
	23	4			18 + 9 –		T cells			Donor HLA: no association	
Selva-O'Callagahan et al. (2003)	47	40	Male	Nested PCR	4/47 2/40	NA	PBMC		Spain		SSc
Burastero et al. (2003)	43	30 with sons, 20 without son	Male	Real time-Y (SRY) PCR	0/43 0/30 0/20		Plasma		Italy	ND	SSc
				Real time-Y (SRY) PCR	3/43 0/30 0/20		Blood				
				Nested PCR	29/43 16/30 0/20		Blood				
Lambert et al. (2004)	18	32	Maternal	HLA Q-PCR	13/18; 7/32	[0–54.5] [0–68.6] per 10^6	PBMC	Freq: S Levels: NS	North America	ND	SSc
	1		Maternal				10 tissues bone marrow	NA			
Tanaka et al. (1999)	37	39	Male	PCR WAVE technology	26/37 28/39	Ratio Y/X 0.402 +/– 0.14 vs. 0.271 +/ –0.05	Liver	NS	Japan	ND	PBC
Rubbia-Brandt et al. (1999)	10	3	Male	FISH	0/10; 0/3		Liver	NS	Switzerland	NA	PBC
Fanning et al. (2000)	18	18	Male	Nest. Y (DYZ3 PCR)	0/18 1/18	ND	PBMC	NS	Australia	ND	PBC
	19	20 Other liver diseases			8/19 0/20	ND	Liver biopsies	S		ND	

Table 1 (*continued*)

Reference	No of cases included	No of controls included	Type of Mc detected	Detection technique	No of + for Mc/ total No cases; controls	Levels of Mc [cases]; [controls][a]	Specimen studied	Difference between controls and cases[b]	Origin of the populations	HLA association	Disease studied[c]
Corpechot et al. (2000)	20	20	Male	Nest Y (DYS1) PCR	9/20 5/20	NA	PBMC	NS	France	ND	PBC
	15	25			5/15 8/25		Liver				
Schoniger-Hekele et al. (2002)	28	77 Other liver diseases	Male	Y chrS PCR FISH	5/28; 4/77 3/21; 1/13	ND ND	Liver biopsies	NS	Austria	ND	PBC
Toda et al. (2001)	18	12 5 NP	Male	Nested Y (TSPY) PCR	0/18 0/12		PBMC		Japan	ND	SS
	10	5 3 NP			0/10 0/5	NA	CD34 enriched cells	NA			
Miyashita et al. (2000)	18	41	Male	Nest Y (DYZ1) PCR	6/18 8/41	NA	Blood	NS	Japan	ND	SS
Aractingi et al. (2002)	16	11 SSC	Male	Y PCR	0/16; 5/11		Labial tissue	S in SSc NS in SS	France	ND	SS
Kuroki et al. (2002)	27 PBMC 42 labial tissue	ND	Male	Nested Y PCR FISH	0/22 PBMC 10/28 tissue	ND	PBMC Labial tissue	S	Japan	ND	SS
Endo et al. (2002)	29	20	Male	Nested Y PCR	5/29 5/20	ND	PBMC	Freq: S	Japan	ND	SS
	20	8		FISH	11/20 1/8		Salivary biopsy				
Klintschar et al. (2001)	17	25 with nodular goiters	Male	SRY PCR and Y/X seq PCR	8/17 1/25	ND	Thyroid tissue	S	Austria	ND	HAT
Srivatsa et al. (2001)	16	13	Male	FISH	16/29; 0/8	ND	Thyroid tissue	S	North America	ND	TD
Ando et al. (2002)	27	10	Male	Y PCR	10/27; 1/10	ND	Thyroid tissue	S	North America	ND	TD
Reed et al. (1998)	3	7 siblings	Maternal	Nested HLA PCR	3/3; 2/7	NA	PBMC	S	North America	ND	JDM
Reed et al. (2000)	15	35 siblings	Maternal	Nested HLA PCR	13/15; 5/35	NA	PBMC	S	North America	DQA1*0501	JDM
	15	17		FISH	11/15; 5/17		PBMC	S			
	15	10		FISH	12/15; 2/10		Muscle tissue	S			

Artlett et al. (2000a)	9	9	Maternal	PCR	8/9; 0/9	NA	CD4 PBMC CD8 PBMC	S	North America	ND	IIM
	10	10		FISH	10/10; 2/10		1 skin sample; Muscle biopsies				
Selva-O'Callaghan et al. (2001)	18	18	Male	Y DNA PCR	1/18; 0/18	NA	PBMC	NS	Spain	ND	IIM
Artlett et al. (2003)	28	29	Maternal	HLA-Cw PCR	20/28; 2/29	ND	PBMC	S	North America	No DQA1 association	IIM
Reed et al. (2004)	72	48	Maternal	Nested HLA PCR FISH	60/72; 11/48 22/30; 12/39	ND	PBMC	S	North America	DQA1*0501 DQB1*02, 03 DRB1*03,11	JDM
Miyashita et al. (2000)	21	41	Male	Nest Y (DYZ1) PCR	0/21 8/41	ND	Blood	ND	Japan	NA	SLE
Johnson et al. (2001)	1		Fetal	FISH	1/1	ND	Tissue	S	North America	NA	SLE
Stevens et al. (2003)	4	4	Maternal	FISH	15/15 2/8	[0.025–2.2%], [0–0.1%]	Cardiac tissue	S	North America	NA	NLS
Stevens et al. (2005)	2/triplets 1/twins	1/triplets 1/twins	Maternal and sibling	Q-PCR for HLA and DYS14	2/3 1/2	NA	Blood	NA	Italy	NA	NLS-CHB
Khosrotehrani et al. (2005)	6	4	Male	FISH	0/6; 0/4	NA	Skin lesions	NA	North America	NA	SLE
Tanei et al. (2000)	10	1	Male	FISH	0/10; 0/1	NA	Skin biopsies	NA	Japan	NA	LP
Lombardi et al. (2001)	15	0	Male	FISH	0/15	NA	Oral mucosa biopsies	NA	Switzerland	NA	OLP
Vabres et al. (2002)	1 case report	0	Male (twin)	Different Y PCR FISH	1/1 0/1	NA	Blood and skin biopsy		France	NA	LP

CTD: connective tissue disease; NP: nulliparous; ND: not done; NA: not applicable

[a] Levels of microchimerism (Mc) expressed in number of cells for fluorescence in situ hybridization experiments (FISH) or genome equivalent of Mc cells for PCR experiments.

[b] S: significant difference; NS: not significant difference; Freq: frequency.

[c] SSc: systemic sclerosus or scleroderma; PBC: primary biliary cyrrhosis; SS: Sjögren's syndrome; HAT: Hashimoto's thyroiditis; TD: thyroid disease; JDM juvenile dermatomyositis; IIM: idiopathic inflammatory myositis; SLE: systemic lupus erythematosus; NLS: neonatal lupus syndrome; CHB: congenital heart block; LP: lichen planus; OLP: oral lichen planus.

in each woman with SSc, most frequently in spleen, but never in pancreas, but not in non-autoimmune controls (Johnson et al., 2001b). By contrast, a small study using peripheral blood from Japanese women with SSc and controls detected no difference for fetal Mc by nested PCR for DYZ1 (Murata et al., 1999) nor did a Spanish study of women with SSc compared to matched healthy women (Selva-O'Callaghan et al., 2003). Contradictory results could result from different detection and quantification methods (Lambert et al., 2001), illustrating the need for standardized quantitative PCR assays. A recent study (Lambert et al., 2002) using a standardized real-time PCR for a Y-chromosome sequence (DYS14), showed that frequency of any detectable male DNA in peripheral blood mononuclear cells (PBMC) was somewhat higher in SSc patients (51%) compared to controls (31%) but not significant ($p = 0.07$). However, circulating male Mc was quantitatively greater in PBMC from SSc patients ($n = 39$), range: 0.0–12.5 genome equivalents/million of maternal cells, compared to healthy women ($n = 39$), range: 0.0–4.4 ($p = 0.03$). Therefore, fetal Mc per se might be a common phenomenon, but levels may differ between cases and controls.

To understand the immunological implications of Mc in SSc, Evans et al. (1999) studied long-term fetal Mc occurs in T lymphocyte, B lymphocyte, monocyte, and NK cell populations of previously pregnant women. The investigators included women with sons and used a nested PCR for a Y-chromosome-specific sequence to test DNA extracted from PBMC and from CD3 (T cells), CD19 (B cells), CD14 (monocytes), and CD56/16 (NK cells) sorted subsets. Fetal Mc was found in PBMCs from 33% (16 of 48) of healthy women and 60% (12 of 20) women with SSc reaching a marginal significance ($p = 0.046$). Mc was found in some women in CD3, CD19, CD14, and CD56/16 subsets up to 38 years after pregnancy. No specific pattern differentiated patients from healthy subjects (Evans et al., 1999). Artlett et al. (2002) using a quantitative Y-chromosome PCR assay, analyzed Mc in the T-cell population and showed that SSc patients had more microchimeric CD4+ T cells but not CD8+ T cells compared to the controls.

Although microchimeric T lymphocytes may be involved in the pathogenesis of SSc, only a few studies address the hypothesis that fetal Mc might have resulted in a GVH-like reaction in women with SSc (Burastero et al., 2003; Scaletti et al., 2002), possibly because of the rarity of Mc cells persisting in the host peripheral blood. Scaletti et al. were able to identify CD4 positive auto-reactive T- cells by cloning T- cells from skin biopsies and peripheral blood of three women with SSc. Some of the autoreactive T cells exhibited a Y chromosome, presumed to be from a male offspring, suggesting that these microchimeric cells can have an anti-host response. Another study, also of three patients, found cellular Mc in SSc patients and controls, but the absolute amount of male DNA was higher in the patients, and the addition of an anti-CD28 costimulatory signal amplified microchimeric cells of patients with SSc but not controls (Burastero et al., 2003). These results support the hypothesis that Mc cells have characteristics of T lymphocytes specific to maternal allogeneic antigens.

Only few investigations concerning maternal Mc in SSc have been done up to date. Maloney et al. (1999) found that non-shared maternal HLA-specific DNA was found in six of nine SSc patients and in 11 out of 22 healthy individuals. The mean age of all subjects with maternal Mc was 28 years (range 9–49 years). Fluorescent in situ hybridization (FISH) with XY-probe labeling revealed that female cells were present in the peripheral blood samples from two male SSc patients out of three patients and two controls tested. This study, although qualitative and not quantitative, found no significant difference in frequency of maternal Mc between patients and controls.

Lambert et al. (2004) recently quantified the maternal microchimeric HLA-specific DNA using a panel of real-time PCR assays in healthy women and women with SSc and studied 50 proband-mother pairs including 32 healthy women and 18 with SSc. Using PBMC, maternal Mc was seen more frequently in women with SSc [13/18 (72%)] than in healthy women [7/32 (22%)]. However, the levels of Mc expressed as genomic equivalence of maternal cells per million of host cells were not significantly different. Maternal Mc was demonstrated in a bone marrow aspirate from a SSc patient in whom peripheral blood had been negative for maternal Mc on four occasions. Moreover tissue samples from the same patient who died several months after autologous stem cell transplantation had high levels of maternal Mc. Levels of maternal Mc were up to 20-fold more in some tissues compared to peripheral blood mononuclear cells (Lambert et al., 2004).

Whether maternal Mc contributes to SSc is not yet known, but the development of a panel of HLA-specific PCR will allow further studies of maternal Mc in autoimmunity and in normal biology.

2.2.2. Primary biliary cirrhosis

Additional studies of fetal Mc include those in PBC, a disorder seen in women often during child-bearing years, with histological similarity to chronic graft versus host disease. In some studies (Fanning et al., 2000), but not in others (Rubbia-Brandt et al., 1999; Tanaka et al., 1999), Mc occured more commonly in the livers of patients with PBC than in controls. One clear feature of PBC is that it is frequently associated with CREST (*c*alcinosis, *R*aynaud's, *e*sophageal *d*ysmotility, *s*clerodactyly, *t*elangiectasia) syndrome, a variation of SSc. Patients with PBC who have CREST syndrome-associated anti-centromere antibody were more likely to have fetal microchimeric cells (Corpechot et al., 2000). When fetal Mc was no greater in maternal liver tissue from PBC patients compared to that from patients with other hepatic disorders (Schoniger-Hekele et al., 2002).

2.2.3. Sjögren's syndrome

Sjögren's syndrome (SS) develops primarily in females and has clinical similarities to cGVHD. Microchimeric cells occur in the blood and tissue of some patients with SS with a trend for secondary Sjögren (that occurring in patients with other autoimmune diseases) to have fetal Mc cells, possibly as a secondary phenomenon to the underlying autoimmune disease (Aractingi et al., 2002). Other studies, which do not differentiate primary versus secondary Sjögrens, find chimeric cells in the salivary gland biopsies and less often in the PBMCs (Aractingi et al., 2002; Endo et al., 2002; Kuroki et al., 2002; Miyashita et al., 2000).

2.2.4. Autoimmune thyroid disease

Fetal Mc has also been investigated in women with hypo- and hyperthyroidism, in part because of a belief that thyroid disease transiently improves during pregnancy and worsens post-partum. One study found male DNA more often in women with Hashimoto's thyroiditis compared to those with nodular goiters, although pregnancy histories were not clear (Klintschar et al., 2001) A second study found male cells found in females who had thyroiditis but also other conditions, such as carcinomas and goiters (Ando et al., 2002). Mice with thyroiditis had more frequently detectable chimeric cells than did controls (Imaizumi et al., 2002). Interthyroid fetal Mc, determined by thyroid biopsies, was common among patients with Grave's disease compared to thyroid specimens from autopsies (Srivatsa et al., 2001).

2.2.5. Myositis

Maternal Mc was first reported in children with juvenile dermatomyositis (JDM) by Reed et al. (2000). Muscle and skin biopsies in both JDM and cGVHD demonstrate perivascular lymphocytic infiltrates and lymphocytic intradermal infiltrates, suggesting similar pathogenesis. Additional supportive evidence is that subjects undergoing cGVHD from allogeneic hematopoietic stem cell transplant can develop myositis. The initial report involved three unrelated families each including a child with JDM, biological parents, and healthy siblings. Chimerism was identified using PCR amplification of the non-transmitted maternal HLA-DQA1 alleles. The non-transmitted maternal HLA-DQA1 allele was seen in all three JDM subjects compared with 2/7 (28%) of the healthy siblings. Additionally, all the JDM mothers had the paternal DQA1 allele seen in the JDM subject (Reed, 1998).

More extensive studies in children with JDM and juvenile idiopathic inflammatory myositis (JIIM) used PCR amplification of the non-transmitted maternal alleles from PBMC and FISH of the PBMC and muscle tissue of male subjects (Artlett et al., 2000b; Reed et al., 2000). In the first study, 11/15 JDM subjects (73%) PBMCs had maternal cells compared with 5/17 (30%) of their siblings ($p < 0.0001$) (Reed et al., 2000). The non-transmitted maternal allele was amplified in 13/15 boys with JDM compared with 5/35 of their siblings ($p = 0.0001$). In the second study, muscle of 12 of 15 male JDM patients (80%) obtained at the onset of their disease had maternal cells compared with 2 of 10 male controls (20%) who underwent diagnostic biopsy and did not have an inflammatory myositis ($p = 0.005$). A third report described nine male subjects with definite or probable JIIM (7/10 had JDM, mean age 14.3) and nine healthy male control subjects (mean age 15.2) investigated using FISH in magnetically separated CD4 or CD8 peripheral blood cells (Artlett et al., 2000b). Eight of the JIIM subjects were positive for maternal XX cells compared to none of healthy controls ($p < 0.001$). Chimeric cells were seen in 10/10 of biopsy samples (nine muscle and one skin) compared with 2/10 controls ($p = 0.0007$). The same authors later reported PCR amplification of three HLA-Cw alleles, the third band presumably from the chimeric cells, in 19/26 JIIM patients compared with 2/21 healthy controls ($p < 0.001$) (Artlett et al., 2003). The authors determined chimerism based on the detection of a third less intensely staining band presumed to be the non-inherited maternal Cw allele. The maternal Cw alleles, however, were unknown in the majority of the cases and the source of the third band could not be confirmed. Additionally, in cases of Cw allele homozygosity, the JIIM subjects were assumed to have chimerism even when a third band could not be demonstrated.

Fetal Mc in adult idiopathic inflammatory myopathies was investigated in peripheral blood cells from 18 Spanish women with myositis and 18 matched healthy women, all with male offspring. Results demonstrated Y-chromosome DNA in the peripheral blood from one myositis patient and none of 18 healthy controls (Selva-O'Callaghan et al., 2001), a non-significant difference. However, the PCR methods used in this short study are not detailed (Selva-O'Callaghan et al., 2001).

2.2.6. Lupus and autoimmune cardiac diseases

Systemic lupus erythematosus (SLE) patients have less frequent detectable Mc than do healthy controls (Miyashita et al., 2000). In further studies in which pathological and histologically normal tissue samples were examined in autopsies, chimeric cells were only found in diseased tissue (Johnson et al., 2001a). However, a recent study reported absence of fetal cells in skin lesions of lupus erythematosus (Khosrotehrani et al., 2005).

Neonatal lupus is an affection of children of mothers who have anti-Sjögren's (anti-SSA/Ro and skin rash. Neonatal lupus heart tissue demonstrated maternal cells in 15/15 sections, suggesting a direct role in the pathogenesis of congenital heart block (Stevens et al., 2003). The chimeric cells were differentiated, suggesting that the maternal cells might be a target of the immune response or part of the repair process. In another recent study, maternal and sibling Mc was tested with HLA and Y-chromosome (DYS14) specific quantitative PCR in two families with twins and triplets discordant for neonatal lupus congenital heart block (Stevens et al., 2005a). Mc in the blood was not specific for heart block, although in one family levels correlated with disease (Stevens et al., 2005a).

Peripartum cardiomyopathy (PPCM), a life-threatening maternal cardiac condition, may have a Mc component. One group of investigators has found PBMCs from PPCM patients demonstrate a heightened level of fetal Mc (Ansari et al., 2002).

2.2.7. Lichen planus

Lichen planus (LP) is a chronic inflammatory mucocutaneous disease affecting three women for every man. The etiology is unknown, but autoimmunity is one proposed cause, in part because cutaneous and oral lesions resembling LP occur in a fraction of cases with cGVHD and disorders of NK-cell functional activity occur in patients with LP. Three studies have tested this hypothesis. Two studies using a FISH technique reported an absence of fetal Mc in biopsies of patients with sclerodermatous LP and oral LP (Lombardi et al., 2001; Tanei et al., 2000). In a case report, male Mc from a dizygotic twin was found in a 9-year-old girl with a rare ulcerative acral variant of LP (Vabres et al., 2002). In the last study detection of fetal Mc was observed in peripheral blood lymphocytes and affected skin only by Y-chromosome PCR techniques but not by FISH.

3. Human leukocyte antigen (HLA)

3.1. A complicated role during pregnancy

HLA molecules are membrane-bound glycoproteins of central importance in the ability of an individual to distinguish "self" from "non-self" or from "danger". The HLA class I region contains genes that encode for three families of molecules HLA-A, B and C. Similarly, the HLA class II region encodes for three families of molecules: HLA-DR, DQ, and DP. Each HLA-DR, DQ, and DP consists of two chains that are non-covalently associated on the cell surface. The chains are referred to as α and β chains, and the genes encoding the chains are referred to as A and B, respectively. A hallmark characteristic of HLA genes is extensive polymorphism that confers a high number of alleles for each gene, except for DRA1 gene.

The classical HLA genes are not expressed in fetal tissue at the maternal–fetal interface. However, maternal antibodies against paternally derived fetal HLA genes are detectable in the circulation in 20% of first pregnancies and 40% after multiple pregnancies. Maternal–fetal incompatibility has been proposed to be advantageous for a successful pregnancy (Billington, 1964; Finkel and Lilly, 1971). And, a controversial hypothesis holds that HLA gene similarities between the female and male (and thus, fetal) reproductive partners may promote fetal loss, especially recurrent miscarriage. Some murine studies support this hypothesis, finding, for example, larger placental size in mice of MHC incompatible matings (ref) and higher rates of fetal absorption in certain MHC compatible matings (refs). It must be emphasized, however, that classical HLA molecules are not expressed at the feto–maternal interface. The non-classical class I gene HLA-G is expressed by placental cells, as is HLA-C, though to a lesser extent. The roles of these proteins at the maternal–fetal interface is currently the subject of intense study.

Studies of maternal–fetal HLA compatibility in women with RA suggest that HLA incompatibility is advantageous to the mother (Nelson et al., 1993).

3.2. A two-step role in autoimmunity

Susceptibility to autoimmune diseases is linked to HLA alleles, i.e., HLA DRB1*01 and DRB1*04 to rheumatoid arthritis, HLA DQA1*0501 to juvenile dermatomyositis. The associations are mainly with HLA class II alleles and differ depending on ethnic groups. Relationship between a particular allele and the pathogenesis of a disease is complex and not fully understood. Some HLA alleles might predispose to immune abnormalities, consequently susceptibility. The DRB1*03 related haplotype is increased among Caucasians with autoimmune diseases (Thorsby, 1997). Healthy individuals who are HLA DRB1*03-positive exhibit a number of immune abnormalities, including defective apoptosis pathway (Stassi et al., 1997), a modified pattern of cytokine production (Lio et al., 1997), prevalence of circulating autoantibodies (Boehm et al., 1993), and other abnormalities.

In the context of Mc and autoimmune diseases, HLA has probably two distinct or complementary roles: a genetic role as a risk factor for subsequent Mc depending upon the associated HLA and a transplantation-like role where the HLA relationship between host and donor cells is crucial.

3.3. Microchimerism and HLA associations in autoimmune diseases

In a study of SSc subjects, persistent fetal Mc was evaluated by Y-chromosome-specific nested PCR in T lymphocytes sorted for study from 37 women (19 healthy and 12 SSc). HLA DQA1*0501 was associated with more frequent persistent fetal Mc in mothers carrying this allele ($OR = 13.5$,

$p = 0.007$) and even more in mothers who had a son carrying this allele ($OR = \infty$, $p = 0.00002$). Although the host's HLA genotype correlated with T-lymphocyte Mc, the child's genotype was an even stronger factor in determining persistent T-lymphocyte Mc of the mother (Lambert et al., 2000).

Similarly, maternal Mc was detected by PCR amplification of the non-inherited maternal DQA1 antigen in juvenile dermatomyositis patients, their healthy siblings, and unaffected control children. Persistent maternal Mc in JDM patients, healthy siblings and controls was associated with a HLA DQA1*0501 allele in the mother ($p = 0.01, 0.04, 0.008$, respectively) (Reed et al., 2004). Further, maternally transferred chimeric T cells were responsive to the host's (JDM child) lymphocytes (33.75 ± 8.4 IFNγ producing cells from JDM cells versus. 5.0 ± 1.25 from maternal cells). These combined data suggest that chimeric cells play a direct role in the JDM disease process and that the mother's HLA genotype facilitates the transfer and/or persistence of maternal cells in the fetal circulation (Reed et al., 2004).

However, a third study describes no significant association of maternal Mc within the T lymphocytes of the child according to DQA1*0501 of the mother ($n = 10$) or of fetal Mc within maternal T lymphocytes ($n = 27$) according to DQA1*0501 of the child (Artlett et al., 2003). The latter result might contrast with the two other reports because of differences in techniques used to detect Mc (Lambert, 2004).

These preliminary data suggest depending upon the donor's HLA genotype (child for the SSc study and mother for the JDM study) transfer and/or persistence of donor's cells into the host might be facilitated. Moreover, in both studies (SSc and JDM) HLA DQA1*0501 has been shown to be the allele involved in this phenomenon. This is interesting in regard to previous work showing that the HLA DQα1*0501/DQβ*0301 molecule might have access to peptides earlier in the processing pathway, due to a decreased class II-associated Li peptide binding, and so might encounter endogenous peptides that would induce autoimmunity (Reed et al., 1997).

3.4. HLA compatibility between donor and host cells in autoimmune disease

Another major role played by HLA molecules is seen in transfusion-associated graft-versus-host disease (TA-GVHD). TA-GVHD mostly occurs in immunologically impaired recipients, where the recipient cannot recognize or destroy engrafted viable donor T lymphocytes. Although rare, TA-GVHD has also been described in immunocompetent recipient after transfusion of cellular components from HLA homozygous donor to recipients heterozygous for that HLA haplotype (Wagner and Flegel, 1995) (Fig. 1). This phenomenon is not dependent upon a specific HLA allele (Takahashi et al., 1994). In this particular donor/recipient HLA relationship, the recipient lymphocytes would perceive the donor cells as self and thus would not respond to donor cells, whereas donor cells would recognize the recipient as foreign and generate a response.

As described above, some autoimmune diseases such as SSc, PBC, and SS have clinical similarities with chronic GVHD. A similar HLA relationship between host and non-host cells has been observed in SSc families. Most of the time the HLA gene a child inherits from the father differs from the mother's HLA genes and thus is HLA-incompatible (Table 2). Sometimes, the HLA gene a child inherits from the father is the same as one of the mother's and thus is HLA-compatible. Fetal Mc is a risk factor for SSc and prior birth of a child who is compatible for DRB1 genes increases the risk of

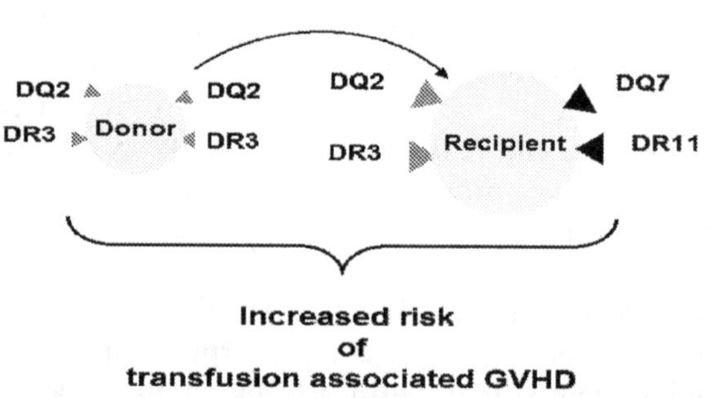

Figure 1. HLA relationship between donor and recipients in transfusion-associated GVHD.

Table 2
HLA relationship between mother and child's cells

	Case 1	Case 2	Case 3	Case 4
Mother (host)	A, B	A, B	A, A	A, B
Child (donor)	A, B	A, A	A, B	A, C
	Bi-directional compatibility	Compatibility from host's perspective	Compatibility from donor's perspective	Incompatibility

SSc in the mother almost ninefold ($p = 0.001$). The association is further strengthened if the child is HLA-compatible due to homozygosity ($OR = 19$, $p = 0.003$) (Nelson et al., 1998). Moreover, maternal Mc commonly persists into adult life (Maloney et al., 1999) and is more frequent in women with SSc than healthy women (Lambert et al., 2004). A significant increased risk of SSc occurs in women for whom the patient's mother was DQA1- and/or DRB1-compatible from the perspective of the patient, which triggers to a trans-generational HLA compatibility between the patient's mother and the patient's child (unpublished data). A woman may become a long-term host to cells from her mother and also her children that would trigger to "auto" immunity under particular HLA relationship between microchimeric sources and the host, specific genetic susceptibility, etc.

In women with inflammatory bowel disease (IBD), disease activity during pregnancy is variable and factors influencing the course of the disease remain unclear. Forty-two of the 50 (84%) pregnancies studied were incompatible at the DRB1 loci and 68% at the DQ loci (Kane et al., 2004). Disease activity scores improved between women who were incompatible at both loci compared with one or neither loci, suggesting that improvement in IBD symptoms during pregnancy many be related to HLA compatibility.

In an experimental murine model, transfusion of homozygous parental lymphocytes into heterozygous progeny results in disease that resembles human SLE (Portanova and Kotzin, 1988). This argues for a possible role in the HLA relationship between donor and host cells triggering autoimmunity. A very recent study has shown that indeed an increased bi-directional HLA class II compatibility was observed in SLE males and their mothers compared to healthy males (Stevens et al., 2005b). Sons with SLE were bi-directionally HLA DRB1 compatible (HLA-identical) with mothers more often than healthy sons ($OR = 5.0$, $p = 0.006$). No increase in uni-directional compatibility of the mother from the son's perspective (Table 2) was observed at any locus.

Although SSc studies have shown increase of HLA compatibility between host and donors' cells and increase levels of fetal Mc in SSc women, there is no clear correlation of HLA compatibility with quantitative Mc and/or presence of Mc. One recent study shows an association between maternal chimerism in the fetus and maternal compatibility at the class II DRB1 and/or DQB1 loci (Berry et al., 2004). However the number of mother/child pairs tested is too small (30) to draw strong conclusions.

In conclusion, it is not Mc alone that triggers autoimmunity, since healthy individuals are also microchimeric, but the relationship between Mc and HLA in the host. Both in SLE and in SSc the increase of HLA compatibility observed is from the host's perspective but not from the donor's perspective, possibly of immunological significance in different diseases in which microchimeric T cells are responsive to the host's lymphocytes (Burastero et al., 2003; Reed et al., 2004; Scaletti et al., 2002).

4. Maternal antibodies

Maternal IgG antibodies are selectively transferred into the fetal circulation through Fcγ receptors expressed on trophoblast. This passive transfer of antibodies plays a role in the protection of the fetus from maternal infection during pregnancy and the newborn from infection after delivery. However, passively transferred antibodies also can result in fetal damage via either alloimmune or autoimmune mechanisms. Examples of antibody-mediated alloimmune disease affecting the fetus-newborn include Rh disease and fetal–neonatal alloimmune thrombocytopenia. The best known in antibody-mediated autoimmune disease affecting the fetus–newborn is known as neonatal lupus syndrome, in which anti-SSA/SSB antibodies appear to cause the immune damage (Boutjdir et al., 1997; Lee LA and Harnon, 1982; Miranda-Carus et al., 1998; Reichlin et al., 1994; Scott et al., 1983; Watson et al., 1984). Current hypotheses state that apoptosis results in SSA/SSB translocation to the cell surface where they bind maternal antibodies. The bound maternal antibodies trigger a release of TGF-β, which promotes scarring, and a profibrotic milieu. This scenario also promotes tissue release of TGF-β and scarring occurs (Clancy and Buyon, 2003, 2004; Nield et al., 2002).

Transfer of maternal antibodies triggers neonatal autoreactive T-cell responses and T-cell mediated organ-specific autoimmune disease in mice (Setiady et al., 2003). Other studies show that fetal islet cell autoantibody exposure protects against the development of diabetes in a 11-year follow-up (Koczwara et al., 2004): offspring who are GAD or IA-2 autoantibody positive at birth have significantly lower risks for developing multiple islet autoantibodies (5-year risk) and diabetes (8-year risk) than do offspring negative at birth. Protection occurred in offspring with the HLA DRB1*03/DRB1*04-DQB1*0302 genotype. In an earlier study of non-obese diabetic (NOD) mice, maternal transmission of antibodies during development influenced T-cell destruction of the islet β cells (Greeley et al., 2002).

5. In summary

Mammalian pregnancy being foreign to the host stimulates a localized tolerant state. Immunological tolerance has to be achieved without compromising the ability of the individual to survive. However, could this same system that promotes tolerance, which for species survival is mandatory, also be the system that triggers or aids in the development of autoimmune disorders? This is suggested by experiments of cell transfer in which HLA similarity or identity adds to the development of disease. The changes that occur as the result of pregnancy represent an immunological challenge that can promote great insights into our understanding of the immune system.

Key points

- The maternal–fetal aspects of autoimmune disease are clearly complex and as yet not fully understood.
- The transfer of fetal and maternal cells during pregnancy may be related to autoimmune disease and to a lesser extent disease flare or remission.
- The transfer or persistence of these cells may be related to the HLA antigens present on both the fetal and maternal cells.
- The placental interface, originally thought to be an immunologically privileged site, appears to be more complex, participating in the transfer of cells and antibodies and potentially playing a role in altering the immune response.

References

Ando, T., Imaizumi, M., Graves, P.N., Unger, P., Davies, T.F. 2002. Intrathyroidal fetal microchimerism in Graves' disease. J. Clin. Endocrinol. Metab. 87, 3315–3320.

Ansari, A.A., Fett, J.D., Carraway, R.E., Mayne, A.E., Onlamoon, N., Sundstrom, J.B. 2002. Autoimmune mechanisms as the basis for human peripartum cardiomyopathy. Clin. Rev. Allergy Immunol. 23, 301–324.

Aractingi, S., Sibilia, J., Meignin, V., Launay, D., Hachulla, E., Le Danff, C., Janin, A., Mariette, X. 2002. Presence of microchimerism in labial salivary glands in systemic sclerosis but not in Sjögren's syndrome. Arthritis Rheum. 46, 1039–1043.

Artlett, C.M., Cox, L.A., Jimenez, S.A. 2000a. Detection of cellular microchimerism of male or female origin in systemic sclerosis patients by polymerase chain reaction analysis of HLA-Cw antigens. Arthritis Rheum. 43, 1062–1067.

Artlett, C.M., Cox, L.A., Ramos, R.C., Dennis, T.N., Fortunato, R.A., Hummers, L.K., Jimenez, S.A., Smith, J.B. 2002. Increased microchimeric CD4+ T lymphocytes in peripheral blood from women with systemic sclerosis. Clin. Immunol. 103, 303–308.

Artlett, C.M., O'Hanlon, T.P., Lopez, A.M., Song, Y.W., Miller, F.W., Rider, L.G. 2003. HLA-DQA1 is not an apparent risk factor for microchimerism in patients with various autoimmune diseases and in healthy individuals. Arthritis Rheum. 48, 2567–2572.

Artlett, C.M., Ramos, R., Jiminez, S.A., Patterson, K., Miller, F.W., Rider, L.G. 2000b. Chimeric cells of maternal origin in juvenile idiopathic inflammatory myopathies. Childhood Myositis Heterogeneity Collaborative Group. Lancet 356, 2155–2156.

Artlett, C.M., Smith, J.B., Jimenez, S.A. 1998. Identification of fetal DNA and cells in skin lesions from women with systemic sclerosis. N. Engl. J. Med. 338, 1186–1191.

Ashkar, A.A., Di Santo, J.P., Croy, B.A. 2000. Interferon gamma contributes to initiation of uterine vascular modification, decidual integrity, and uterine natural killer cell maturation during normal murine pregnancy. J. Exp. Med. 192, 259–270.

Barakonyi, A., Polgar, B., Szekeres-Bartho, J. 1999. The role of gamma/delta T-cell receptor-positive cells in pregnancy: part II. Am. J. Reprod. Immunol. 42, 83–87.

Berry, S.M., Hassan, S.S., Russell, E., Kukuruga, D., Land, S., Kaplan, J. 2004. Association of maternal histocompatibility at class II HLA loci with maternal microchimerism in the fetus. Pediatr. Res. 56, 73–78.

Bianchi, D.W., Zickwolf, G.K., Weil, G.J., Sylvester, S., DeMaria, M.A. 1996. Male fetal progenitor cells persist in maternal blood for as long as 27 years postpartum. Proc. Natl. Acad. Sci. USA 93, 705–708.

Billington, W.D. 1964. Influence of immunological dissimilarity of mother and foetus on size of placenta in mice. Nature 202, 317–318.

Boehm, B.O., Kuhnl, P., Loliger, C., Ketzler-Sasse, U., Holzberger, G., Seidl, S., Bauerle, R., Schifferdecker, E., Usadel, K.H. 1993. HLA-DR3 and HLA-DR5 confer risk for autoantibody positivity against the thyroperoxidase (mic-TPO) antigen in healthy blood donors. Clin. Investig. 71, 221–225.

Borish, L.C., Steinke, J.W. 2003. 2. Cytokines and chemokines. J. Allergy Clin. Immunol. 111, S460–S475.

Boutjdir, M., Chen, L., Zhang, Z.H., Tseng, C.E., DiDonato, F., Rashbaum, W., Morris, A., el-Sherif, N., Buyon, J.P. 1997. Arrhythmogenicity of IgG and anti-52-kD SSA/Ro affinity-purified antibodies from mothers of children with congenital heart block. Circ. Res. 80, 354–362.

Burastero, S.E., Galbiati, S., Vassallo, A., Sabbadini, M.G., Bellone, M., Marchionni, L., Smid, M., Ferrero, E., Ferrari, A., Ferrari, M., Cremonesi, L. 2003. Cellular microchimerism as a lifelong physiologic status in parous women: an immunologic basis for its amplification in patients with systemic sclerosis. Arthritis Rheum. 48, 1109–1116.

Check, J.H., Ostrzenski, A., Klimek, R. 1997. Expression of an immunomodulatory protein known as progesterone induced blocking factor (PIBF) does not correlate with first trimester spontaneous abortions in progesterone supplemented women. Am. J. Reprod. Immunol. 37, 330–334.

Clancy, R.M., Buyon, J.P. 2003. Clearance of apoptotic cells: TGF-beta in the balance between inflammation and fibrosis. J. Leukoc. Biol. 74, 959–960.

Clancy, R.M., Buyon, J.P. 2004. Autoimmune-associated congenital heart block: dissecting the cascade from immunologic insult to relentless fibrosis. Anat. Rec. 280A, 1027–1035.

Corpechot, C., Barbu, V., Chazouilleres, O., Poupon, R. 2000. Fetal microchimerism in primary biliary cirrhosis. J. Hepatol. 33, 696–700.

Endo, Y., Negishi, I., Ishikawa, O. 2002. Possible contribution of microchimerism to the pathogenesis of Sjögren's syndrome. Rheumatology (Oxford) 41, 490–495.

Evans, P.C., Lambert, N., Maloney, S., Furst, D.E., Moore, J.M., Nelson, J.L. 1999. Long-term fetal microchimerism in peripheral blood mononuclear cell subsets in healthy women and women with scleroderma. Blood 93, 2033–2037.

Fanning, P.A., Jonsson, J.R., Clouston, A.D., Edwards-Smith, C., Balderson, G.A., Macdonald, G.A., Crawford, D.H., Kerlin, P., Powell, L.W., Powell, E.E. 2000. Detection of male DNA in the liver of female patients with primary biliary cirrhosis. J. Hepatol. 33, 690–695.

Finkel, S.I., Lilly, F. 1971. Influence of histoincompatibility between mother and foetus on placental size in mice. Nature 234, 102–103.

Greeley, S.A., Katsumata, M., Yu, L., Eisenbarth, G.S., Moore, D.J., Goodarzi, H., Barker, C.F., Naji, A., Noorchashm, H. 2002. Elimination of maternally transmitted autoantibodies prevents diabetes in nonobese diabetic mice. Nat. Med. 8, 399–402.

Imaizumi, M., Pritsker, A., Unger, P., Davies, T.F. 2002. Intrathyroidal fetal microchimerism in pregnancy and postpartum. Endocrinology 143, 247–253.

Johnson, K.L., McAlindon, T.E., Mulcahy, E., Bianchi, D.W. 2001a. Microchimerism in a female patient with systemic lupus erythematosus. Arthritis Rheum. 44, 2107–2111.

Johnson, K.L., Nelson, J.L., Furst, D.E., McSweeney, P.A., Roberts, D.J., Zhen, D.K., Bianchi, D.W. 2001b. Fetal cell microchimerism in tissue from multiple sites in women with systemic sclerosis. Arthritis Rheum. 44, 1848–1854.

Jonsson, Y., Ekerfelt, C., Berg, G., Nieminen, K., Sharma, S., Ernerudh, J., Matthiesen, L. 2004. Systemic Th1/Th2 cytokine responses to paternal and vaccination antigens in preeclampsia: no differences compared with normal pregnancy. Am. J. Reprod. Immunol. 51, 302–310.

Kane, S., Kisiel, J., Shih, L., Hanauer, S. 2004. HLA disparity determines disease activity through pregnancy in women with inflammatory bowel disease. Am. J. Gastroenterol. 99, 1523–1526.

Khosrotehrani, K., Mery, L., Aractingi, S., Bianchi, D.W., Johnson, K.L. 2005. Absence of fetal cell microchimerism in cutaneous lesions of lupus erythematosus. Ann. Rheum. Dis. 64, 159–160.

Klintschar, M., Schwaiger, P., Mannweiler, S., Regauer, S., Kleiber, M. 2001. Evidence of fetal microchimerism in

Hashimoto's thyroiditis. J. Clin. Endocrinol. Metab. 86, 2494–2498.

Koczwara, K., Bonifacio, E., Ziegler, A.G. 2004. Transmission of maternal islet antibodies and risk of autoimmune diabetes in offspring of mothers with type 1 diabetes. Diabetes 53, 1–4.

Kuroki, M., Okayama, A., Nakamura, S., Sasaki, T., Murai, K., Shiba, R., Shinohara, M., Tsubouchi, H. 2002. Detection of maternal–fetal microchimerism in the inflammatory lesions of patients with Sjögren's syndrome. Ann. Rheum. Dis. 61, 1041–1046.

Lambert, N.C. 2004. HLA-DQA1 as a risk factor for microchimerism: comment on the article by Artlett et al. Arthritis Rheum. 50, 2713.

Lambert, N.C., Erickson, T.D., Yan, Z., Pang, J.M., Guthrie, K.A., Furst, D.E., Nelson, J.L. 2004. Quantification of maternal microchimerism by HLA-specific real-time polymerase chain reaction: studies of healthy women and women with scleroderma. Arthritis Rheum. 50, 906–914.

Lambert, N.C., Evans, P.C., Hashizumi, T.L., Maloney, S., Gooley, T., Furst, D.E., Nelson, J.L. 2000. Cutting edge: persistent fetal microchimerism in T lymphocytes is associated with HLA-DQA1*0501: implications in autoimmunity. J. Immunol. 164, 5545–5548.

Lambert, N.C., Lo, Y.M., Erickson, T.D., Tylee, T.S., Guthrie, K.A., Furst, D.E., Nelson, J.L. 2002. Male microchimerism in healthy women and women with scleroderma: cells or circulating DNA? A quantitative answer. Blood 100, 2845–2851.

Lambert, N.C., Stevens, A.M., Tylee, T.S., Erickson, T.D., Furst, D.E., Nelson, J.L. 2001. From the simple detection of microchimerism in patients with autoimmune diseases to its implication in pathogenesis. Ann. NY Acad. Sci. 945, 164–171.

Le Bouteiller, P. 1994. HLA class I chromosomal region, genes, and products: facts and questions. Crit. Rev. Immunol. 14, 89–129.

Lee LA, R.B., Harnon, C. 1982. Autoantibodies to SS-A/Ro in congenital heart block. Arthritis Rheum. 20, S24.

Lio, D., Candore, G., Romano, G.C., D'Anna, C., Gervasi, F., Di Lorenzo, G., Modica, M.A., Potestio, M., Caruso, C. 1997. Modification of cytokine patterns in subjects bearing the HLA-B8,DR3 phenotype: implications for autoimmunity. Cytokines Cell Mol. Ther. 3, 217–224.

Lo, E.S., Lo, Y.M., Hjelm, N.M., Thilaganathan, B. 1998. Transfer of nucleated maternal cells into fetal circulation during the second trimester of pregnancy. Br. J. Haematol. 100, 605–606.

Lo, Y.M., Lau, T.K., Chan, L.Y., Leung, T.N., Chang, A.M. 2000. Quantitative analysis of the bidirectional fetomaternal transfer of nucleated cells and plasma DNA. Clin. Chem. 46, 1301–1309.

Lombardi, T., Philippeaux, M.M., Hadengue, A., Samson, J., Borisch, B., Rubbia-Brandt, L. 2001. Absence of leukocyte microchimerism in oral lichen planus (OLP): an in situ hybridisation study. J. Oral Pathol. Med. 30, 398–401.

Maloney, S., Smith, A., Furst, D.E., Myerson, D., Rupert, K., Evans, P.C., Nelson, J.L. 1999. Microchimerism of maternal origin persists into adult life. J. Clin. Invest. 104, 41–47.

Matthiesen, L., Ekerfelt, C., Berg, G., Ernerudh, J. 1998. Increased numbers of circulating interferon-gamma- and interleukin-4-secreting cells during normal pregnancy. Am. J. Reprod. Immunol. 39, 362–367.

Mellor, A.L., Munn, D.H. 1999. Tryptophan catabolism and T-cell toleransb: immunosuppression by starvation?. Immunol. Today 20, 469–473.

Miranda-Carus, M.E., Boutjdir, M., Tseng, C.E., DiDonato, F., Chan, E.K., Buyon, J.P. 1998. Induction of antibodies reactive with SSA/Ro-SSB/La and development of congenital heart block in a murine model. J. Immunol. 161, 5886–5892.

Miyashita, Y., Ono, M., Ueki, H., Kurasawa, K. 2000. Y chromosome microchimerism in rheumatic autoimmune disease. Ann. Rheum. Dis. 59, 655–656.

Morales, P.J., Pace, J.L., Platt, J.S., Phillips, T.A., Morgan, K., Fazleabas, A.T., Hunt, J.S. 2003. Placental cell expression of HLA-G2 isoforms is limited to the invasive trophoblast phenotype. J. Immunol. 171, 6215–6224.

Munn, D.H., Zhou, M., Attwood, J.T., Bondarev, I., Conway, S.J., Marshall, B., Brown, C., Mellor, A.L. 1998. Prevention of allogeneic fetal rejection by tryptophan catabolism. Science 281, 1191–1193.

Murata, H., Nakauchi, H., Sumida, T. 1999. Microchimerism in Japanese women patients with systemic sclerosis. Lancet 354, 220.

Nagaeva, O., Jonsson, L., Mincheva-Nilsson, L. 2002. Dominant IL-10 and TGF-beta mRNA expression in gamma deltaT cells of human early pregnancy decidua suggests immunoregulatory potential. Am. J. Reprod. Immunol. 48, 9–17.

Nakagome, Y., Nagafuchi, S., Nakahori, Y. 1990. Prenatal sex determination. Lancet 335, 291.

Nakagome, Y., Nagafuchi, S., Seki, S., Nakahori, Y., Tamura, T., Yamada, M., Iwaya, M. 1991. A repeating unit of the DYZ1 family on the human Y chromosome consists of segments with partial male-specificity. Cytogenet. Cell Genet. 56, 74–77.

Nelson, J.L. 1996. Maternal–fetal immunology and autoimmune disease: is some autoimmune disease auto-alloimmune or allo-autoimmune?. Arthritis Rheum. 39, 191–194.

Nelson, J.L., Furst, D.E., Maloney, S., Gooley, T., Evans, P.C., Smith, A., Bean, M.A., Ober, C., Bianchi, D.W. 1998. Microchimerism and HLA-compatible relationships of pregnancy in scleroderma. Lancet 351, 559–562.

Nelson, J.L., Hughes, K.A., Smith, A.G., Nisperos, B.B., Branchaud, A.M., Hansen, J.A. 1993. Maternal–fetal disparity in HLA class II alloantigens and the pregnancy-induced amelioration of rheumatoid arthritis. N. Engl. J. Med. 329, 466–471.

Nield, L.E., Silverman, E.D., Taylor, G.P., Smallhorn, J.F., Mullen, J.B., Silverman, N.H., Finley, J.P., Law, Y.M., Human, D.G., Seaward, P.G., Hamilton, R.M., Hornberger, L.K. 2002. Maternal anti-Ro and anti-La antibody-associated endocardial fibroelastosis. Circulation 105, 843–848.

Ober, C. 1998. HLA and pregnancy: the paradox of the fetal allograft. Am. J. Hum. Genet. 62, 1–5.

Ohtsuka, T., Miyamoto, Y., Yamakage, A., Yamazaki, S. 2001. Quantitative analysis of microchimerism in systemic sclerosis skin tissue. Arch. Dermatol. Res. 293, 387–391.

Østensen, M., Forger, F., Nelson, J.L., Schuhmacher, A., Hebisch, G., Villiger, P.M. 2005. Pregnancy in patients with rheumatic disease: anti-inflammatory cytokines increase in pregnancy and decrease post partum. Ann. Rheum. Dis. 64, 839–844.

Pazmany, L., Mandelboim, O., Vales-Gomez, M., Davis, D.M., Reyburn, H.T., Strominger, J.L. 1996. Protection from natural killer cell-mediated lysis by HLA-G expression on target cells. Science 274, 792–795.

Piccinni, M.P., Giudizi, M.G., Biagiotti, R., Beloni, L., Giannarini, L., Sampognaro, S., Parronchi, P., Manetti, R., Annunziato, F., Livi, C., et al. 1995. Progesterone favors the development of human T helper cells producing Th2-type cytokines and promotes both IL-4 production and membrane CD30 expression in established Th1 cell clones. J. Immunol. 155, 128–133.

Pollack, M.S., Kirkpatrick, D., Kapoor, N., Dupont, B., O'Reilly, R.J. 1982. Identification by HLA typing of intrauterine-derived maternal T cells in four patients with severe combined immunodeficiency. N. Engl. J. Med. 307, 662–666.

Poole, J.A., Claman, H.N. 2004. Immunology of pregnancy. Implications for the mother. Clin. Rev. Allergy Immunol. 26, 161–170.

Portanova, J.P., Kotzin, B.L. 1988. Lupus-like autoimmunity in murine graft-versus-host disease. Concepts Immunopathol 6, 119–140.

Rajagopalan, S., Long, E.O. 1999. A human histocompatibility leukocyte antigen (HLA)-G-specific receptor expressed on all natural killer cells. J. Exp. Med. 189, 1093–1100.

Reed, A.M., Collins, E.J., Shock, L.P., Klapper, D.G., Frelinger, J.A. 1997. Diminished class II-associated Ii peptide binding to the juvenile dermatomyositis HLA-DQ alpha 1*0501/DQ beta 1*0301 molecule. J. Immunol. 159, 6260–6265.

Reed, A.M., McNallan, K., Wettstein, P., Vehe, R., Ober, C. 2004. Does HLA-dependent chimerism underlie the pathogenesis of juvenile dermatomyositis?. J. Immunol. 172, 5041–5046.

Reed, A.M., Picornell, Y.J., Harwood, A., Kredich, D.W. 2000. Chimerism in children with juvenile dermatomyositis. Lancet 356, 2156–2157.

Reed, A.M., Shock, L.P., Picornell, J. 1998. Microchimerism in children with juvenile dermatomyositis. Arthritis Rheum. 41, S264.

Reichlin, M., Brucato, A., Frank, M.B., Maddison, P.J., McCubbin, V.R., Wolfson-Reichlin, M., Lee, L.A. 1994. Concentration of autoantibodies to native 60-kd Ro/SS-A and denatured 52-kd Ro/SS-A in eluates from the heart of a child who died with congenital complete heart block. Arthritis Rheum. 37, 1698–1703.

Roberts, C.W., Walker, W., Alexander, J. 2001. Sex-associated hormones and immunity to protozoan parasites. Clin. Microbiol. Rev. 14, 476–488.

Rubbia-Brandt, L., Philippeaux, M.M., Chavez, S., Mentha, G., Borisch, B., Hadengue, A. 1999. FISH for Y chromosome in women with primary biliary cirrhosis: lack of evidence for leukocyte microchimerism. Hepatology 30, 821–822.

Rukavina, D., Gill, T.J., III 1997. Immunobiology and immunopathology of early pregnancy. Early Pregnancy 3, 141–145.

Sanchez-Ramon, S., Navarro, A.J., Aristimuno, C., Rodriguez-Mahou, M., Bellon, J.M., Fernandez-Cruz, E., Andres, C. 2005. Pregnancy-induced expansion of regulatory T-lymphocytes may mediate protection to multiple sclerosis activity. Immunol. Lett. 96, 195–201.

Scaletti, C., Vultaggio, A., Bonifacio, S., Emmi, L., Torricelli, F., Maggi, E., Romagnani, S., Piccinni, M.P. 2002. Th2-oriented profile of male offspring T cells present in women with systemic sclerosis and reactive with maternal major histocompatibility complex antigens. Arthritis Rheum. 46, 445–450.

Schoniger-Hekele, M., Muller, C., Ackermann, J., Drach, J., Wrba, F., Penner, E., Ferenci, P. 2002. Lack of evidence for involvement of fetal microchimerism in pathogenesis of primary biliary cirrhosis. Dig. Dis. Sci. 47, 1909–1914.

Schrocksnadel, H., Baier-Bitterlich, G., Dapunt, O., Wachter, H., Fuchs, D. 1996. Decreased plasma tryptophan in pregnancy. Obstet. Gynecol. 88, 47–50.

Scott, J.S., Maddison, P.J., Taylor, P.V., Esscher, E., Scott, O., Skinner, R.P. 1983. Connective-tissue disease, antibodies to ribonucleoprotein, and congenital heart block. N. Engl. J. Med. 309, 209–212.

Selva-O'Callaghan, A., Boeckh-Behrens, T.M., Balada-Prades, E., Solans-Laque, R., Vilardell-Tarres, M. 2001. Fetal microchimerism and inflammatory myopathies. Lancet 357, 887.

Selva-O'Callaghan, A., Mijares-Boeckh-Behrens, T., Prades, E.B., Solans-Laque, R., Simeon-Aznar, C.P., Fonollosa-Pla, V., Vilardell-Tarres, M. 2003. Lack of evidence of foetal microchimerism in female Spanish patients with systemic sclerosis. Lupus 12, 15–20.

Setiady, Y.Y., Samy, E.T., Tung, K.S. 2003. Maternal autoantibody triggers de novo T cell-mediated neonatal autoimmune disease. J. Immunol. 170, 4656–4664.

Shevach, E.M. 2000. Regulatory T cells in autoimmmunity*. Annu. Rev. Immunol. 18, 423–449.

Shevach, E.M., McHugh, R.S., Thornton, A.M., Piccirillo, C., Natarajan, K., Margulies, D.H. 2001. Control of autoimmunity by regulatory T cells. Adv. Exp. Med. Biol. 490, 21–32.

Srivatsa, B., Srivatsa, S., Johnson, K.L., Bianchi, D.W. 2003. Maternal cell microchimerism in newborn tissues. J. Pediatr. 142, 31–35.

Srivatsa, B., Srivatsa, S., Johnson, K.L., Samura, O., Lee, S.L., Bianchi, D.W. 2001. Microchimerism of presumed fetal origin in thyroid specimens from women: a case-control study. Lancet 358, 2034–2038.

Stassi, G., Todaro, M., De Maria, R., Candore, G., Cigna, D., Caruso, C., Galluzzo, A., Giordano, C. 1997. Defective expression of CD95 (FAS/APO-1) molecule suggests apoptosis impairment of T and B cells in HLA-B8, DR3-positive individuals. Hum. Immunol. 55, 39–45.

Stevens, A.M., Hermes, H.M., Lambert, N.C., Nelson, J.L., Meroni, P.L., Cimaz, R. 2005a. Maternal and sibling microchimerism in twins and triplets discordant for neonatal lupus syndrome-congenital heart block. Rheumatology (Oxford) 44, 187–191.

Stevens, A.M., Hermes, H.M., Rutledge, J.C., Buyon, J.P., Nelson, J.L. 2003. Myocardial-tissue-specific phenotype of maternal microchimerism in neonatal lupus congenital heart block. Lancet 362, 1617–1623.

Stevens, A.M., Tsao, B.P., Hahn, B.H., Guthrie, K., Lambert, N.C., Porter, A.J., Tylee, T.S., Nelson, J.L. 2005b. Maternal HLA class II compatibility in men with systemic lupus erythematosus. Arthritis Rheum. 52, 2768–2773.

Szekeres-Bartho, J. 2002. Immunological relationship between the mother and the fetus. Int. Rev. Immunol. 21, 471–495.

Takahashi, K., Juji, T., Miyamoto, M., Uchida, S., Akaza, T., Tadokoro, K., Shibata, Y., Ino, T., Hidano, A. 1994. Analysis of risk factors for post-transfusion graft-versus-host disease in Japan. Japanese Red Cross PT-GVHD Study Group. Lancet 343, 700–702.

Tanaka, A., Lindor, K., Gish, R., Batts, K., Shiratori, Y., Omata, M., Nelson, J.L., Ansari, A., Coppel, R., Newsome, M., Gershwin, M.E. 1999. Fetal microchimerism alone does not contribute to the induction of primary biliary cirrhosis. Hepatology 30, 833–838.

Tanei, R., Yokono, H., Motoori, T., Katsuoka, K. 2000. Microchimerism seems uninvolved in the pathogenesis of idiopathic lichen planus. Dermatology 201, 373–374.

Thorsby, E. 1997. Invited anniversary review: HLA associated diseases. Hum. Immunol. 53, 1–11.

Toda, I., Kuwana, M., Tsubota, K., Kawakami, Y. 2001. Lack of evidence for an increased microchimerism in the circulation of patients with Sjögren's syndrome. Ann. Rheum. Dis. 60, 248–253.

Vabres, P., Malinge, M.C., Larregue, M., Bonneau, D. 2002. Microchimerism from a dizygotic twin in juvenile ulcerative lichen planus. Lancet 359, 1861–1862.

van der Meer, A., Lukassen, H.G., van Lierop, M.J., Wijnands, F., Mosselman, S., Braat, D.D., Joosten, I. 2004. Membrane-bound HLA-G activates proliferation and interferon-gamma production by uterine natural killer cells. Mol. Hum. Reprod. 10, 189–195.

Vassiliadis, S., Ranella, A., Papadimitriou, L., Makrygiannakis, A., Athanassakis, I. 1998. Serum levels of pro- and anti-inflammatory cytokines in non-pregnant women, during pregnancy, labour and abortion. Mediators Inflamm 7, 69–72.

Wagner, F.F., Flegel, W.A. 1995. Transfusion-associated graft-versus-host disease: risk due to homozygous HLA haplotypes. Transfusion 35, 284–291.

Watson, R.M., Lane, A.T., Barnett, N.K., Bias, W.B., Arnett, F.C., Provost, T.T. 1984. Neonatal lupus erythematosus. A clinical, serological and immunogenetic study with review of the literature. Medicine (Baltimore) 63, 362–378.

Wegmann, T.G., Lin, H., Guilbert, L., Mosmann, T.R. 1993. Bidirectional cytokine interactions in the maternal–fetal relationship: is successful pregnancy a TH2 phenomenon? Immunol. Today 14, 353–356.

Handbook of Systemic Autoimmune Diseases, Volume 4
Reproductive and Hormonal Aspects of Systemic Autoimmune Diseases
Michael Lockshin and D. Ware Branch, editors

CHAPTER 4

Fertility and Autoimmune Disease

Shawn Gurtcheff[a], Harry Hatasaka[b,*]

[a]*General Division of Obstetrics and Gynecology, Department of Obstetrics and Gynecology, University of Utah Health Sciences Center, Salt Lake City, UT, USA*

[b]*Division of Reproductive Endocrinology, Department of Obstetrics and Gynecology, University of Utah Health Sciences Center, Salt Lake City, UT, USA*

1. Introduction

Autoimmune diseases have a predilection for women of reproductive age. In the United States, approximately 8.5 million people are affected by autoimmune disease. Eighty-five percent of these are women [1]. Fertility and fecundity in women with these conditions are of obvious importance. When considering infertility in women with autoimmune disease, one must consider three aspects of the issue. First, does autoimmune disease contribute to infertility in affected women? Second, what is the impact of therapy for autoimmune disease on fertility? Lastly, what are the effects of infertility therapy on women with autoimmune disease?

Autoimmunity is an immune reaction to self, usually due to a loss of tolerance. The pathologic mechanisms may be cellular or humoral, involving autoreactive T lymphocytes, autoantibodies, or immune complexes containing autoantigens. A variety of human tissues are susceptible to attack by autoimmune mechanisms. How the human reproductive tract tissues avoid disruption by the normally functioning immune system is as yet unknown. One might surmise that breeches in the immunologic refuge given to a conceptus or spermatozoa might lead to infertility or recurrent pregnancy loss (RPL); indeed immunologic mechanisms have been ascribed to both. Both direct and indirect immune effects potentially lead to reproductive failure. Direct effects of antibodies against reproductive tissues, such as ovaries, sperm, and endometrium could damage reproductive tissue. Indirect effects such as immune-mediated endocrine abnormalities, vascular abnormalities, and inflammation could play a significant role. In this chapter, we will explore potential mechanisms of immune-mediated infertility, the roles that the systemic autoimmune diseases and autoimmunity might play in infertility, the effects of infertility therapy on autoimmune diseases, and how treatment of autoimmune disease may relate to infertility in women.

2. The epidemiology and etiology of infertility

Infertility is defined as 1 year of unprotected coitus without conception. Approximately 10–15% of the reproductive age couples are affected [2]. This number has been increasing; in 1995 one in six women reported that they had sought professional help because of infertility [3]. Potential causes of infertility include tubal and pelvic pathology, male factor, and ovulatory dysfunction. Infertility is

*Corresponding author.
Division of Reproductive Endocrinology, Department of Obstetrics and Gynecology, University of Utah Health Sciences Center, 30 N 1900 East, Rm 2B-200, Salt Lake City, UT 84132, USA.
Tel.: +1-801-581-3834; fax: +1-801-585-2388.
E-mail address: harry.hatasaka@hsc.utah.edu (H. Hatasaka).

DOI: 10.1016/S1571-5078(05)04004-3

unexplained in 10–20% of infertile couples [4]. A major contributor to infertility is the advancing age in women who desire to conceive. With the availability of safe and effective contraception, changing roles and aspirations for women, and resultant older ages at marriage, the average age of women seeking pregnancy is increasing. In the United States, births to women aged 35–44 have been steadily increasing over the past several years despite relatively stable overall birth rates [5,6]. Tietze's studies of fertility rates within the Hutterite colonies in the 1950s helped quantitate the relationship between maternal age and fecundity [7]. This was a healthy, stable population of men and women not using contraception. Tietze found that in Hutterite women, 33% were infertile at age 40, and 87% were infertile at age 45.

Advancing maternal age correlates with an increasing likelihood of maternal health concerns. Systemic autoimmune diseases are no exception with an average age of onset in women of 30–49 and depending on the diagnosis, an increasing incidence with increasing age [8,9]. Therefore, the age-related decrease in fecundity will be an additional concern to many women with autoimmune diseases who are hoping to conceive.

A particularly troublesome form of reproductive failure is RPL. This is traditionally defined as three pregnancy losses of early (< 20 weeks) but clinically recognized (postimplantation) pregnancies. It is a clinical entity distinct from that of primary (unable to conceive) infertility. It occurs in approximately 1% of women. Potential causes are varied and include genetic abnormalities, environmental factors, anatomic anomalies, infectious etiologies, thrombophilias, and endocrine dysfunction. Unfortunately, after evaluation, etiologies remain unexplained in over 50% of couples with RPL. As with infertility, autoimmunity has been proposed as a potential cause of RPL.

3. Treatment of infertility

Effects of autoimmune disease on fecundity, and infertility treatments on the outcomes of women with autoimmune diseases would best be studied when isolated autoimmune disease was the only detectable factor contributing to infertility. Unfortunately there typically are multiple confounding issues involved in conception, as well as numerous infertility therapies (both specific and empiric), making it difficult to isolate correlations between autoimmunity and infertility. Two types of fertility therapy have been pertinent to the study of autoimmunity and infertility, ovulation induction (OI) and in vitro fertilization (IVF).

OI is accomplished by administering exogenous follicle stimulating hormone (FSH) to induce multiple ovarian egg-containing follicles to develop. When used in a woman who ovulates normally, the process is termed "superovulation" or "controlled ovarian hyperstimulation." The principal rationale of this empiric therapy is to increase the probability of gamete encounters.

The other infertility therapy is IVF. Reporting of statistics for IVF procedures is mandated for all reproductive centers through the Centers for Disease Control. Although autoimmune diseases of women undergoing assisted reproductive technologies are not officially tabulated, the age-related fertility outcome from the national statistics database represent a good source of assessing baseline age-related fertility expectations for each treatment. IVF offers the highest per-attempt success rates of all infertility treatments and theoretically serves to bypass the most common infertility factors (such as male and tubal factors). The attributable risk for infertility among women with autoimmune diseases can be extrapolated better when the major confounding factors are controlled via Assisted Reproductive Technologies.

Although specific techniques vary by center, the fundamental process of IVF is universal. Analogues of gonadotropin-releasing hormone are given to the oocyte donor to suppress the release of endogenous gonadotropins. The ovaries are then stimulated with FSH. Oocyte maturation is induced with human chorionic gonadotropin, and then an outpatient procedure is performed using local analgesia whereby ultrasound guidance directs follicular puncture and retrieval of oocytes. Spermatozoa are isolated from the seminal fluid and capacitation is induced in vitro. Spermatozoa are then added to oocytes and allowed to fertilize. If indicated, micromanipulation may be performed and sperm can be injected into the cytoplasm in the process known as intracytoplasmic sperm injection. Induction and maintenance of a mature luteal phase endometrium is achieved with progesterone or human chorionic gonadotropin. Once embryonic cleavage has occurred, embryos are transferred to the uterus via the cervix.

Couples at risk for offspring with detectable serious genetic abnormalities (such as cystic fibrosis) may opt for prenatal genetic diagnosis to select unaffected embryos for uterine transfer. Single blastomeres are biopsied for genetic testing during the early totipotent cleaving stages of embryonic development.

Several common physiologic effects of these two therapies may impact the activity of autoimmune diseases. For example, the use of FSH stimulates follicular development and thus increases serum estrogen concentrations that may acutely surpass normal pregnancy levels [10–12]. Also, the number of embryos implanted directly affects risk of multiple gestation and thus further complications of pregnancy that could interact with an underlying autoimmune condition.

Indeed, women with autoimmune disease seem to be at additional risk when undergoing assisted reproductive technologies. In a retrospective chart review of 19 women with antiphospholipid antibody syndrome (APS) or systemic lupus erythematosus (SLE) who underwent 68 cycles of OI or IVF, Guballa et al. [13] found a high rate of complications. These included osteopenia, lupus flare, hemorrhage, diabetes, multiple gestation, nephritis flare, costochondritis, and suicidal depression. Unfortunately, reports of the outcomes of assisted reproductive therapies in women with systemic autoimmune diseases are retrospective, uncontrolled, and few, but will be addressed later in relation to specific diseases.

4. Fertility issues in women with specific autoimmune diseases

4.1. Systemic lupus erythematosus

Systemic lupus erythematosus (SLE) is an autoimmune disease that predominantly affects women of reproductive age. Fertility in patients with SLE is thought to be equivalent to that of the general population [14]. Interestingly, Geva and coworkers noted a 1.5% prevalence of undiagnosed SLE in a population of women with infertility [15]. Pregnancy rates of 2.0–2.4 pregnancies per patient have been described and seem to be unaltered by disease activity [16,17]. In a retrospective analysis of 138 women with SLE and 276 age-matched controls, Hardy et al. [18] found that women with SLE are at greater risk of pregnancy loss by spontaneous miscarriage (OR 2.21, 95% CI 1.46–3.35, $P<.01$) and elected surgical termination (OR 2.44, 95% CI 1.22–4.87, $P=.01$). In their study, more important determinants of family size than fecundity were race, as well as social and cultural identifiers.

Although the disease itself does not seem to cause infertility, other factors related to the treatment of SLE may contribute to lowered fertility rates. Women undergoing treatment of lupus nephritis with intravenous cyclophosphamide pulse therapy have a high incidence of premature ovarian failure [19,20]. The incidence ranges from 12% to 62% and is dependent on the patient's age at the time of therapy (with older women at higher risk), and number of doses of cyclophosphamide [21,22]. Oral cyclophosphamide use in women with SLE has also been associated with ovarian dysfunction and ovarian failure [23]. In other studies, the use of low-dose intravenous cyclophosphamide therapy does not seem to increase incidence of premature ovarian failure [24,25]. Women with SLE are often given long-term non-steroidal anti-inflammatory medications (NSAIDs) as therapy for pain and inflammation. While the most common adverse events related to NSAID therapy involve the renal and gastrointestinal systems, NSAIDs also interfere with ovulation [26,27]. Case reports of women with infertility on long-term NSAID therapy reveal successful pregnancies after withdrawal of these medications [28]. Chronic renal disease, a complication of SLE, has also been associated independently with ovarian failure [29]. However, in the absence of renal failure, cyclophosphamide therapy, or active disease, women with SLE have normal fertility.

For women with SLE seeking infertility therapy, there is little reported regarding outcomes of assisted reproduction. Huong et al. [30] recently reported outcomes of 114 OI cycles in 21 women with SLE. Eighteen pregnancies led to 9 live births, 4 fetal deaths, and 5 embryonic losses. The higher than expected fetal death rate is concerning.

Techniques for ovulation induction stimulate follicular development and thus increase serum estrogen concentrations [10–12]. For women with SLE, serum estrogen concentrations may be associated with disease activity. Complications from lupus flares have been reported after ovulation induction therapy [11,30]. Onset of SLE (as well as antiphospholipid antibody syndrome and insulin-dependent diabetes) has occurred in association with the initiation of ovulation induction therapy [31,32]. Women with SLE who require OI or IVF may be counseled that the risk of inducing a flare from the treatment exists but the more pertinent concern is not fertility or its treatment, but rather the potential effects of the SLE on a pregnancy and a pregnancy on the SLE. Fertility therapy should be restricted to women with longstanding inactive disease.

4.2. Thyroid disorders

Between 2.3 and 5.1% of patients in an infertile population will have thyroid dysfunction [33,34]. Thyroid disease may lead to ovulatory dysfunction as a source of infertility. Also, because of the common concurrence of autoimmune thyroiditis, screening of thyroid function is indicated in all women with ovulatory dysfunction during infertility evaluations.

4.2.1. Hypothyroidism

Hypothyroidism may be a result of autoimmune (Hashimoto's) thyroiditis, primary failure, ablation for treatment of Grave's disease, or iodine deficiency. Hypothyroidism is associated with polymenorrhea, oligomenorrhea, amenorrhea, and anovulation. These menstrual abnormalities have been reported in 68.2% of hypothyroid women compared to 12.2% of euthyroid controls [35]. Subclinical hypothyroidism may also manifest as menstrual irregularities and has been associated with subfertility and infertility [36]. Regular ovulation and thus menses usually normalize within 3–6 months of thyroid replacement therapy [37]. Fertility can be restored with treatment and normalization of thyroid function [38].

4.2.2. Hyperthyroidism

Menstrual irregularities are features of hyperthyroidism as well, typically clinical evident as oligomenorrhea or amenorrhea (58% in one study) [39]. The mechanism of abnormal menstrual function associated with thyroid disease appears to involve changes in the metabolism of the key menstrual regulatory hormones. For instance, amenorrhea in hyperthyroidism is associated with elevated LH and FSH and loss of the LH surge [40]. Subclinical hyperthyroidism may not be associated with anovulation, as ovulation has been confirmed by endometrial biopsy in a subset of these women [39]. Restoration of a euthyroid state results in resumption of ovulatory cycles and thus improved fertility. Treatments include radioactive iodine treatment, carbimazole, methimazole, propylthiouracil, and surgical resection. While radioactive iodine is contraindicated in pregnancy or in those seeking pregnancy, the other treatments have not been found to have adverse effects on fertility [41].

4.2.3. Antithyroid antibodies

Thyroglobulin assists in retention and storage of thyroid hormones. Thyroid peroxidase is involved in iodination and coupling of thyroid residues. Antithyroglobulin and antithyroid peroxidase are major autoantibodies present in women with autoimmune thyroid disorders. Antithyroid antibodies (ATAs) are five times more common in women than in men, and are present sometimes in healthy (not infertile) populations of women of reproductive age [42].

Women with autoimmune thyroid disease may be at increased risk for unexplained infertility, recurrent early pregnancy loss, and IVF failure [43,44]. However, the data are conflicting. One study found only 9% of infertile women have ATAs, compared to 15% of controls [44]. The prevalence of antithyroid antibodies is elevated in women with RPL (20–25%) versus normal pregnant women (15%) [45]. However, Rushworth et al. [46] found that the future risk of miscarriage in women with RPL was not explained by their thyroid antibody status.

An increased incidence of antithyroid antibodies was found in euthyroid women with multiple IVF failures [47], but other investigators found no difference in pregnancy outcomes after IVF comparing women with ATAs versus controls [48]. In a prospective study of 173 women undergoing IVF, Muller [49] found that women who tested positive for ATAs had a miscarriage rate of 33%, and women who tested negative had a miscarriage rate of 19%, but this difference was not significant. Thus, routine screening of women undergoing IVF or with RPL for ATAs is not currently recommended.

There are two working hypotheses regarding fertility and ATAs: (1) there is direct action between hormones and ATAs. (2) ATAs are a secondary marker and thus not directly related to pregnancy loss or IVF failure. A high proportion of women with SLE (45%) have thyroid autoantibodies [50]. However, these women also have a high prevalence of non-organ-specific autoantibodies, suggesting systemic immune dysfunction, thereby confounding conclusions regarding autoimmune thyroid disease and fertility.

4.3. *Insulin-dependent diabetes*

Oligomenorrhea, amenorrhea, and polymenorrhea occur in approximately 30% of women with insulin-dependent diabetes mellitus (IDDM). The incidence of hypogonadotropic amenorrhea is high in diabetic women [51]. Onset of diabetes prior to menarche and other complications of diabetes result in delayed menarche and a higher chance of menstrual irregularities [52] thought to be hypothalamic in origin, and possibly related to abnormal pulsatile GnRH activity [53]. Insulin resistance with compensatory hyperinsulinemia and hyperandrogenism correlates with ovulatory dysfunction in women with polycystic ovary syndrome [54]. Insulin resistance may also contribute to ovulatory dysfunction in some diabetic women; thus menstrual dysfunction may not be a direct function of autoimmunity, but rather a secondary consequence of insulin resistance.

A diabetic woman's ability to conceive equals that of a non-diabetic woman. In a survey of 245 unselected diabetic women and 253 age-matched non-diabetic controls, rates of involuntary infertility were equivalent at 17% [55]. The same study showed fewer pregnancies overall and fewer births per pregnancy in women with diabetes; this finding was possibly due to negative attitudes in diabetic women regarding pregnancy.

Miscarriage risk in women with diabetes is traditionally thought to be high, although a large meta-analysis of 50 studies reviewing 8041 diabetic pregnancies found no increased risk of spontaneous abortion [56]. The data are marred by lack of controls and proper attention to the level of diabetic control. Studies considering glycosylated hemoglobin levels (and thus general diabetic control at the time of conception) find a higher incidence of miscarriage in poorly controlled diabetics with glycosylated hemoglobin levels greater than 12% [57,58]. Preconception counseling reduces this risk [59]. For diabetic women seeking evaluation for recurrent miscarriage or infertility, glycemic control is essential.

4.4. *Rheumatoid arthritis*

Approximately 2% of women will develop rheumatoid arthritis (RA) during their lifetime. The literature regarding infertility and RA is incomplete; however, several case-control studies have been published. The first mention that women with RA might be "subfertile" was in 1965, when Kay and Bach published an analysis of the number of live births prior to disease onset in women with RA. A mean of 1.40 live births was reported in 54 women with RA versus a mean of 2.29 live births in the controls. Unfortunately this study was limited by confounding variables, including a potential voluntary desire to limit family size. In 1993, Nelson et al. [60] performed a prospective, population-based case-controlled study of 259 women with recent onset RA and 1258 women without RA. They found an increased incidence of altered fecundity in women with RA prior to actual onset of the disease, defining altered fecundity as unprotected intercourse for $\geqslant 12$ months without pregnancy, with an odds ratio of 1.44 (95% CI 1.10–1.91). Thirteen percent of cases and 10% of controls had sought treatment for infertility, and 2–3% of both cases and controls had taken medications for infertility. An increased time to conception has also been reported for women with RA in other studies [60,61].

However, others have found no significant difference between patients with RA and controls. Through a mailed questionnaire in a case controlled study of 34 women with recent onset RA and 68 healthy controls, Pope et al. reported an odds ratio for infertility of 0.7 with a 95% confidence interval of 0.3–1.7. Kaplan et al. [62] also reported no significant difference between the number of pregnancies prior to disease onset in 89 women with RA versus 113 controls.

In 1997, Brennan et al. [63] found "reduced fecundity" in a population-based study of 115 women with RA versus 115 controls, with an odds ratio of 1.8, but again confidence intervals crossed one (0.7–5.0). Also, the definition of "reduced fecundity" was not clarified. Finally, Steen et al. [64] found no difference in 167 women with RA versus 105 healthy controls in regards to the frequency of never being pregnant or evaluations for infertility after adjusting for contributing factors. Though the data conflict, if an association between infertility and RA exists, it is relatively minor and more likely to be a decrease in fecundity rather than true infertility.

4.5. Systemic sclerosis

The frequency of systemic sclerosis (scleroderma) and pregnancy is low due to the fact that mean age of onset of disease is in the early 40 s. However, the disease affects women three times more commonly than men; thus reproductive aspects of the disease are important. There does not seem to be an increase in infertility in patients with systemic sclerosis, nor does there seem to be an increase in miscarriage rates [64–66]. However, in one study involving 150 case–control pairs and using a postal questionnaire, Silman et al. [67] found that women with systemic sclerosis had a poor reproductive history—a higher incidence of infertility and spontaneous miscarriage even before the onset of the disease. Another study found a lower birth rate for women with systemic sclerosis prior to first hospitalization for the disease compared to aged-matched controls [68]. This suggests that an abnormality may antedate clinical diagnosis.

Low doses of cyclophosphamide may be used for the treatment of systemic sclerosis. Despite reports that high-dose cyclophosphamide has been associated with ovulatory failure in women with SLE [23], low-dose cyclophosphamide therapy in patients with systemic sclerosis does not apparently increase the incidence of ovarian failure [69].

4.6. Addison's disease and the autoimmune polyglandular syndromes

The most common cause of primary adrenal failure (Addison's disease) in developed countries is autoimmunity, and more than half of patients with Addison's disease will have other autoimmune disorders [70]. There may be a rising incidence of autoimmune adrenal failure [71]. Adrenal failure and other endocrine dysfunctions are classified as the autoimmune polyglandular syndromes (APGS), or autoimmunity against two or more endocrine organs. APGS type I is an autosomal recessive disease that includes hypoparathyroidism, adrenal failure, and mucocutaneous candidiasis. It usually occurs in children, and premature ovarian failure (POF) (manifested as primary amenorrhea) occurs in 60% of patients with APGS type I. APGS type II, also known as Schmidt's syndrome, is characterized by adrenal failure and either autoimmune thyroid disease or IDDM. The incidence of ovarian failure is variable, but 10% of women with Addison's disease may develop POF several years prior to adrenal dysfunction [72]. Autoimmune adrenal dysfunction is by definition absent from patients with APGS type III, which includes autoimmune thyroid disease and at least one other organ affected. Autoimmune POF occurs in up to 60% of these women [73].

The steroidogenic enzyme 21-hydoxylase (21-OH) is thought to be the major autoantigen in autoimmune adrenal insufficiency, although antibodies to several other enzymes important in steroid biosynthesis have also been detected [74]. Other antibodies that may also contribute to autoimmune POF include adrenocortical antibodies (ACA), 17α-hydroxylase, P450-ssc (side-chain cleavage enzyme), and ovarian steroid cell antibodies (StCA) against the theca or granulosa cells [73]. Among patients with adrenal failure and normal ovarian function, 40% of women with antibodies to steroid-producing cells will develop ovarian failure within 10–15 years [75]. However, it is not practical to screen for these serum autoantibodies in all women with infertility and autoimmune disease unless the diagnosis of Addison's disease is present.

4.7. Autoimmune premature ovarian failure

The annual incidence rates of natural menopause are reported to be 10/100,000 person-years for women aged 15–29, 76/100,000 person-years for women aged 30–39, and 881/100,000 person-years in women aged 40–44 [76]. However, the designation of POF has been arbitrarily restricted to women <40 years of age. The incidence of POF is 1% by age 40. Autoimmunity is one of several causes of POF. (Table 1).

In women with POF, the true incidence of coexisting autoimmune disease is unknown but may be anywhere from 0 to 57%, the variability possibly being a reflection of population bias [77]. The variability also reflects the lack of a uniformly accepted definition of autoimmune POF. The diagnosis of POF is clinical and non-specific. One definition is: amenorrhea for a minimum of 4 months, and elevated gonadotropins >40 IU/L on two occasions at least 1 month apart in women below the age of 40 [78]. POF is characterized by sex steroid deficiency and infertility. To designate POF as "autoimmune" depends upon further clinical, histological, and immunological findings. The autoimmune company that the POF keeps supports the diagnosis. In a prospective evaluation of 119 women with karyotypically normal spontaneous premature ovarian failure, 32 had hypothyroidism (27%), 3 had adrenal insufficiency consistent with Addison's (2.5%), and 3 had diabetes mellitus (2.5%) [79]. A more objective although less practical criterion to diagnose autoimmune POF is documentation of lymphocytic and plasma cell infiltration of the ovary, first described in a woman with autoimmune adrenal insufficiency [80]. Other criteria rely on the detection of altered serum ratios of immune cells and the presence of antibodies to a variety of ovarian immune targets. Unfortunately, reproducible assays for antiovarian antibodies have not been uniformly accepted. The prevalence and mechanism of initiation of autoimmune POF remain unknown.

Table 1
Etiologies of premature ovarian failure

Idiopathic (karyotypically normal spontaneous premature ovarian failure)
Autoimmunity
Autoimmune polyglandular syndromes
Gonadotropin and gonadotropin-receptor abnormalities (signal defects)
Enzyme deficiencies (cholesterol desmolase, 17α-hydroxylase, 17–20 desmolase)
Iatrogenic (chemotherapy, radiation)
X-chromosome abnormalities
Galactosemia
Viral agents

Adapted from Kalantaridou et al. [78].

Initially, POF was thought to cause irreversible infertility. However, several reports have documented spontaneous pregnancies after the diagnosis of POF [81,82]; 20% of young women with POF have ovulated spontaneously in 4 months of observation [83]. Women with a diagnosis of autoimmune POF have a 5–10% cumulative chance of spontaneous pregnancy [84]; thus POF is not premature menopause (which by definition consists of irreversible oocyte depletion and sterility) [78].

Therapy to restore fertility to women diagnosed with POF of all etiologies has been disappointing. Case reports and uncontrolled studies have noted occasional ovulation after immunosuppressive treatment with corticosteroids [85,86]. A randomized controlled trial of prednisone treatment is underway. Unfortunately, corticosteroid treatment in a woman with POF can cause iatrogenic Cushing's syndrome, osteonecrosis, and osteoporosis [87]. Van Kasteren et al. [88] examined the utility of corticosteroids in the ovarian response to exogenous gonadotropins in 100 women with idiopathic POF in a placebo-controlled, double-blinded randomized controlled trial of dexamethasone given at the time of gonadotropin therapy. No ovulations were documented and the study was therefore discontinued after 36 patients were studied.

Future directions for study may include further evaluation of plasmapheresis, thymectomy, and intravenous immunoglobulin. However, in the absence of treatments with demonstrated safety and efficacy, the key to reproductive success in these women may be early identification (perhaps prior to the onset of POF). Then, cryopreservation of ovarian tissue that harbors oocytes (although not yet perfected), and cryopreservation of fertilized eggs (pre-embryos) would be possible solutions in the event of future infertility due to POF [89]. Egg donation appears to be the one current reliable means of helping women with POF conceive [90,91]. However, no reports have focused on the outcome of egg donation attempts for the subgroup with autoimmune POF. If pathogenic anti-oocyte antibodies are operative in this group, then successful conception by donor eggs may be compromised.

4.8. Antiphospholipid antibody syndrome

Antiphospholipid antibodies [APAs, a group comprised of lupus anticoagulant (LAC) and anticardiolipin (ACLA) antibodies] have such a strong correlation with fetal loss that they are now routinely screened for in the evaluation of RPL. Also, treatment of women with APS with heparin and aspirin improves live birth rates and is now routine [92]. Extrapolation of RPL data has led some to hypothesize that perhaps the same autoimmune dysfunction would affect earlier unrecognized pregnancies, leading to infertility.

Phospholipids are a broad and ubiquitous class of biologically active molecules composed of a glycerin backbone, phosphorous, and fatty acid residues. Phospholipids are critical components of the coagulation cascade as well as integral components of the lipid bilayer of plasma membranes. Two prominent examples are lecithins and sphingomyelins. Negatively charged phospholipids, primarily phosphatidylserine, are exposed on activated or apoptotic cell membranes and are the likely targets of APAs, primarily through phospholipid-binding proteins such as β_2-glycoprotein I or prothrombin. APAs are clinically associated with a prolongation of phospholipid-dependent coagulation tests (activated partial thromboplastin time; dilute Russell's viper venom time) and paradoxical thrombosis. Some investigators have proposed that pelvic tissue damage related to endometriosis, pelvic inflammatory disease, or egg retrievals during IVF may be related to the development of antiphospholipid antibodies, although this remains unsubstantiated.

When APAs do form, the most prevalent are the lupus anticoagulant (LAC) and anticardiolipin (ACL). Others include antiphosphatidylserine, antiphosphatidylcholine, antiphosphatidylglycerol, antiphosphatidylethanolamine, antiphosphatidylinositol, anti- β_2-glycoprotein I, and anti-prothrombin. Proposed mechanisms by which these antibodies might affect fertility or IVF success include abnormal implantation, impaired placentation, and embryonic vascular compromise. Laboratories across the globe disagree whether APAs (as well as other immunologic anomalies) contribute to infertility [93]. Panel testing women with infertility for APA has been professed to predict infertility. Certainly several studies have found increased incidences of ACA in women with unexplained infertility [44,94,95]. However, positive APA status has not been found to influence pregnancy outcome in most studies; thus, this approach to diagnosing immune-mediated infertility is still the subject of much debate. Standardized assays for LAC and ACL are available but notable for substantial interlaboratory variation. Studies attempting to show an association between infertility and APA lack consistency in assay methodology. Another major problem is the lack of comparable controls. Yet some laboratories and infertility centers offer desensitization and immunomodulation therapies despite the lack of proven benefit and positive benefit to risk ratio. In a 2004 article in Lupus, Lockshin commented on the multitude of highly charged facets surrounding this issue by noting "this field is contentious, litigious, and lucrative for the participants" [96].

Hornstein et al. [97] performed a meta-analysis to evaluate the relationship between APA and infertility, evaluating seven studies that used APA panels for evaluation of IVF outcome. None of the seven studies identified a statistically lower pregnancy outcome in women who were positive for APA. In addition, the 95% confidence intervals of the odds ratios representing the relative likelihood of clinical pregnancy in women positive for APA compared with women negative for APA all crossed 1.0, indicating lack of statistically significant differences (Table 2). The conclusion of this analysis was that assessment of APA and therapy for couples undergoing IVF is not warranted on the basis of current data. This same position was taken in an October 1999 Practice Committee Report for the American Society for Reproductive Medicine.

Table 2
The odds ratios of studies attempting to detect the impact of APA on IVF pregnancy rates do not identify a significant relationship

Authors	Odds ratio	95% Confidence intervals
Birdsall et al.	1.65	(0.50, 5.46)
Denis et al.	0.91	(0.42, 1.97)
El-Roiey et al.	0.26	(0.04, 1.83)
Gleicher et al.	1.34	(0.36, 4.95)
Kowalik et al.	1.38	(0.52, 3.64)
Kutteh et al.	0.85	(0.21, 3.5)
Sher et al.	0.55	(0.13, 2.34)
Average	0.99	(0.64, 1.53)

Adapted from Hornstein et al. [97].

Intravenous immunoglobulin and antithrombogenic therapies including aspirin and heparin have been shown to improve pregnancy outcome in women with antiphospholipid antibodies and RPL [98]. The same has been purported for women with antiphospholipid antibodies undergoing IVF [99,100]; however, the later data are much more tenuous. Stern et al. [101] performed a randomized, double-blinded placebo-controlled trial of heparin and aspirin for women with a history of IVF implantation failure and documented presence of APA, antinuclear antibody, or glycoprotein autoantibody. In their study of 300 embryo transfers in 143 women, no difference was noted in pregnancy or implantation rates in women treated with heparin and aspirin versus placebo. Of the other studies reported, none have been randomized and some were uncontrolled (Table 3). Unfortunately varying combinations of treatments and varying populations of women with infertility as well as differing definitions of APA positivity have made for poor systematic study. In 1996, a pregnancy-related death associated with heparin and aspirin treatment for infertility was reported by the Centers for Disease Control [102]. Available data simply do not justify the use of these treatments except in approved protocols, especially considering the risk of associated morbidity and mortality.

5. The effects of immunosuppressive and anti-inflammatory medications on fertility

Tubal motility and blastocyst implantation are mediated by the local action of prostaglandins. NSAIDs commonly used in women suffering from the rheumatic systemic autoimmune diseases act by inhibiting prostaglandin synthesis, and have been associated with reversible infertility in case reports [28]. Corticosteroids, hydroxychloroquine, sulfasalazine, azathioprine, cyclosporine, gold, methotrexate, etanercept, and heparinoids are thought not to adversely affect fertility [103]. Effects of these medications on the pregnancy itself are varying and discussed elsewhere in this book. Successful pregnancy after ovulation induction in a woman on chronic etanercept therapy has been reported [104]. The cytotoxic agents cyclophosphamide

Table 3
Empiric treatment for presumed antibody-mediated infertility

Authors	Number of APA positive subjects treated	Treatment	Treatment Criteria	Outcome
Birkenfield et al. [107]	15	Aspirin + prednisone and IVF	⩾1 of 4 autoantibody assays positive; last embryo transfer unsuccessful	7/15 (46.6%) ongoing pregnancies, no differences from previous untreated cycles for # of ova or transferred embryos
Sher et al. [99]	169	Heparin + aspirin and IVF	⩾1 of 18 APA assays positive; organic pelvic pathology	82/169 (49%) clinical pregnancies
Schenk et al. [108]	35	Heparin + aspirin and IVF	⩾2 of 12 APA assays positive; unselected IVF candidates	10/35 (51.4%) clinical pregnancies versus 12/40 (30%) for untreated seronegatives [NS]. No differences between the groups for peak estradiol, # of eggs, # or quality of embryos transferred, # of cryopreserved embryos. Implantation rates were 28/140 (20%) when seropositive/treated and 9.7% when seronegative/untreated ($P = .014$)
Kutteh et al. [109]	19	Heparin + aspirin and IVF	⩾1 of 3 assays for ACL isotypes positive, no history of RPL	No differences for clinical pregnancies: 10/19 (52.6%), ongoing pregnancies: 8/19 (42.1%), or implantation rates versus untreated cycles
Sher et al. [110]	52	Heparin + aspirin and IVF	⩾4 IVF failures	42% APA positive and 19% APA negative delivered ($P = .02$)
Geva et al. [111]	52	Prednisone + aspirin and IVF	⩾1 of 4 autoantibody or rheumatoid factor positive and ⩾1 previous IVF failure	17/52 (32.7%) clinical pregnancy rate, uncontrolled
Stern et al. [101]	143	Heparin + aspirin and IVF	⩾1 APA, ANA, or β-2 glycoprotein autoantibodies and unsuccessful transfer of ⩾10 embryos	Implantation rates 20/296 (6.8%) for treated cycles and 22/259 (8.5%) for placebo cycles

IVF, in vitro fertilitzation; APA, antiphospholipid antibody; ANA, antinuclear antibody; RPL, recurrent pregnancy loss. Adapted from Hatasaka. [106].

(as discussed previously) and chlorambucil have been associated with impaired fertility. GnRH-a co-treatment has been reported to possibly decrease this risk [105].

6. Conclusion

Antibodies against reproductive tissues such as ovaries, sperm, and endometrium, and immune-mediated endocrine abnormalities, vascular abnormalities, and inflammation have all been hypothesized to play a role in infertility. The possibility that these immune effects could lead to reproductive failure coupled with the fact that autoimmune diseases have a predilection for reproductive age women predict that widespread impaired fertility should be observed in women with autoimmune diseases. With the exception of autoimmune-mediated premature ovarian failure, it is fortunate to note that much of the hypothesized reproductive compromise is not clinically realized. The majority of women afflicted with a systemic autoimmune disease, and certainly all women in remission or good control, may be offered reassurance and support during preconception counseling that their ability to conceive should not be lowered appreciably by their autoimmune condition.

Key points

- In general, the systemic autoimmune diseases do not seem to be associated with high rates of primary infertility.
- Autoimmune thyroid and adrenal disorders are likely associated with infertility due to influences on the endocrine system.
- RPL is more frequent in women with poorly controlled diabetes and APS than in women in the general population.
- Screening couples with infertility for APA and treating them with costly and potentially risky therapies are not justified by the current evidence.
- Therapeutic regimens involving the cytotoxic agents cyclophosphamide and chlorambucil have been associated with POF and thus infertility.
- Use of NSAIDs may be associated with reversible infertility.
- When evaluating a woman with systemic autoimmune disease for the use of assisted reproductive technologies, considerations must be given to potential effects on her underlying disease—only women with stable or inactive disease should be candidates for assisted reproductive technologies.

References

1. McCarthy, M. 2000. The gender gap in autoimmune disease. Lancet 356 (9235), 1088.
2. Mosher, W.D., Pratt, W.F. 1991. Fecundity and infertility in the United States: incidence and trends. Fertil. Steril. 56 (2), 192–193.
3. Abma, J.C., et al. 1997. Fertility, family planning, and women's health: new data from the 1995 National Survey of Family Growth. Vital. Health Stat. 23 (19), 1–114.
4. Isaksson, R., Tiitinen, A. 2004. Present concept of unexplained infertility. Gynecol. Endocrinol. 18 (5), 278–290.
5. Martin, J.A., et al. 2002. Births: final data for 2000. Natl. Vital. Stat. Rep. 50 (5), 1–101.
6. Martin, J.A., et al. 2003. Births: final data for 2002. Natl. Vital. Stat. Rep. 52 (10), 1–113.
7. Tietze, C. 1957. Reproductive span and rate of reproduction among Hutterite women. Fertil. Steril. 8 (1), 89–97.
8. Alamanos, Y., et al. 2003. Epidemiology of systemic lupus erythematosus in northwest Greece 1982–2001. J. Rheumatol. 30 (4), 731–735.
9. Lind, P., et al. 1998. Epidemiology of thyroid diseases in iodine sufficiency. Thyroid 8 (12), 1179–1183.
10. Meirow, D., Laufer, N., Schenker, J.G. 1992. Ovulation induction in in vitro fertilization. Gynecol. Endocrinol. 6 (3), 211–224.
11. Huong, D.L., et al. 1996. Risks of ovulation-induction therapy in systemic lupus erythematosus. Br. J. Rheumatol. 35 (11), 1184–1186.
12. Speroff, L., Glass, R.H., Kase, N.G. 1989. Clinical gynecologic endocrinology and infertility. In: L. Speroff (Ed.), Induction of Ovulation. Williams and Wilkins, Baltimore, Fourth edition.
13. Guballa, N., et al. 2000. Ovulation induction and in vitro fertilization in systemic lupus erythematosus and antiphospholipid syndrome. Arthritis. Rheum. 43 (3), 550–556.

14. Khamashta, M.A., Hughes, G.R. 1996. Pregnancy in systemic lupus erythematosus. Curr. Opin. Rheumatol. 8 (5), 424–429.
15. Geva, E., et al. 2004. Undiagnosed systemic lupus erythematosus in a cohort of infertile women. Am. J. Reprod. Immunol. 51 (5), 336–340.
16. Nossent, H.C., Swaak, T.J. 1990. Systemic lupus erythematosus. VI. Analysis of the interrelationship with pregnancy. J. Rheumatol. 17 (6), 771–776.
17. Kaufman, R.L., Kitridou, R.C. 1982. Pregnancy in mixed connective tissue disease: comparison with systemic lupus erythematosus. J. Rheumatol. 9 (4), 549–555.
18. Hardy, C.J., et al. 1999. Pregnancy outcome and family size in systemic lupus erythematosus: a case–control study. Rheumatology (Oxford) 38 (6), 559–563.
19. Park, M.C., et al. 2004. Risk of ovarian failure and pregnancy outcome in patients with lupus nephritis treated with intravenous cyclophosphamide pulse therapy. Lupus 13 (8), 569–574.
20. Langevitz, P., et al. 1992. The effect of cyclophosphamide pulses on fertility in patients with lupus nephritis. Am. J. Reprod. Immunol. 28 (3–4), 157–158.
21. Mok, C.C., Lau, C.S., Wong, R.W. 1998. Risk factors for ovarian failure in patients with systemic lupus erythematosus receiving cyclophosphamide therapy. Arthritis. Rheum. 41 (5), 831–837.
22. Boumpas, D.T., et al. 1993. Risk for sustained amenorrhea in patients with systemic lupus erythematosus receiving intermittent pulse cyclophosphamide therapy. Ann. Intern. Med. 119 (5), 366–369.
23. Wang, C.L., Wang, F., Bosco, J.J. 1995. Ovarian failure in oral cyclophosphamide treatment for systemic lupus erythematosus. Lupus 4 (1), 11–14.
24. Martin-Suarez, I., et al. 1997. Immunosuppressive treatment in severe connective tissue diseases: effects of low dose intravenous cyclophosphamide. Ann. Rheum. Dis. 56 (8), 481–487.
25. D'Cruz, D., et al. 1997. Immunosuppressive therapy in lupus nephritis. Clin. Exp. Rheumatol. 15 (3), 275–282.
26. Akil, M., Amos, R.S., Stewart, P. 1996. Infertility may sometimes be associated with NSAID consumption. Br. J. Rheumatol. 35 (1), 76–78.
27. Smith, G., et al. 1996. Reversible ovulatory failure associated with the development of luteinized unruptured follicles in women with inflammatory arthritis taking nonsteroidal anti-inflammatory drugs. Br. J. Rheumatol. 35 (5), 458–462.
28. Mendonca, L.L., et al. 2000. Non-steroidal anti-inflammatory drugs as a possible cause for reversible infertility. Rheumatology (Oxford) 39 (8), 880–882.
29. Cochrane, R., Regan, L. 1997. Undetected gynaecological disorders in women with renal disease. Hum. Reprod. 12 (4), 667–670.
30. Le Thi Huong, D., Wechsler, B., Piette, J.C. 2003. Ovulation induction therapy and systemic lupus erythematosus. Ann. Med. Interne. (Paris) 154 (1), 45–50.
31. Ben-Chetrit, A., Ben-Chetrit, E. 1994. Systemic lupus erythematosus induced by ovulation induction treatment. Arthritis Rheum. 37 (11), 1614–1617.
32. Macut, D., et al. 2000. Ovulation induction and early pregnancy loss in a woman susceptible to autoimmune diseases: a possible interrelationship. Gynecol. Endocrinol. 14 (3), 153–157.
33. Stratford, G.A., et al. 2000. Value of thyroid function tests in routine screening of women investigated for infertility. Hum. Fertil. (Cambridge) 3 (3), 203–206.
34. Lincoln, S.R., Ke, R.W., Kutteh, W.H. Screening for hypothyroidism in infertile women. J. Reprod. Med. 44 (5), 455–457.
35. Joshi, J.V., et al. 1993. Menstrual irregularities and lactation failure may precede thyroid dysfunction or goiter. J. Postgrad. Med. 39 (3), 137–141.
36. Strickland, D.M., Whitted, W.A., Wians, F.H., Jr. 1990. Screening infertile women for subclinical hypothyroidism. Am. J. Obstet. Gynecol. 163 (1.1), 262–263.
37. Brenner, P.F. 1996. Differential diagnosis of abnormal uterine bleeding. Am. J. Obstet. Gynecol. 175 (3.2), 766–769.
38. Louvet, J.P., et al. 1979. Hypothyroidism and anovulation. Lancet 1 (8124), 1032.
39. Goldsmith, R.E., et al. 1952. The menstrual pattern in thyroid disease. J. Clin. Endocrinol. Metab. 12 (7), 846–855.
40. Thomas, R., Reid, R.L. 1987. Thyroid disease and reproductive dysfunction: a review. Obstet. Gynecol. 70 (5), 789–798.
41. Wing, D.A., et al. 1994. A comparison of propylthiouracil versus methimazole in the treatment of hyperthyroidism in pregnancy. Am. J. Obstet. Gynecol. 170 (1.1), 90–95.
42. Geva, E., et al. 1997. Autoimmunity and reproduction. Fertil. Steril. 67 (4), 599–611.
43. Matalon, S.T., et al. 2001. The association between antithyroid antibodies and pregnancy loss. Am. J. Reprod. Immunol. 45 (2), 72–77.
44. Roussev, R.G., et al. 1996. Laboratory evaluation of women experiencing reproductive failure. Am. J. Reprod. Immunol. 35 (4), 415–420.
45. Kutteh, W.H., et al. 1999. Increased prevalence of antithyroid antibodies identified in women with recurrent pregnancy loss but not in women undergoing assisted reproduction. Fertil. Steril. 71 (5), 843–848.
46. Rushworth, F.H., et al. 2000. Prospective pregnancy outcome in untreated recurrent miscarriers with thyroid autoantibodies. Hum. Reprod. 15 (7), 1637–1639.
47. Bussen, S., Steck, T., Dietl, J. 2000. Increased prevalence of thyroid antibodies in euthyroid women with a history of recurrent in-vitro fertilization failure. Hum. Reprod. 15 (3), 545–548.
48. Kutteh, W.H., Schoolcraft, W.B., Scott, R.T., Jr. 1999. Antithyroid antibodies do not affect pregnancy outcome in women undergoing assisted reproduction. Hum. Reprod. 14 (11), 2886–2890.

49. Muller, A.F., et al. 1999. Thyroid autoimmunity and abortion: a prospective study in women undergoing in vitro fertilization. Fertil. Steril. 71 (1), 30–34.
50. Magaro, M., et al. 1992. The association of silent thyroiditis with active systemic lupus erythematosus. Clin. Exp. Rheumatol. 10 (1), 67–70.
51. Kjaer, K., et al. 1992. Epidemiology of menarche and menstrual disturbances in an unselected group of women with insulin-dependent diabetes mellitus compared to controls. J. Clin. Endocrinol. Metab. 75 (2), 524–529.
52. Yeshaya, A., et al. 1995. Menstrual characteristics of women suffering from insulin-dependent diabetes mellitus. Int. J. Fertil. Menopausal. Stud. 40 (5), 269–273.
53. Griffin, M.L., et al. 1994. Insulin-dependent diabetes mellitus and menstrual dysfunction. Ann. Med. 26 (5), 331–340.
54. Lord, J.M., Flight, I.H., Norman, R.J. 2003. Insulin-sensitising drugs (metformin, troglitazone, rosiglitazone, pioglitazone, D-chiro-inositol) for polycystic ovary syndrome. Cochrane Database Syst. Rev. (3), CD003053.
55. Kjaer, K., et al. 1992. Infertility and pregnancy outcome in an unselected group of women with insulin-dependent diabetes mellitus. Am. J. Obstet. Gynecol. 166 (5), 1412–1418.
56. Kalter, H. 1987. Diabetes and spontaneous abortion: a historical review. Am. J. Obstet. Gynecol. 156 (5), 1243–1253.
57. Miodovnik, M., et al. 1984. Spontaneous abortion among insulin-dependent diabetic women. Am. J. Obstet. Gynecol. 150 (4), 372–376.
58. Miodovnik, M., et al. 1985. Elevated maternal glycohemoglobin in early pregnancy and spontaneous abortion among insulin-dependent diabetic women. Am. J. Obstet. Gynecol. 153 (4), 439–442.
59. Dicker, D., et al. 1988. Spontaneous abortion in patients with insulin-dependent diabetes mellitus: the effect of preconceptional diabetic control. Am. J. Obstet. Gynecol. 158 (5), 1161–1164.
60. Nelson, J.L., et al. 1993. Fecundity before disease onset in women with rheumatoid arthritis. Arthritis Rheum. 36 (1), 7–14.
61. Del Junco, D.J., et al. 1989. The relationship between rheumatoid arthritis and reproductive function. Br. J. Rheumatol. 28 (Suppl. 1) 33; discussion 42–45.
62. Kaplan, D. 1986. Fetal wastage in patients with rheumatoid arthritis. J. Rheumatol. 13 (5), 875–877.
63. Brennan, P., et al. 1997. Oral contraceptives and rheumatoid arthritis: results from a primary care-based incident case-control study. Semin. Arthritis Rheum. 26 (6), 817–823.
64. Steen, V.D., Medsger, T.A., Jr. 1999. Fertility and pregnancy outcome in women with systemic sclerosis. Arthritis Rheum. 42 (4), 763–768.
65. Launay, D., et al. 2002. Systemic sclerosis and pregnancy. Rev. Med. Interne. 23 (7), 607–621.
66. Rabhi, M., et al. 2002. Scleroderma and pregnancy. Ann. Med. Interne. (Paris) 153 (3), 193–200.
67. Silman, A.J., Black, C. 1988. Increased incidence of spontaneous abortion and infertility in women with scleroderma before disease onset: a controlled study. Ann. Rheum. Dis. 47 (6), 441–444.
68. Lambe, M., et al. 2004. Childbearing and the risk of scleroderma: a population-based study in Sweden. Am. J. Epidemiol. 159 (2), 162–166.
69. D'Angelo, S., et al. 2003. Low-dose intravenous cyclophosphamide in systemic sclerosis: a preliminary safety study. Clin. Rheumatol. 22 (6), 393–396.
70. Betterle, C., Volpato, M. 1998. Adrenal and ovarian autoimmunity. Eur. J. Endocrinol. 138 (1), 16–25.
71. Lovas, K., Husebye, E.S. 2002. High prevalence and increasing incidence of Addison's disease in western Norway. Clin. Endocrinol. (Oxford) 56 (6), 787–791.
72. Anasti, J.N. 1998. Premature ovarian failure: an update. Fertil. Steril. 70 (1), 1–15.
73. Betterle, C., et al. 2002. Autoimmune adrenal insufficiency and autoimmune polyendocrine syndromes: autoantibodies, autoantigens, and their applicability in diagnosis and disease prediction. Endocr. Rev. 23 (3), 327–364.
74. Chen, S., et al. 1996. Autoantibodies to steroidogenic enzymes in autoimmune polyglandular syndrome, Addison's disease, and premature ovarian failure. J. Clin. Endocrinol. Metab. 81 (5), 1871–1876.
75. Betterle, C., et al. 1993. Premature ovarian failure: autoimmunity and natural history. Clin. Endocrinol. (Oxford) 39 (1), 35–43.
76. Coulam, C.B., Adamson, S.C., Annegers, J.F. 1986. Incidence of premature ovarian failure. Obstet. Gynecol. 67 (4), 604–606.
77. LaBarbera, A.R., et al. 1988. Autoimmune etiology in premature ovarian failure. Am. J. Reprod. Immunol. Microbiol. 16 (3), 115–122.
78. Kalantaridou, S.N., Nelson, L.M. Premature ovarian failure is not premature menopause. Ann. N. Y. Acad. Sci. 900, 393–402.
79. Kim, T.J., et al. 1997. Routine endocrine screening for patients with karyotypically normal spontaneous premature ovarian failure. Obstet. Gynecol. 89 (5.1), 777–779.
80. Irvine, W.J., et al. 1968. Immunological aspects of premature ovarian failure associated with idiopathic Addison's disease. Lancet 2 (7574), 883–887.
81. Alper, M.M., Jolly, M.M., Garner, P.R. 1986. Pregnancies after premature ovarian failure. Obstet. Gynecol. 67 (Suppl. 3), 59S–62S.
82. Kreiner, D., et al. 1988. Spontaneous and pharmacologically induced remissions in patients with premature ovarian failure. Obstet. Gynecol. 72 (6), 926–928.
83. Nelson, L.M., et al. 1994. Development of luteinized graafian follicles in patients with karyotypically normal spontaneous premature ovarian failure. J. Clin. Endocrinol. Metab. 79 (5), 1470–1475.
84. Kalantaridou, S.N., Davis, S.R., Nelson, L.M. 1998. Premature ovarian failure. Endocrinol. Metab. Clin. N. Am. 27 (4), 989–1006.

85. Morris, R.S., Sauer, M.V. 1993. New advances in the treatment of infertility in women with ovarian failure. Curr. Opin. Obstet. Gynecol. 5 (3), 368–377.
86. Corenblum, B., Rowe, T., Taylor, P.J. 1993. High-dose, short-term glucocorticoids for the treatment of infertility resulting from premature ovarian failure. Fertil. Steril. 59 (5), 988–991.
87. Kalantaridou, S.N., et al. 1999. Treatment of autoimmune premature ovarian failure. Hum. Reprod. 14 (7), 1777–1782.
88. van Kasteren, Y.M., et al. 1999. Corticosteroids do not influence ovarian responsiveness to gonadotropins in patients with premature ovarian failure: a randomized, placebo-controlled trial. Fertil. Steril. 71 (1), 90–95.
89. Kauffman, R.P., Castracane, V.D. 2003. Premature ovarian failure associated with autoimmune polyglandular syndrome: pathophysiological mechanisms and future fertility. J. Womens Health (Larchmt) 12 (5), 513–520.
90. Sauer, M.V., et al. 1994. Three hundred cycles of oocyte donation at the University of Southern California: assessing the effect of age and infertility diagnosis on pregnancy and implantation rates. J. Assist. Reprod. Genet. 11 (2), 92–96.
91. Lydic, M.L., et al. 1996. Success of donor oocyte in in vitro fertilization-embryo transfer in recipients with and without premature ovarian failure. Fertil. Steril. 65 (1), 98–102.
92. Kutteh, W.H., Rote, N.S., Silver, R. 1999. Antiphospholipid antibodies and reproduction: the antiphospholipid antibody syndrome. Am. J. Reprod. Immunol. 41 (2), 133–152.
93. Gleicher, N., Vidali, A., Karande, V. 2002. The immunological Wars of the Roses: disagreements amongst reproductive immunologists. Hum. Reprod. 17 (3), 539–542.
94. Balasch, J., et al. 1996. Antiphospholipid antibodies and human reproductive failure. Hum. Reprod. 11 (10), 2310–2315.
95. Radojcic, L., et al. 2004. Anticardiolipin antibodies in women with unexplained infertility. Physiol. Res. 53 (1), 91–96.
96. Lockshin, M.D. 2004. Autoimmunity, infertility and assisted reproductive technologies. Lupus 13 (9), 669–672.
97. Hornstein, M.D., et al. 2000. Antiphospholipid antibodies and in vitro fertilization success: a meta-analysis. Fertil. Steril. 73 (2), 330–333.
98. Kutteh, W.H. 1996. Antiphospholipid antibody-associated recurrent pregnancy loss: treatment with heparin and low-dose aspirin is superior to low-dose aspirin alone. Am. J. Obstet. Gynecol. 174 (5), 1584–1589.
99. Sher, G., et al., High fecundity rates following in-vitro fertilization and embryo transfer in antiphospholipid antibody seropositive women treated with heparin and aspirin. Hum. Reprod. 9 (12), 2278–2283.
100. Coulam, C.B., Krysa, L.W., Bustillo, M. 1994. Intravenous immunoglobulin for in-vitro fertilization failure. Hum. Reprod. 9 (12), 2265–2269.
101. Stern, C., et al. 2003. A randomized, double-blind, placebo-controlled trial of heparin and aspirin for women with in vitro fertilization implantation failure and antiphospholipid or antinuclear antibodies. Fertil. Steril. 80 (2), 376–383.
102. Pregnancy-related death associated with heparin and aspirin treatment for infertility, 1996 MMWR. Morb. Mortal. Wkly. Rep. 1998. 47 (18) 368–371.
103. Janssen, N.M., Genta, M.S. 2000. The effects of immunosuppressive and anti-inflammatory medications on fertility, pregnancy, and lactation. Arch. Intern. Med. 160 (5), 610–619.
104. Sills, E.S., et al. 2001. Successful ovulation induction, conception, and normal delivery after chronic therapy with etanercept: a recombinant fusion anti-cytokine treatment for rheumatoid arthritis. Am. J. Reprod. Immunol. 46 (5), 366–368.
105. Blumenfeld, Z., et al. 2000. Preservation of fertility and ovarian function and minimizing gonadotoxicity in young women with systemic lupus erythematosus treated by chemotherapy. Lupus 9 (6), 401–405.
106. Hatasaka, H. 2000. Immunologic factors in infertility. Clin. Obstet. Gynecol. 43 (4), 830–843.
107. Birkenfeld, A., et al. 1994. Incidence of autoimmune antibodies in failed embryo transfer cycles. Am. J. Reprod. Immunol. 31 (2–3), 65–68.
108. Schenk, L.M., Butler, L., Monis, J.P., Cox, B., Leete, J., Abuhamed, A., Oehninger, S., Muasher, S. 1996. Heparin and aspirin treatment yields higher implantation rates in IVF patients with antiphospholipid antibody seropositivity compared to untreated seronegative patients. In: 52nd Annual Meeting of the American Society for Reproductive Medicine [Abstract O-076] (data updated from presentation). November 2–6, Boston.
109. Kutteh, W.H., et al. 1997. Effect of antiphospholipid antibodies in women undergoing in-vitro fertilization: role of heparin and aspirin. Hum. Reprod. 12 (6), 1171–1175.
110. Sher, G., et al. 1998. The selective use of heparin/aspirin therapy, alone or in combination with intravenous immunoglobulin G, in the management of antiphospholipid antibody-positive women undergoing in vitro fertilization. Am. J. Reprod. Immunol. 40 (2), 74–82.
111. Geva, E., et al. 2000. Prednisone and aspirin improve pregnancy rate in patients with reproductive failure and autoimmune antibodies: a prospective study. Am. J. Reprod. Immunol. 43 (1), 36–40.

Handbook of Systemic Autoimmune Diseases, Volume 4
Reproductive and Hormonal Aspects of Systemic Autoimmune Diseases
Michael Lockshin and D. Ware Branch, editors

CHAPTER 5

Pregnancy and Systemic Lupus Erythematosus

Megan E.B. Clowse*, Michelle Petri
Division of Rheumatology, Johns Hopkins School of Medicine, Baltimore, MD, USA

1. Introduction

Systemic lupus erythematosus (SLE) primarily affects women during their reproductive years. As fertility is maintained in women with lupus, the dilemma of managing lupus during pregnancy, and vice versa, is common. Fortunately, most lupus pregnancies are successful, and the effect of pregnancy on lupus activity and damage is manageable.

Several subsets of women, however, may have significant difficulties carrying pregnancy. Women with active lupus at onset or early in the pregnancy course have a high rate of pregnancy loss (Clowse et al., 2005; Wong et al., 1991; Carmona et al., 1999; Urowitz et al., 1993). Women taking teratogenic medications, including cyclophosphamide, methotrexate, leflunomide, mycophenolate mofetil, and thalidomide, should protect against pregnancy (Janssen and Genta, 2000; Karim et al., 2001). Women with lupus, antiphospholipid syndrome (APS), and a history of prior arterial thrombosis are at increased risk for stroke during pregnancy despite adequate anticoagulation (Petri, 1997).

2. Prevalence of pregnancy in SLE

Women with SLE have a similar overall fertility rate to that of normal women. Several studies comparing women with SLE to healthy controls show a similar mean number of pregnancies, between 2.15 and 3.6 (Petri and Allbritton, 1993; Hardy et al., 1999; Fraga et al., 1974), with two-thirds of pregnancies in SLE patients occurring prior to diagnosis of the disease (Petri and Allbritton, 1993).

3. Epidemiology

3.1. Maternal outcomes

3.1.1. Maternal mortality

Few women with lupus who become pregnant die. A study of pregnancy outcomes in lupus patients in California in 1993–1994 found no maternal deaths in 555 deliveries (Yasmeen et al., 2001). However, the rate of maternal mortality may still be increased over that of the general population. The Hopkins Lupus Cohort identified three deaths occurring within 2 months of delivery, due to pregnancy-related illness, among 267 pregnancies in 203 women (Clowse et al., 2005). Maternal deaths occur because of pre-eclampsia, severe lupus flares, opportunistic infections, or thrombosis from associated APS (Georgiou et al., 2000; Varner et al., 1983; Clowse et al., 2005).

3.1.2. Gestational diabetes and hypertension

The incidence of gestational diabetes is low, but hyperglycemia requiring treatment with either diet modification or medication may occur in lupus patients taking high-dose prednisone during pregnancy

*Corresponding author.
Duke University Medical Center, Box 3535, Durham, NC 27710.
E-mail address: megan.clowse@duke.edu (M.E.B. Clowse).

DOI: 10.1016/S1571-5078(05)04005-5

(Tossounian and Petri, 1994). Women with lupus also are at increased risk for hypertension during pregnancy. From 20 to 30% of women with lupus will develop hypertension during pregnancy, a much higher incidence than in healthy women (Petri et al., 1992). Particular risk factors include renal insufficiency and pre-existing hypertension.

3.1.3. *Pre-eclampsia*

Women with lupus are at increased risk for pre-eclampsia, especially if they are on high dose prednisone during pregnancy (Tossounian and Petri, 1994). The rate of pre-eclampsia varies in different studies and ranges from 2.7 to 30% (Petri, 1997; Clark et al., 2003; Rubbert et al., 1992). Women with lupus are up to 5.6 times more likely to have pre-eclampsia than are other women (Petri, 1997; Wolfberg et al., 2004). Nephritis, renal insufficiency, and preexisting hypertension also raise the risk for pre-eclampsia. There are several reports of eclampsia and HELLP syndrome (*h*emolysis, *e*levated *l*iver tests, *l*ow *p*latelets) in lupus patients, some of them lethal to mother and child. Due to the infrequency of eclampsia and HELLP syndrome, it is not clear if they occur more commonly in lupus patients (Clowse et al., 2005; Clark et al., 2003; Lima et al., 1995).

3.1.4. *Cesarean sections*

The cesarean section rate of lupus pregnancies is higher than normal, ranging between 26 and 48% in recent studies (Petri, 1997; Carmona et al., 1999), compared to a rate of 26.1% in all pregnancies in the United States in 2002. In California between 1993 and 1994, the cesarean section rate was 38.2% in lupus pregnancies versus 19.7% in non-lupus pregnancies. The single biggest reason for cesarean section was fetal distress. More cesarean sections were performed for hypertension in lupus patients than in non-lupus patients (23.5 vs. 5.3%) (Yasmeen et al., 2001).

3.2. *Pregnancy outcomes*

3.2.1. *Live births*

The majority of pregnancies in lupus patients result in a live birth; though the rate of live births is lower than in the general population. A comparison of women with lupus to healthy friends and relatives demonstrated a pregnancy loss rate after the diagnosis of lupus of 27%, while 7–14% of the pregnancies in healthy women ended without a live birth (Petri and Allbritton, 1993). A population-based study in the United Kingdom found that 23.4% of the pregnancies after lupus diagnosis were lost compared to 8.3% in healthy women (Hardy et al., 1999). Although, the rate of pregnancy loss varies between 15–59% in different lupus cohorts across the world, most studies report a pregnancy loss rate of 15–30% (see Table 1). On the other hand, pregnancy outcomes in women with other rheumatic diseases, such as rheumatoid arthritis and scleroderma, are roughly equivalent to pregnancy outcomes in a healthy population (Steen, 1999; Steen et al., 1989).

The majority of pregnancy losses occur in the first trimester; however the rate of loss in the second and third trimesters remains higher than that expected in a healthy population (Varner et al., 1983; Lima et al., 1995). Some centers report high rates of elective and therapeutic abortions (Wong et al., 1991; Kiss et al., 2002; Georgiou et al., 2000). Risk factors for pregnancy loss include active lupus during pregnancy, lupus nephritis, anti-phospholipid antibody syndrome, and a history of prior pregnancy losses (Lima et al., 1995; Varner et al., 1983; Martinez-Rueda et al., 1996). Increased lupus activity doubles the risk of pregnancy loss (Clowse et al., 2003).

3.2.2. *Preterm births*

Lupus pregnancies have a high rate of complications. Preterm birth, defined most frequently as a delivery before 37 weeks gestation, is almost six times more common in pregnancies affected by lupus than in pregnancies in healthy women (Yasmeen et al., 2001). Preterm-birth rates range from less than 10% to over 50%, averaging about one-third (see Table 1) (Clark et al., 2003; Georgiou et al., 2000; Rubbert et al., 1992; Wong et al., 1991). The rate of preterm premature rupture of membranes is high and is a major contributor to the high rate of preterm deliveries (Johnson et al., 1995). Labor is frequently induced in lupus patients in order to take advantage of stable disease and to avoid the complications of an unplanned

Table 1
Pregnancy outcomes in lupus patients

References	Pregnancy loss	Preterm birth (% of live births)
Varner et al. (1983)	11/38 (29%)	9/27 (33%)
Wong et al. (1991)	12/29 (41%)[a]	9/17 (53%)
Tincani et al. (1992)	4/25 (16%)	6/21 (29%)
Buchanan et al. (1992)	28/100 (28%)	Not reported
Rubbert et al. (1992)	2/21 (10%)	13/19 (68%)
Petri et al. (1992)	11/74 (15%)	33/63 (52%)
Urowitz et al. (1993)	37/79 (47%)[a]	Not reported
Ramsey-Goldman et al. (1993)	33/136 (24%)	Not reported
Lima et al. (1995)	19/108 (18%)	38/89 (43%)
Martinez-Rueda et al. (1996)	22/73 (30%)	7/51 (14%)
Carmona et al. (1999)	7/60 (12%)	11/53 (21%)
Georgiou et al. (2000)	20/59 (34%)	3/39 (8%)
Yasmeen et al. (2001)	Not reported	116/555 (21%)
Kiss et al. (2002)	36/61 (59%)[a]	10/25 (40%)
Cortes-Hernandez et al. (2002)	35/103 (34%)	19/68 (28%)
Clark et al. (2003)	15/88 (17%)	28/73 (38%)
Clowse et al. (2003)	38/267 (14%)	90/228 (39%)

[a] Over 20% of pregnancies ended with an induced abortion.

birth. More often, however, preterm delivery occurs because of fetal distress or pre-eclampsia (Lima et al., 1995; Clark et al., 2003).

Risk factors for preterm birth include increased lupus activity during pregnancy, anti-phospholipid antibodies, hypertension, increased prednisone dose, and the use of anti-rheumatic medications at the onset of pregnancy (Clowse et al., 2003; Clark et al., 2003; Cortes-Hernandez et al., 2002). Not all studies found an association between preterm birth and lupus activity, most likely because some negative studies included mild flares of dermatologic or arthritis lupus as increased activity, diluting the overall population (Wong et al., 1991; Lima et al., 1995; Carmona et al., 1999). Moderate to severe lupus activity doubles the risk for preterm delivery (Clowse et al., 2003).

3.2.3. Low birth weight

Low birth weight, defined as <2500 g, and small for gestational age (SGA), defined as birth weight less than the 10th percentile for gestational age, are more common in lupus pregnancies (Witter and Petri, 2000). The rate for small infants ranges between 10 and 30% (Carmona et al., 1999; Cortes-Hernandez et al., 2002; Clowse et al., 2003). Risk factors for low birth weight include increased lupus activity during pregnancy, maternal age over 35, low complement, and hypertension (Clowse et al., 2003; Cortes-Hernandez et al., 2002).

3.2.4. Neonatal lupus

Neonatal lupus is discussed at length elsewhere in this book. In women with positive anti-Ro/SSA or anti-La/SSB antibodies, 2–5% of offspring will be affected with either congenital heart block (CHB) or dermatologic manifestations of neonatal lupus. CHB can be diagnosed in utero with a fetal echocardiogram. Once CHB is identified, the mother may receive therapy with β-methasone, a corticosteroid that transfers through the placenta. Once established, CHB is not reversible.

3.3. Special circumstances

3.3.1. SLE diagnosed during pregnancy

When lupus is diagnosed during pregnancy, the risk of poor pregnancy outcomes is increased (Varner et al., 1983). In a series of 11 pregnancies with gestational-onset lupus, the fetal loss rate was 45%, markedly worse than the fetal loss rate of 13% in women with established lupus at the time of conception (Bobrie et al., 1987). In the Hopkins

Lupus Cohort, 36 of 267 pregnancies coincided with the diagnosis of lupus. These pregnancies had similar rates of live births and preterm births, but a higher rate of small for gestational age babies compared to women diagnosed prior to pregnancy (Clowse et al., 2005).

3.3.2. *SLE active at conception*

Conception within 6 months of significant lupus activity is associated with an increased rate of adverse pregnancy outcome (Bobrie et al., 1987; Moroni and Ponticelli, 2003). In the Hopkins Lupus Cohort, activity within 6 months of conception was associated with a four-fold increase in the pregnancy loss rate. Increased lupus activity during pregnancy occurred in seven times as many of these pregnancies compared to pregnancies beginning in the absence of lupus activity (Clowse et al., 2005).

3.3.3. *Lupus nephritis*

The rate of pregnancy loss, pre-eclampsia, and preterm birth is increased in women with renal disease during pregnancy compared to lupus patients without renal disease. The majority of women with active renal lupus during pregnancy have a return to normal renal function with aggressive therapy after delivery. There are, however, reports of maternal death and permanently damaged renal function in a few women who suffered renal flares during pregnancy (Rubbert et al., 1992; Cortes-Hernandez et al., 2002; Georgiou et al., 2000).

In women with a prior history of lupus nephritis, pregnancy is usually successful as long as the lupus activity is in remission at conception. A small study more than 20 years ago reported a live birth rate of 87% in 26 pregnancies in women with prior lupus nephritis. Six of these pregnancies were complicated by a recurrence of renal disease, two of which resulted in renal failure (Jungers et al., 1982). More recent reports of lupus nephritis during pregnancy report rare cases of permanent renal failure. Three reports in the 1990's combine for a total of 143 pregnancies in women with prior lupus nephritis. Of these, only one woman developed permanent renal failure after pregnancy (Julkunen, 2001). The pregnancies affected by lupus nephritis in the Hopkins Lupus Cohort had similar results, with just 2% of women having persistent renal dysfunction after pregnancy (Petri, 1997).

4. Pathogenesis

SLE contributes to poor pregnancy outcomes by affecting placental function. The placenta resulting from a pregnancy affected by lupus is likely to be small, with over a quarter of them being less than 2 standard deviations below normal size (Magid et al., 1998). Placental perfusion may be decreased by poor development of maternal-fetal circulation early in pregnancy or vessel occlusion later in pregnancy (Salafia and Parke, 1997). Placental cells (trophoblasts) invade and prompt remodeling of maternal uterine wall (spiral) arteries to provide sufficient blood flow to the developing placenta and embryo. In vitro studies have shown that antiphospholipid antibodies can impair the ability of the trophoblast to invade normally into a collagen gel matrix similar to that of the uterine wall (Di Simone et al., 2000). Human placental studies have shown an increase in vasculopathy, including the occlusion of arteries. Occlusion may be from thrombosis, particularly in women with antiphospholipid antibodies or the lupus anticoagulant. Increased atherosis, with lipid-laden cells invading the walls of blood vessels, is also seen in increased levels in the placentas of women with lupus (Abramowsky, 1981). As all pregnancies near term, the placental vessels have an increase in perivillous fibrin, which can lead to small local infarcts. The amount of perivillous fibrin deposits in lupus patients is far greater than in normal pregnancy, a condition that may lead to increased areas of infarction earlier in pregnancy (Magid et al., 1998).

Chronic inflammation and deposition of immune complexes may also play a role in preterm delivery and fetal loss in lupus patients. Some studies show that immune complex and C3 deposition on the trophoblastic basement membrane is increased in women with active lupus during pregnancy (Abramowsky, 1981; Grennan et al., 1978). It is also postulated that the chronic inflammatory milieu may prompt a change in the cytokine composition in the uterus to a state similar to that during chorioamnionitis. Such uterine inflammation is touted as a major cause of premature rupture of membranes and preterm delivery (Salafia and Parke, 1997).

5. Clinical manifestations

5.1. *Lupus flares*

The effect of pregnancy on lupus activity is debated (see Table 2). Several studies have shown that pregnancy increases lupus activity compared to the same patient when she is not pregnant or to other non-pregnant women with lupus (Petri, 1997; Lima et al., 1995; Ruiz-Irastorza et al., 1996). Other studies have found that the rate of flare during pregnancy is unchanged (Urowitz et al., 1993; Tincani et al., 1992; Lockshin et al., 1984; Lockshin, 1989). The inclusion of different populations and varying definitions of flare may explain conflicting results.

Women are at increased risk for lupus flare during pregnancy if they have active disease at conception (Urowitz et al., 1993; Clowse et al., 2005; Lima et al., 1995). Stopping anti-malarial medications can also increase the risk of lupus flare during pregnancy (Clowse et al., 2004; Cortes-Hernandez et al., 2002; Levy et al., 2001). For this reason, we recommend that women on hydroxychloroquine continue the drug throughout pregnancy. Women with a prior history of three or more lupus flares prior to pregnancy are also at increased risk for lupus activity during pregnancy (Cortes-Hernandez et al., 2002).

The timing of lupus flares in pregnancy is quite variable. Different studies show a predominance of lupus activity in different trimesters, but the risk persists throughout pregnancy and in the weeks following delivery. The importance of a lupus flare on pregnancy success is greatest in the first trimester; a flare early in pregnancy triples the risk for pregnancy loss (Clowse et al., 2005).

Lupus activity during pregnancy is usually mild. Constitutional symptoms, arthritis, and skin disease are the most common manifestations of lupus during pregnancy. These generally respond to a temporary increase in prednisone dose (Lima et al., 1995; Rubbert et al., 1992; Cortes-Hernandez et al., 2002; Petri et al., 1991). Serositis, both pericarditis and pleuritis, can complicate pregnancy. Although there are several reports of neuro-psychiatric lupus during pregnancy (Petri et al., 1992; Georgiou et al., 2000; Tincani et al., 1992; Varner et al., 1983), this occurrence is uncommon.

Renal disease occurs in from 4 to 43% of lupus pregnancies (Petri et al., 1991; Cortes-Hernandez et al., 2002; Wong et al., 1991), depending on the series and definition of renal disease. Biopsy is generally deferred until after delivery.

5.2. *Blood pressure*

During the first and second trimesters of a healthy pregnancy, the diastolic blood pressure drops to

Table 2
Lupus flare rate in pregnant vs. non-pregnant patients

References	Flare rate during pregnancy	Flare rate during non-pregnancy
Tincani et al. (1992)	11/25 (40%) 0.07 flares per patient month	Similar rate (data not shown)
Urowitz et al. (1993)	43/61 (70%)	47/59 (80%)
Lima et al. (1995)	62/108 (57%) 0.073 flares per patient month	Fewer flares post-pregnancy and in controls (data not shown)
Petri (1997)	60% 1.6 flares per patient year	0.64 flares per patient year
Georgiou et al. (2000)	8/59 (13.5%)	13/59 (22%)
Cortes-Hernandez et al. (2002)	33% 1.2 flares per patient year	0.4 flares per patient year

approximately 10 mmHg below pre-pregnancy levels as systemic vascular resistance falls. The diastolic blood pressure then slowly increases during the third trimester, but rarely rises above pre-pregnancy readings (Gordon, 2002). A similar pattern is seen in most lupus patients, unless a renal flare or pre-eclampsia induces an elevation in blood pressure.

Hypertension during pregnancy affects almost a third of all lupus pregnancies, particularly those with renal insufficiency (Petri et al., 1992). Frequent blood pressure monitoring is very important, as pre-eclampsia can develop quickly. In the Hopkins Lupus Cohort, the mean diastolic blood pressure in pregnancies that delivered preterm was 90 mmHg, while it was 78 mmHg in those that delivered at term (Petri, 1997). Hypertension during pregnancy is associated with placental insufficiency, which puts the fetus at risk for delayed growth, preterm delivery, and even death (Branch, 2004).

5.3. *Renal changes*

In normal pregnancy, the glomerular filtration rate increases by 30–50% and creatinine clearance to over 100 ml/min, causing a normal decrease in blood urea nitrogen and serum creatinine. Tubular reabsorption of protein is decreased during pregnancy, leading to an increase in the normal amount of proteinuria to 150–180 mg/24 h urine collection.

The American College of Obstetrics and Gynecology considers over 300 mg of protein per 24 h urine collection as pathologic. Fixed renal lesions, in particular membranous nephritis, can appear to worsen during pregnancy with marked increases in proteinuria because of these normal physiologic changes.

6. Diagnostic investigations

All pregnancies in women with lupus should be considered high risk and followed by an obstetrician trained in maternal–fetal medicine. A rheumatologist also should follow every pregnancy to ensure that any signs or symptoms of lupus flare are identified early and treated appropriately. These pregnancies require close monitoring of the health of the mother and the fetus.

6.1. *Radiology*

6.1.1. *Fetal ultrasound*

A thorough fetal ultrasound for anatomy should be performed in all pregnancies between 18 and 20 weeks' gestation (see Table 3). Thereafter, fetal ultrasound should be performed every 3–4 weeks to assess fetal growth and amniotic fluid level. Placental insufficiency, a significant problem in lupus pregnancies, results in slow fetal growth and oligohydramnios (Branch, 2004). Each of these signs is a marker for preterm birth and fetal death.

Table 3
Radiologic testing in lupus pregnancy

Test	Who to test	Gestational age to start	Frequency
Fetal ultrasound:			
Establish dates	Any pregnancy with unknown gestational age	7 weeks or as early as possible	Once
Anatomy screen	All pregnancies	18–20 weeks	Once
For fetal growth	All lupus pregnancies and any pregnancy with uterine size over 2 weeks behind dates	18 weeks	3–4 weeks and as needed
Fetal ECHO	Any mother with a history of positive Ro or La antibodies	16–28 weeks	Weekly
Biophysical profile	All lupus pregnancies	28	Weekly until delivery

6.1.2. Fetal surveillance testing

Periodic assessment of the fetus for evidence of hypoxemia is an important part of lupus pregnancy management. Several acceptable methods may be used, including the non-stress test, the biophysical profile, umbilical artery Doppler velocimetry waveform analysis, and others. In most cases, fetal surveillance testing is started at 28–32 weeks' gestation and is performed once or twice a week until delivery. Earlier fetal surveillance is warranted in some clinical situations (Druzin et al., 1987). Perhaps the most commonly employed method of fetal surveillance testing in the United States is the "modified" biophysical profile consisting of a non-stress test and an amniotic fluid measurement performed twice weekly. Umbilical artery Doppler velocimetry waveform analysis allows assessment of placental vascular resistance, which is low in normal pregnancy but is increased in the setting of placental insufficiency, as might be seen in lupus pregnancy. Markedly increased vascular resistance results in absent or reverse diastolic flow in the umbilical artery. Absent or reverse diastolic flow is associated with fetal growth restriction, fetal hypoxemia, and, eventually, fetal death. Abnormal fetal surveillance results, i.e., test results suggesting fetal hypoxemia, should prompt strong consideration of delivery.

6.1.3. Fetal echocardiography

A four-chamber fetal echocardiogram should be obtained weekly between 16 and 28 weeks in all pregnant mothers with a history of anti-Ro/SSA and/or anti-La/SSB antibodies. First, second, and third degree CHB may be identified through this test, allowing for therapy with β-methasone, and possibly correcting the conduction abnormality if the CHB is not complete. This test is not required if the mother does not have these antibodies.

6.2. Functional testing

Iatrogenic preterm delivery may be indicated in cases of severe preeclampsia or fetal distress. In some less obvious situations, however, testing for fetal lung maturity may guide the decision to proceed to delivery or prolong gestation. Otherwise stable mild-to-moderate maternal hypertension at 34 weeks' gestation serves as one such example. Fetal lung maturity testing of the amniotic fluid assesses fetal lung production of surfactant phospholipids associated with normal, mature alveoli function. Several different tests can be used, including thin-layer chromatography to determine the lecithin-to-sphingomyelin ratio, fluorescence polarization determinations of the amount of surfactant per gram of albumin, and the lamellar body count. "Mature" test results indicate a very low likelihood of respiratory distress syndrome of the newborn and would encourage care providers to move to delivery as opposed to continuing intrauterine care of the fetus.

In the clinical situation wherein early delivery is considered to be likely, but is not urgent, and the fetal lungs are immature, as indicated either by amniotic fluid testing or merely an early gestational age (e.g., <34 weeks' gestation), administration of β-methasone to the mother will enhance fetal lung maturity. The optimal effect of glucocorticoids on fetal lung function is seen no earlier than 24 hours after the first dose of β-methasone. Recent research has suggested that β-methasone may be safer than dexamethasone in terms of fetal neuro-cognitive development.

6.3. Biochemistry, serologic, immunology

Initial visit: If possible, a full laboratory analysis to assess for pregnancy risk should be completed prior to pregnancy, and may bear repeating at the first visit during pregnancy (see Table 4). Laboratory tests should include evaluation of anti-phospholipid antibody status with anti-cardiolipin antibodies, anti-β2 glycoprotein 1 antibodies, and the lupus anticoagulant according to international recommendations. (If any one of these tests is known to be repeatedly positive, the others need not be done.) The risk for neonatal lupus should be assessed with anti-Ro/SSA and anti-La/SSB antibodies. Laboratory tests that provide clues about disease activity, including anti-dsDNA antibodies, complement levels, and C-reactive protein (CRP) also should be evaluated. A complete urinalysis and 24 h urine protein and creatinine should be obtained to look for active renal disease. Finally, complete

Table 4
Laboratory testing in lupus pregnancy

Laboratory test	Initial pregnancy visit	Monthly during pregnancy	To distinguish lupus flare from pre-eclampsia
Complete blood count with differential	X	X	X
Complete chemistries with liver and kidney function tests	X	X	X
Uric acid level	X		X
Anti-cardiolipin antibodies	X[a]		
Lupus anticoagulant: dilute Russell viper venom time and sensitive PTT	X[a]		
Anti-Ro (SSA) and anti-La (SSB) antibodies	X		
Anti-dsDNA antibodies	X	X	X
Complement levels: C3 and C4	X	X	X
Complete urinalysis	X	X	X
24 h urine for protein and creatinine	X	X	X
24 h urine for calcium	X		X

[a] If positive, repeat in 6–8 weeks.

chemistries and a complete blood count should be tested to assess liver, kidney, and hematologic status at the onset of pregnancy. These laboratory tests may suggest active lupus and will serve as a baseline for comparison later in pregnancy.

The human chorionic gonadotropin (hCG) level can be used to confirm pregnancy. The gestational age is determined by menstrual history and fetal ultrasound. Note that the maternal serum alpha-fetal protein (AFP) level, commonly measured to assess the risk for fetal neural tube defects and Down syndrome, may be falsely elevated in women with lupus. This elevation is associated with high prednisone dose, positive anticardiolipin antibody, and preterm birth (Petri et al., 1995) and not necessarily with fetal abnormalities. Of course, an elevated maternal serum AFP always requires thorough fetal evaluation.

Follow-up visits: Each woman should have re-evaluation of anti-dsDNA, complement levels, urinalysis with 24 h urine protein collection, complete chemistries, and a complete blood count every month of pregnancy to monitor lupus acitivity.

If anti-phospholipid antibodies or the lupus anticoagulant is positive on initial testing, it should be repeated at least 6 weeks later to ensure it is not a transient elevation.

7. Differential diagnosis

Pregnancy is associated with dramatic physiologic changes, which can lead to signs and symptoms reminiscent of lupus activity. It is important to distinguish between the symptoms of pregnancy and a lupus flare (see Table 5).

Signs and symptoms of increased lupus activity during pregnancy include lupus-associated rashes, lymphadenopathy, inflammatory arthritis, and serositis. Laboratory tests that may indicate active lupus include lymphopenia, hemolytic anemia, and moderate to marked thrombocytopenia. Hypocomplementemia and a rising titer of anti-dsDNA antibodies indicate increased serologic and possibly clinical lupus activity (see Table 6).

Table 5
Symptoms of pregnancy that can mimic lupus activity

Constitutional	• Fatigue that can be debilitating, all trimesters
Skin	• Palmar erythema and non-specific facial blush from increased estrogen
Face	• Melasma: 'Mask of Pregnancy.' Macular, hyperpigmented, photosensitive, over cheeks and forehead
Hair	• Increased hair growth and thickness during pregnancy • Hair loss in the weeks to months post-partum
Pulmonary	• Increased respiratory rate early in pregnancy from progesterone • Dyspnea from enlarging uterus late in pregnancy

Musculoskeletal	• Back pain in second and third trimesters
	  ○ Relaxin loosens SI joint and symphysis pubis
	  ○ Gravid uterus increases lumbar lordosis
	
	• Joint effusions: noninflammatory in lower extremities

CNS	• Headache can be part of normal pregnancy or associated with hypertension • Seizures occur in eclampsia • Cerebral vascular accidents can be caused by pre-eclampsia or APS

Table 6
Laboratory changes of pregnancy

Anemia	• Due to volume expansion during pregnancy • Diagnosed in up to 50% of healthy pregnant women (Samuels, 2002) • Hemolytic anemia is not usually found in pregnancy: Test LDH, Coombs' tests, and a peripheral blood smear for diagnosis
Leukocytosis	• The neutrophil count increases, leading to a rise in the overall WBC count to 9000–15,000/mm^2 • The absolute lymphocyte count remains unchanged (Buyon et al., 1999) • Lymphopenia $<1000/mm^2$ may be an indication of active lupus
Thrombocytopenia	• In 8% of normal pregnancies, the platelet count falls to between 100,000 and 130,000 unassociated with any disease process • Thrombocytopenia during pregnancy can be from a lupus flare, or from pre-eclampsia, HELLP syndrome, APS, intrauterine fetal demise, or placental abruption
Complement	• Complement production is increased in the liver by estrogen, leading to an increase of 10–50% in the levels of C3, C4 and CH50 • Lupus pregnancy: increasing, stable, or low complement levels
Erythrocyte sedimentation rate (ESR)	• The ESR often increases dramatically during normal pregnancy • It is not clinically helpful in determining lupus activity in pregnancy
C-reactive protein	• The CRP can be mildly elevated during normal pregnancy • Its predictive value has not been evaluated for lupus flare and pregnancy outcomes

Pre-eclampsia is the combination of hypertension (blood pressure over 140/90) and proteinuria (over 300 mg of protein in a 24 h urine collection) occurring after 20 weeks gestation (see Table 7). Severe pre-eclampsia is defined by having higher blood pressure ($\geqslant$160/110), proteinuria $\geqslant$5 g/24 h urine collection, oliguria <500 ml in 24 h, pulmonary edema, liver dysfunction, cerebral or visual changes, abdominal pain, or thrombocytopenia. The occurrence of new-onset grand mal seizures in addition to the hypertension and proteinuria defines eclampsia (Schroeder, 2002).

Distinguishing lupus activity from pre-eclampsia can be challenging (see Table 7). The timing of the onset of symptoms can be helpful, as pre-eclampsia does not occur prior to 20 weeks gestation, and not usually until the third trimester. The presence of other lupus symptoms, such as arthritis, malar rash, or serositis can be a helpful indicator of lupus activity. Laboratory markers can also be helpful. Pre-eclampsia does not increase levels of anti-dsDNA antibodies. Complement is typically normal, but may fall with pre-eclampsia. The ratio of complement to complement split products (CH50:Ba) may be useful; if this ratio is elevated, with high complement and low split products, pre-eclampsia is more likely. Low-complement with high-split products signify complement activation and indicate lupus activity (Abramson and Buyon, 1992). In HELLP syndrome, complement split products may increase (Haeger et al., 1990). Pre-eclampsia also is associated with a low urine calcium level (<195 mg/24 h), but during a lupus flare the urine calcium level would be normal to high (Taufield et al., 1987). The serum uric acid may increase in pre-eclampsia, but it generally remains normal during a lupus flare.

8. Treatment

The treatment of lupus during pregnancy necessitates balancing the benefits of a medication in controlling lupus with the risks of the medication to the developing fetus (see Table 8) (Please refer to the chapter on Anti-Rheumatic Medication in Pregnancy in this book for further information about the medications discussed here).

Table 7
Comparison of active lupus, pre-eclampsia, severe pre-eclampsia, and HELLP syndrome

Signs and symptoms	Active Lupus	Pre-eclampsia	Severe Pre-eclampsia	HELLP syndrome
Timing	Any trimester	Third trimester	Third trimester	Third trimester
Proteinuria	Normal or elevated	>300 mg/24 h urine collection	>5000 mg/24 h urine collection	Normal or elevated
Blood pressure	Normal or high	High $\geqslant$140/90	High $\geqslant$160/110	Normal or high
Complement levels	Normal or low	Usually normal	Usually normal	Not characterized
Complement split products	Low CH50:Ba ratio	High CH50:Ba ratio	High CH50:Ba ratio	High C3a, C5a, C5b-9
Other SLE symptoms	Present	Absent	Absent	Absent
CNS dysfunction	Possible	Headache	Headache, confusion, stroke	Uncommon
Platelets	Low or normal	Normal	Low	<100,000
Hemolysis	Possible	No	No	Microangiopathic hemolytic anemia LDH>600
Serum creatinine	Stable or rising	Stable	Stable or rising	Stable
Liver function tests	Normal or high	Normal	Normal or high	High AST and ALT>1000
Anti-dsDNA antibody	Negative or high	Negative or stable	Negative or stable	Negative or stable
Uric acid	Normal or high	High (>5.0 mg/dl)	High	High
Urine calcium	Normal or high	Low	Low	Not characterized

Table 8
Treatment plan for lupus during pregnancy

Lupus activity	Treatment
All pregnant lupus patients	Pre-natal multivitamin Hydroxychloroquine (if on it previously)
No activity	None needed
Mild activity	Low dose prednisone (under 20 mg a day) NSAID's—only in the first trimester
Moderate activity	High dose prednisone (up to 60 mg a day) IV methylprednisolone (up to 1 g a day for 3 days) Azathioprine
Severe activity	High dose prednisone IV methylprednisolone Azathioprine Cyclophosphamide—high risk of fetal loss

8.1. All pregnant women

A daily pre-natal multivitamin with at least 800 μg of folic acid and 27 mg of iron should be started prior to or as early as possible in pregnancy. Women who are on hydroxychloroquine or azathioprine prior to pregnancy should continue these medications. The increased likelihood of lupus exacerbation if these medications are stopped places the fetus and mother at greater risk than the medications themselves. ACE-inhibitors are stopped as soon as pregnancy is recognized. Mycophenolate mofetil, methotrexate, and cyclophosphamide are stopped 3 months before conception.

8.2. No lupus activity

If a woman conceives after a prolonged period of lupus inactivity and has no signs or symptoms of lupus activity, she may not require any specific medical therapy during her pregnancy. Prednisone prophylaxis during pregnancy has not been shown to be helpful, and prednisone is associated with increased rates of preterm delivery, hypertension, and diabetes (Carmona et al., 1999).

8.3. Mild lupus activity

Low-dose prednisone is the first-line therapy for mild lupus flares during pregnancy. Hydroxychloroquine also can be started during pregnancy with recent evidence suggesting an acceptably low risk of teratogenesis or associated adverse pregnancy outcomes (Clowse et al., 2004; Costedoat-Chalumeau et al., 2003; Klinger et al., 2001; Motta et al., 2002). Non-steroidal anti inflammatory drug (NSAID) can be used intermittently during the first and second trimesters to treat mild inflammatory arthritis, serositis, and pain. They probably should be avoided in the third trimester because of untoward fetal renal and vascular effects.

Women on hydroxychloroquine prior to pregnancy should be continued on it during pregnancy. The risk for lupus flare doubles when hydroxychloroquine is stopped in non-pregnant patients (Tsakonas et al., 1998). In the Hopkins Lupus Cohort, we found an increase in high activity lupus and the need for prednisone in women who stopped hydroxychloroquine upon discovering pregnancy. This rise in lupus activity did not occur in women who continued hydroxychloroquine throughout pregnancy, or in women never on the drug (Clowse et al., 2004). The half-life of hydroxychloroquine is between 32 to 50 days. Therefore, stopping it once pregnancy is discovered may still result in significant fetal exposure.

8.4. Moderate lupus activity

Lupus activity that does not respond to low dose prednisone can be treated with higher doses of prednisone and/or azathioprine. Intravenous pulse methylprednisolone of 1 g/day for 3 days can be very effective in bringing active lupus, including lupus nephritis and CNS lupus, under control quickly during pregnancy. When it is administered, close monitoring for hypertension and hyperglycemia is warranted. Whether this form of administration affects the fetus is unknown.

Azathioprine is the first choice as a steroid-sparing medication for lupus flares during pregnancy: many reported pregnancies had azathioprine exposure for renal transplant maintenance or inflammatory bowel disease (Petri, 2003). These pregnancies had no increase in pregnancy loss or congenital abnormalities over the general population (Katz and Pore, 2001). Rare cases of transient thrombocytopenia and leukopenia in infants exposed to azathioprine in utero have been reported (Ramsey-Goldman and Schilling, 1997).

8.5. Severe lupus activity

Severe, life or organ threatening lupus during pregnancy puts the success of the pregnancy in great jeopardy. Therapy with high dose oral steroid, pulse IV methylprednisolone, or azathioprine is warranted.

Cyclophosphamide should be avoided during pregnancy because it can cause fetal abnormalities during the first trimester. Three cases of its use during the second and third trimesters for severe lupus activity have been published, one resulting in the birth of a healthy, preterm infant (Kart Koseoglu et al., 2001). Two cases from our institution were associated with fetal demise within days of starting cyclophosphamide (Clowse et al., 2005). Thus, we do not recommend its use unless the life of the mother is at risk. When cyclophosphamide is required, a frank discussion about the high risk for fetal loss should be undertaken with the mother.

8.6. Hypertension

Hypertension during pregnancy needs to be aggressively managed in order to protect the health of the mother and fetus. The cure for severe gestational hypertension, pre-eclampsia, and HELLP syndrome is delivery of the fetus. Magnesium sulfate should be used to prevent seizures in a woman with pre-eclampsia.

To treat acute severe hypertension, IV labetalol is recommended. Chronic blood pressure control can be obtained safely during pregnancy with hydralazine, methyldopa, or other agents. Oral labetalol and long-acting nifedipine are also used during pregnancy and do not appear to cause problems in fetal growth or development (Gregg, 2004). ACE-inhibitors should be avoided.

Key points

- Most pregnancies in women with lupus are successful.
- Pregnancy is most successful if conception occurs during a period of lupus inactivity.
- A rheumatologist and a high-risk obstetrician should closely monitor all pregnancies in women with lupus.
- Increased lupus activity, in particular lupus nephritis, is associated with increased preterm birth and more fetal losses.
- Signs and symptoms of lupus flare can mimic those of pregnancy, and vice versa.
- A woman with lupus who presents with hypertension and proteinuria in the latter part of pregnancy may have either a lupus flare or pre-eclampsia. It is important to distinguish between the two, as therapies are very different.
    - Check the complement levels, anti-dsDNA titer, uric acid, and urine calcium.
    - Look for other signs of a lupus flare, such as arthritis or a malar rash.
- Women on hydroxychloroquine prior to pregnancy should continue this medication throughout pregnancy.
- Women on azathioprine at the time of conception should continue it if it is required to treat active lupus.
- Prednisone is the medication of choice to treat a lupus flare during pregnancy.
- Cyclophosphamide, mycophenolate mofetil, methotrexate, leflunomide, thalidomide, and ACE-inhibitors should be avoided during pregnancy.

References

Abramowsky, C.R. 1981. Lupus erythematosus, the placenta, and pregnancy: a natural experiment in immunologically mediated reproductive failure. Prog. Clin. Biol. Res. 70, 309–320.

Abramson, S.B., Buyon, J.P. 1992. Activation of the complement pathway: comparison of normal pregnancy, preeclampsia, and systemic lupus erythematosus during pregnancy. Am. J. Reprod. Immunol. 28, 183–187.

Bobrie, G., Liote, F., Houillier, P., Grunfeld, J.P., Jungers, P. 1987. Pregnancy in lupus nephritis and related disorders. Am. J. Kidney Dis. 9, 339–343.

Branch, D.W. 2004. Pregnancy in patients with rheumatic diseases: obstetric management and monitoring. Lupus 13, 696–698.

A current review of obstetrical management for women with lupus, rheumatoid arthritis, scleroderma, and antiphospholipid antibody syndrome.

Buchanan, N.M., Khamashta, M.A., Morton, K.E., Kerslake, S., Baguley, E.A., Hughes, G.R. 1992. A study of 100 high risk lupus pregnancies. Am. J. Reprod. Immunol. 28, 192–194.

Buyon, J.P., Kalunian, K.C., Ramsey-Goldman, R., Petri, M.A., Lockshin, M.D., Ruiz-Irastorza, G., Khamashta, M. 1999. Assessing disease activity in SLE patients during pregnancy. Lupus 8, 677–684.

A review of the signs and symptoms of pregnancy that can mimic lupus activity. Outlines several instruments to measure lupus activity during pregnancy.

Carmona, F., Font, J., Cervera, R., Munoz, F., Cararach, V., Balasch, J. 1999. Obstetrical outcome of pregnancy in patients with systemic Lupus erythematosus. A study of 60 cases. Eur. J. Obstet. Gynecol. Reprod. Biol. 83, 137–142.

A prospective study of 60 pregnancies in lupus patients. The majority of the patients had inactive lupus at conception, leading to good pregnancy outcomes.

Clark, C.A., Spitzer, K.A., Nadler, J.N., Laskin, C.A. 2003. Preterm deliveries in women with systemic lupus erythematosus, J. Rheumatol. 30, 2127–2132.

A comparison of lupus pregnancies that resulted in preterm versus fullterm deliveries that identifies multiple risk factors for preterm delivery.

Clowse, M., Magder, L.C., Petri, M. 2003. Impact of the intensity and timing of lupus activity on pregnancy outcomes [abstract #1085]. Arthritis Rheum. 48, S435.

Clowse, M., Magder, L.C., Petri, M. 2004. The effect of hydroxychloroquine on pregnancy outcomes and disease activity in lupus patients [abstract #1846]. Arthritis Rheum. 50 .

Clowse, M.E., Magder, L., Petri, M. 2005. Cyclophosphamide for lupus during pregnancy. Lupus 14, 593–597.

Clowse, M., Witter, F. R., Magder, L. C., Petri, M. 2005. The impact of increased lupus activity on obstetrical outcomes. Arthritis Rheum. 52, 514–521.

A report of 267 pregnancies in lupus patients in the Hopkins Lupus Pregnancy Cohort from 1987 to 2002.

Cortes-Hernandez, J., Ordi-Ros, J., Paredes, F., Casellas, M., Castillo, F., Vilardell-Tarres, M. 2002. Clinical predictors of fetal and maternal outcome in systemic lupus erythematosus: a prospective study of 103 pregnancies. Rheumatology (Oxford) 41, 643–650.

A prospective cohort study of 103 pregnancies in lupus patients that identifies risk factors for fetal loss, prematurity, and intrauterine growth restriction.

Costedoat-Chalumeau, N., Amoura, Z., Duhaut, P., Huong du, L.T., Sebbough, D., Wechsler, B., Vauthier, D., Denjoy, I., Lupoglazoff, J.M., Piette, J.C. 2003. Safety of hydroxychloroquine in pregnant patients with connective tissue diseases: a study of one hundred thirty-three cases compared with a control group. Arthritis Rheum. 48, 3207–3211.

Di Simone, N., Meroni, P.L., de Papa, N., et al. 2000. Antiphospholipid antibodies affect trophoblast gonadotropin secretion and invasiveness by binding directly and through adhered beta2-glycoprotein I. Arithritis Rheum. 43, 140–150.

Druzin, M.L., Lockshin, M., Edersheim, T.G., Hutson, J.M., Krauss, A.L., Kogut, E. 1987. Second-trimester fetal monitoring and preterm delivery in pregnancies with systemic lupus erythematosus and/or circulating anticoagulant. Am. J. Obstet. Gynecol. 157, 1503–1510.

Fraga, A., Mintz, G., Orozco, J., Orozco, J. 1974. Sterility and fertility rates, fetal wastage and maternal morbidity in systemic lupus erythematosus. J. Rheumatol. 1, 293–298.

Georgiou, P.E., Politi, E.N., Katsimbri, P., Sakka, V., Drosos, A.A. 2000. Outcome of lupus pregnancy: a controlled study. Rheumatology (Oxford) 39, 1014–1019.

Gordon, M.C. 2002. Maternal Physiology in Pregnancy. In: S.G. Gabbe (Ed.), Obstetrics: Normal and Problem Pregnancies, fourth edition, Chapter 3. Churchill Livingstone, New York.

Gregg, A.R. 2004. Hypertension in pregnancy. Obstet. Gynecol. Clin. N. Am. 31, 223–241. v.

Grennan, D.M., McCormick, J.N., Wojtacha, D., Carty, M., Behan, W. 1978. Immunological studies of the placenta in systemic lupus erythematosus. Ann. Rheum. Dis. 37, 129–134.

Haeger, M., Unander, M., Bengtsson, A. 1990. Enhanced anaphylatoxin and terminal C5b-9 complement complex formation in patients with the syndrome of hemolysis, elevated liver enzymes, and low platelet count. Obstet. Gynecol. 76, 698–702.

Hardy, C.J., Palmer, B.P., Morton, S.J., Muir, K.R., Powell, R.J. 1999. Pregnancy outcome and family size in systemic lupus erythematosus: a case–control study. Rheumatology (Oxford) 38, 559–563.

Janssen, N.M., Genta, M.S. 2000. The effects of immunosuppressive and anti-inflammatory medications on fertility, pregnancy, and lactation. Arch. Intern. Med. 160, 610–619.

Johnson, M.J., Petri, M., Witter, F.R., Repke, J.T. 1995. Evaluation of preterm delivery in a systemic lupus erythematosus pregnancy clinic. Obstet. Gynecol. 86, 396–399.

Julkunen, H. 2001. Pregnancy and lupus nephritis. Scand. J. Urol. Nephrol. 35, 319–327.

Jungers, P., Dougados, M., Pelissier, C., Kuttenn, F., Tron, F., Lesavre, P., Bach, J.F. 1982. Lupus nephropathy and pregnancy. Report of 104 cases in 36 patients. Arch. Intern. Med. 142, 771–776.

Karim, M.Y., Ruiz-Irastorza, G., Khamashta, M.A., Hughes, G.R. 2001. Update on therapy—thalidomide in the treatment of lupus. Lupus 10, 188–192.

Kart Koseoglu, H., Yucel, A.E., Kunefeci, G., Ozdemir, F.N., Duran, H. 2001. Cyclophosphamide therapy in a serious case of lupus nephritis during pregnancy. Lupus 10, 818–820.

Katz, J.A., Pore, G. 2001. Inflammatory bowel disease and pregnancy. Inflamm. Bowel. Dis. 7, 146–157.

Kiss, E., Bhattoa, H.P., Bettembuk, P., Balogh, A., Szegedi, G. 2002. Pregnancy in women with systemic lupus erythematosus. Eur. J. Obstet. Gynecol. Reprod. Biol. 101, 129–134.

Klinger, G., Morad, Y., Westall, C.A., Laskin, C., Spitzer, K.A., Koren, G., Ito, S., Buncic, R.J. 2001. Ocular toxicity and antenatal exposure to chloroquine or hydroxychloroquine for rheumatic diseases. Lancet 358, 813–814.

Levy, R.A., Vilela, V.S., Cataldo, M.J., Ramos, R.C., Duarte, J.L., Tura, B.R., Albuquerque, E.M., Jesus, N.R. 2001. Hydroxychloroquine (HCQ) in lupus pregnancy: double-blind and placebo-controlled study. Lupus 10, 401–404.
A randomized trial of hydroxychloroquine use in pregnancy that shows improvement in lupus activity and pregnancy outcomes with the medication.

Lima, F., Buchanan, N.M., Khamashta, M.A., Kerslake, S., Hughes, G.R. 1995. Obstetric outcome in systemic lupus erythematosus. Semin. Arthritis Rheum. 25, 184–192.

Lockshin, M.D. 1989. Pregnancy does not cause systemic lupus erythematosus to worsen. Arthritis Rheum. 32, 665–670.

Lockshin, M.D., Reinitz, E., Druzin, M.L., Murrman, M., Estes, D. 1984. Lupus pregnancy. Case-control prospective study demonstrating absence of lupus exacerbation during or after pregnancy. Am. J. Med. 77, 893–898.

Magid, M.S., Kaplan, C., Sammaritano, L.R., Peterson, M., Druzin, M.L., Lockshin, M.D. 1998. Placental pathology in systemic lupus erythematosus: a prospective study. Am. J. Obstet. Gynecol. 179, 226–234.

Martinez-Rueda, J.O., Arce-Salinas, C.A., Kraus, A., Alcocer-Varela, J., Alarcon-Segovia, D. 1996. Factors associated with fetal losses in severe systemic lupus erythematosus. Lupus 5, 113–119.

Moroni, G., Ponticelli, C. 2003. The risk of pregnancy in patients with lupus nephritis. J. Nephrol. 16, 161–167.

Motta, M., Tincani, A., Faden, D., Zinzini, E., Chirico, G. 2002. Antimalarial agents in pregnancy. Lancet 359, 524–525.

Petri, M. 1997. Hopkins lupus pregnancy center: 1987 to 1996. Rheum. Dis. Clin. N. Am. 23, 1–13.

Petri, M. 2003. Immunosuppressive drug use in pregnancy. Autoimmunity 36, 51–56.

Petri, M., Allbritton, J. 1993. Fetal outcome of lupus pregnancy: a retrospective case-control study of the Hopkins Lupus Cohort. J. Rheumatol. 20, 650–656.
A comparison of pregnancy rates and outcomes in a large number of women with lupus versus their healthy friends and relatives.

Petri, M., Ho, A.C., Patel, J., Demers, D., Joseph, J.M., Goldman, D. 1995. Elevation of maternal alpha-fetoprotein in systemic lupus erythematosus: a controlled study. J. Rheumatol. 22, 1365–1368.

Petri, M., Howard, D., Repke, J. 1991. Frequency of lupus flare in pregnancy. The Hopkins Lupus Pregnancy Center experience. Arthritis Rheum. 34, 1538–1545.

Petri, M., Howard, D., Repke, J., Goldman, D.W. 1992. The Hopkins Lupus Pregnancy Center: 1987–1991 update. Am. J. Reprod. Immunol. 28, 188–191.

Ramsey-Goldman, R., Mientus, J.M., Kutzer, J.E., Mulvihill, J.J., Medsger, T.A., Jr. 1993. Pregnancy outcome in women with systemic lupus erythematosus treated with immunosuppressive drugs. J. Rheumatol. 20, 1152–1157.
A retrospective study of the impact of the prior use of immunosuppressive drugs on pregnancy outcomes.

Ramsey-Goldman, R., Schilling, E. 1997. Immunosuppressive drug use during pregnancy. Rheum. Dis. Clin. N. Am. 23, 149–167.

Rubbert, A., Pirner, K., Wildt, L., Kalden, J.R., Manger, B. 1992. Pregnancy course and complications in patients with systemic lupus erythematosus. Am. J. Reprod. Immunol. 28, 205–207.

Ruiz-Irastorza, G., Lima, F., Alves, J., Khamashta, M.A., Simpson, J., Hughes, G.R., Buchanan, N.M. 1996. Increased rate of lupus flare during pregnancy and the puerperium: a prospective study of 78 pregnancies. Br. J. Rheumatol. 35, 133–138.

Salafia, C.M., Parke, A.L. 1997. Placental pathology in systemic lupus erythematosus and phospholipid antibody syndrome. Rheum. Dis. Clin. N. Am. 23, 85–97.

Samuels, P. 2002. Hematologic Complications of Pregnancy. In: S.G. Gabbe (Ed.), Obstetrics: Normal and Problem Pregnancies, fourth edition, Chapter 34. Churchill Livingstone, New York.

Schroeder, B.M. 2002. ACOG practice bulletin on diagnosing and managing preeclampsia and eclampsia. American College of Obstetricians and Gynecologists. Am. Fam. Physician 66, 330–331.

Steen, V.D. 1999. Pregnancy in women with systemic sclerosis. Obstet. Gynecol. 94, 15–20.

Steen, V.D., Conte, C., Day, N., Ramsey-Goldman, R., Medsger, T.A., Jr. 1989. Pregnancy in women with systemic sclerosis. Arthritis Rheum. 32, 151–157.

Taufield, P.A., Ales, K.L., Resnick, L.M., Druzin, M.L., Gertner, J.M., Laragh, J.H. 1987. Hypocalciuria in preeclampsia. N. Eng. J. Med. 316, 715–718.

Tincani, A., Faden, D., Tarantini, M., Lojacono, A., Tanzi, P., Gastaldi, A., Di Mario, C., Spatola, L., Cattaneo, R., Balestrieri, G. 1992. Systemic lupus erythematosus and pregnancy: a prospective study. Clin. Exp. Rheumatol. 10, 439–446.

Tossounian, S., Petri, M. 1994. Maternal morbidity of SLE pregnancy: a case-control study [abstract]. Arthritis Rheum. 37, S216.

Tsakonas, E., Joseph, L., Esdaile, J.M., Choquette, D., Senecal, J.L., Cividino, A., Danoff, D., Osterland, C.K., Yeadon, C., Smith, C.D. 1998. A long-term study of hydroxychloroquine withdrawal on exacerbations in systemic lupus erythematosus. The Canadian Hydroxychloroquine Study Group. Lupus 7, 80–85.

Urowitz, M.B., Gladman, D.D., Farewell, V.T., Stewart, J., McDonald, J. 1993. Lupus and pregnancy studies. Arthritis Rheum. 36, 1392–1397.

A case-control study of pregnant versus non-pregnant lupus patients. Assesses the risk of lupus flare during pregnancy and the importance of pre-pregnancy disease activity.

Varner, M.W., Meehan, R.T., Syrop, C.H., Strottmann, M.P., Goplerud, C.P. 1983. Pregnancy in patients with systemic lupus erythematosus. Am. J. Obstet. Gynecol. 145, 1025–1040.

Witter, F.R., Petri, M. 2000. Antenatal detection of intrauterine growth restriction in patients with systemic lupus erythematosus. Int. J. Gynaecol. Obstet. 71, 67–68.

Wolfberg, A.J., Lee-Parritz, A., Peller, A.J., Lieberman, E.S. 2004. Association of rheumatologic disease with preeclampsia. Obstet. Gynecol. 103, 1190–1193.

Wong, K.L., Chan, F.Y., Lee, C.P. 1991. Outcome of pregnancy in patients with systemic lupus erythematosus. A prospective study. Arch. Intern. Med. 151, 269–273.

Yasmeen, S., Wilkins, E.E., Field, N.T., Sheikh, R.A., Gilbert, W.M. 2001. Pregnancy outcomes in women with systemic lupus erythematosus. J. Matern. Fetal. Med. 10, 91–96.

A population study of all deliveries in California in the mid 1990's. A comparison of pregnancy complications and outcomes in women with lupus versus healthy controls.

Handbook of Systemic Autoimmune Diseases, Volume 4
Reproductive and Hormonal Aspects of Systemic Autoimmune Diseases
Michael Lockshin and D. Ware Branch, editors

CHAPTER 6

Antiphospholipid Syndrome

D.W. Branch[a,*], M. Lockshin[b]

[a]*Department of Obstetrics and Gynecology, Division of Maternal Fetal Medicine, University of Utah Health Sciences Center, Salt Lake City, UT, USA*

[b]*Department of Rheumatology, Hospital for Special Surgery, New York City, NY, USA*

1. Introduction

Synonyms for the antiphospholipid antibody syndrome (APS) are anticardiolipin antibody, lupus anticoagulant, and Hughes' syndrome. Diagnosis requires that a patient have *both* a clinical event (thrombosis or pregnancy complication) *and* an antiphospholipid antibody (aPL) documented by a solid phase serum assay (anticardiolipin) or by an inhibitor of phospholipid-dependent clotting (lupus anticoagulant), or by both. A false-positive test for syphilis does not fulfill the laboratory criterion. Preliminary 1999 classification criteria for APS (Wilson et al., 1999) are listed in Table 1. A revision proposed in late 2004 will add IgA aPL antibody, antibody to the phospholipid-binding protein β_2 glycoprotein I (β_2GPI), valvular heart disease, thrombocytopenia, and livedo reticularis as associated phenomena (Table 2).

APS occurs as an isolated diagnosis (primary antiphospholipid antibody syndrome, PAPS) and associated with systemic lupus erythematosus (SLE) or another rheumatic disease (secondary APS, sAPS). Positive tests for aPL may precede symptoms for many years (Arbuckle et al., 2001). Estimates of the probability that an asymptomatic person incidentally found to have aPL will eventually develop thromboses are between 0.5 and 2%/year (Erkan et al., 2001).

The anticardiolipin enzyme-linked immunosorbent assay (ELISA) is sensitive, but not specific for the diagnosis of APS (Day et al., 1998). Documentation of a *lupus anticoagulant* requires the four-step process outlined in Table 1. Approximately 80% of patients with lupus anticoagulant have anticardiolipin antibody, and 20% of patients positive for anticardiolipin antibody have lupus anticoagulant.

Negative predictive value is high for β_2GPI-dependent anticardiolipin, lupus anticoagulant, and anti-β_2GPI tests, but positive predictive value is not. Antibodies to prothrombin (factor II), thrombomodulin, and other coagulation proteins sometimes accompany aPLs directed against β_2GPI (Horbach et al., 1998). It is likely that β_2GPI and prothrombin-dependent antibodies will be proven more specific for clinical disease.

2. Prevalence and Epidemiology

Low-titer anticardiolipin antibody occurs in 2–7% of normal blood donors and moderate to high titer anticardiolipin antibody or lupus anticoagulant in 0.2%. The prevalence of positive tests increases with age. Sixty to eighty percent of patients with PAPS are women. Familial disease is frequent, but

*Corresponding author.
Division of Maternal Fetal Medicine, Department of Obstetrics and Gynecology, University of Utah Health Sciences Center, 30 N 1900 East, Rm 2B-200, Salt Lake City, UT 84132, USA.
Tel.: +/-801-581-7260; Fax: +/-801- 585-2594.
E-mail address: wareb@aol.com (D.W. Branch).

DOI: 10.1016/S1571-5078(05)04006-7

Table 1
Preliminary Classification Criteria for Antiphospholipid Antibody Syndrome (Wilson, 1999)

Type	Criteria
Clinical	
Vascular thrombosis	One or more episodes of: • Arterial thrombosis, *or* • Venous thrombosis, *or* • Small vessel thrombosis, in any tissue or organ, confirmed by imaging or Doppler studies or histopathologic studies. For histopathologic confirmation, thrombosis should be present without significant evidence of inflammation in the vessel wall.
Pregnancy morbidity	One or more: • Unexplained deaths of a morphologically normal fetus at or after the 10th week of gestation with fetal morphology documented by ultrasound or by direct examination of the fetus, *or* • Premature birth of a morphologically normal neonate at or before the 34th week of gestation because of severe preeclampsia, eclampsia, or severe placental insufficiency, *or* • Three or more unexplained consecutive miscarriages with anatomic, genetic, or hormonal causes excluded.
Laboratory	
Anticardiolipin antibody (aCL)	• IgG and/or IgM isotype present in medium or high titer, on two or more occasions, 6 weeks or more apart, *and* • Measured by a standardized ELISA for βs glycoprotein I-dependent anticardiolipin antibody • Abnormality present in plasma, on two or more occasions, 6 weeks or more apart, *and* • Detected according to the guidelines of the International Society on Thrombosis and Hemostasis Scientific Subcommittee on Lupus Anticoagulants/phospholipid-dependent antibodies in the following steps: ○ Demonstration of a prolonged phospholipid-dependent coagulation screening test, e.g., activated partial thromboplastin time, kaolin clotting time, dilute Russell viper venom time, dilute prothrombin time ○ Failure to correct the prolonged screening test by mixing with normal platelet poor plasma ○ Shortening or correction of the prolonged screening test by the addition of excess phospholipid ○ Exclusion of other coagulopathies as clinically indicated, e.g., factor VIII inhibitor, heparin

human leukocyte antigen (HLA) typing of patients has not revealed a single consistent profile.

According to a study of normal male physicians followed prospectively for 3 years, those with moderate to high titers of IgG anticardiolipin antibody have a risk for thrombophlebitis or pulmonary embolus eight times higher than do men with negative tests (Ginsburg et al., 1992). Approximately 10% of first-stroke victims have aPL (The APASS Group, 1993), especially those who are young (Levine et al., 1995), as do up to 21% of women who have suffered three or more consecutive fetal losses (Stephenson, 1996). In a retrospective study, 60% of women identified to have aPL after an abnormal pregnancy suffered a thrombotic event in the subsequent 10 years (Erkan, 2001).

3. Etiology/pathogenesis

In experimental animal models, passive or active immunization with viral peptides (Gharavi et al., 2001), bacterial peptides (Blank et al., 2002), and heterologous β_2GPI (Gharavi et al., 1992) induce polyclonal aPL, lupus anticoagulant, and clinical events associated with APS. These data suggest that pathologic aPL is induced in genetically disposed humans by infection.

It is likely that vascular injury and/or endothelial cell activation ('second hit') immediately precede the occurrence of thrombosis in persons bearing the antibody. The role of a second hit or cell activation step in aPL-associated pregnancy loss or morbidity is less certain. A proposed pathogenesis begins with activation or apoptosis of platelets, endothelial cells during which negatively charged phosphatidylserine migrates from the inner to the normally electrically neutral outer cell membrane (Fig. 1). In the placenta, the migration of phosphatidylserine may occur during trophoblast syncytium formation. Circulating β_2GPI then binds to phosphatidylserine. APL then binds to a β_2GPI dimer (Lutters et al., 2003), activating complement and initiating a signaling cascade that induces cell surface tissue factor expression and adhesion molecules, causing platelets to aggregate and initiate thrombosis (Bordron et al., 1998). An alternative, thrombotic hypothesis holds that aPL competes in the placenta for phosphatidylserine with the natural anticoagulant placental anticoagulant protein I (annexin V) (Sammaritano et al., 1992; Rand et al., 1997), possibly interrupting a shield that is thought to protect the fetus from maternal prothrombotic mechanisms (Rand, 2002). Finally, others suggest that aPLs may operate through the signaling cascade and they also inhibit production of placental prolactin, insulin growth factor β-1, and signal transducer and activator of transcription 5 (Stat5) (Mak et al., 2002), and they adversely affect the formation of a trophoblast syncytium, placental apoptosis, and trophoblast invasion, all processes required for normal establishment of placental function. In vitro, pathogenic aPL induces adhesion molecule and tissue factor expression in endothelial cells and expression of GPIIb/IIIa on platelets (reviewed in Pierangeli et al., 2004) and results in enhanced

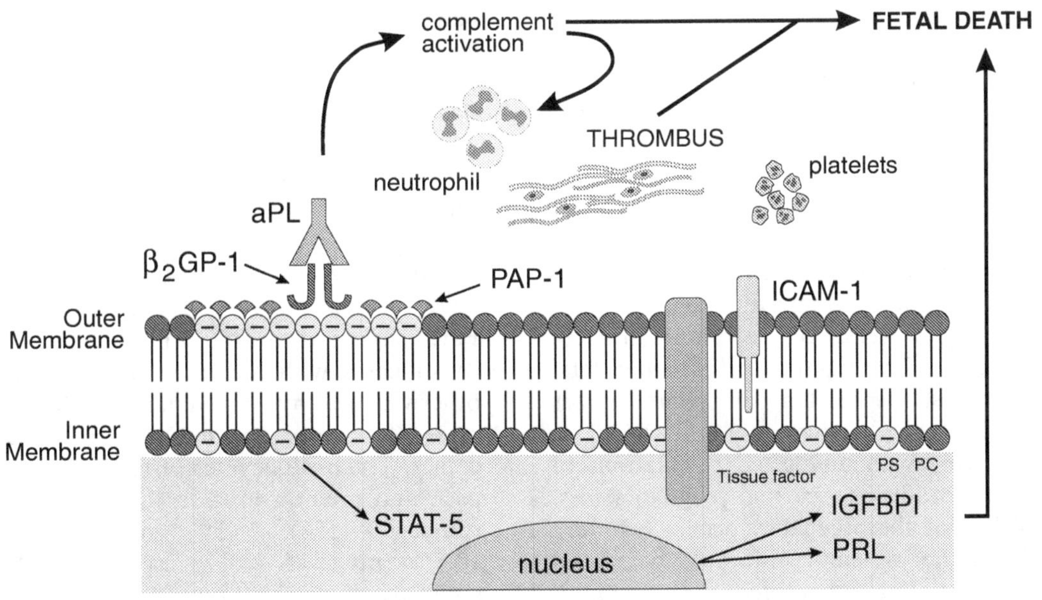

Figure 1. Proposed mechanisms of placental insufficiency leading to fetal death in antiphospholipid syndrome. (A) β_2GPI then binds to syncytial, externalized phosphatidylserine, and, in turn, aPL binds to a β_2GPI dimers. Complement activation initiates a signaling cascade that attracts neutrophils and induces cell surface tissue factor expression and adhesion molecules, causing platelets to aggregate and initiate thrombosis. (B) aPL competes at the surface of the placenta for phosphatidylserine with the natural anticoagulant placental anticoagulant protein I (annexin V), leading to disruption of the protective 'anticoagulant' shield. (C) aPL operate through the signaling cascades to inhibit production of placental prolactin, insulin growth factor β-1, and signal transducer and activator of transcription 5 (Stat5). See text for a more detailed explanation.

adherence of leukocytes to endothelium (Simantov et al., 1996). In experimental animal models, aPL causes fetal resorption (Branch et al., 1990; Holers et al., 2002) and increases size and duration of trauma-induced venous and arterial thrombi (Pierangeli et al., 1995; Jankowski et al., 2002). Inhibiting complement activation by a variety of mechanisms prevents experimental aPL-induced fetal death (Holers et al., 2002); C5 knock-out mice carry pregnancies normally despite aPL (Girardi et al., 2003).

Independent coagulopathies [heritable deficiencies of protein C, protein S, or antithrombin; mutations of factor V (A506G, factor V_{Leiden}), prothrombin (G20210A), or methylene tetrahydrofolate reductase (MTHFR C677T, hyperhomocysteinemia)] may further increase thrombotic risk and pregnancy risk of patients with aPL.

4. Clinical manifestations

4.1. Pregnancy loss

When APS was first formally introduced to the literature, 'fetal loss' was proposed as the obstetric criterion (Harris, 1987). Indeed, obstetric histories detailed in some case series of women with antiphospholipid syndrome suggest that 40% or more of pregnancy losses reported by women with lupus anticoagulant or medium-to-high positive IgG anticardiolipin antibodies occurred in the fetal period. (10 menstrual weeks of gestation) (Branch, 1987), and some investigators believe that fetal death is the most specific type of pregnancy loss associated with APS (Oshiro et al., 1996). This contrasts sharply with unselected populations of women with sporadic or recurrent pregnancy loss, for whom loss of the pregnancy occurs far more commonly in the pre-embryonic (<6 menstrual weeks of gestation) or embryonic (6th through 9th menstrual weeks of gestation) periods. In addition to a high rate of fetal death, prospectively followed pregnancies in several large case series that included women with systemic lupus erythematosus, prior to thrombosis, and other medical conditions have demonstrated high rates of premature delivery for gestational hypertension-preeclampsia and utero-placental insufficiency as manifested by fetal growth restriction, oligohydramnios, and non-reassuring fetal surveillance (Lockshin et al., 1985; Branch et al., 1992; Lima et al., 1996). In such cases, pregnancy is often normal until the second trimester, when fetal growth slows and amniotic fluid volume decreases. APS patients may develop severe, early preeclampsia and HELLP (*h*emolysis, *e*levated *l*iver enzymes, *l*ow *p*latelets) syndrome. Placental infarction would appear to be a cause of fetal growth restriction or death, though non-thrombotic mechanisms of placental dysfunction also occur (Rand et al., 1997, Rand, 2002; Mak et al., 2002).

More recent work focusing on women with recurrent pre-embryonic and embryonic pregnancy loss and without significant past medical history has shown that 10–20% of these more typical cases of recurrent miscarriage have detectable antiphospholipid antibodies (Rai et al., 1995; Yetman and Kutteh, 1996; Stephenson, 1996; Spitzer et al., 2002). Given the incidence of recurrent early pregnancy loss, at approximately 1:100–1:200 women attempting to bear children, the greatest number of obstetric APS cases are likely to be diagnosed in this category. Compared to fetal death after 10 weeks' gestation, however, early pregnancy losses are more commonly due to chromosomal and other etiologies, a factor which may confuse the clinical picture. Most prospective treatment trials (Cowchock et al., 1992; Silver et al., 1993; Kutteh, 1996; Rai et al., 1997; Pattison et al., 2000; Farquharson et al., 2002) have included a majority of cases with recurrent early miscarriages in otherwise healthy women and found relatively low rates of adverse second or third trimester outcomes. The median rates of fetal death, preeclampsia, and preterm birth in these trials were 4.5% (range, 0–15%), 10.5% (range, 0–15%), and 10.5% (range, 5–40%), respectively. Among all six trials, comprising over 300 patients, only one woman suffered a thrombotic event, and there were no neonatal deaths due to complications of prematurity. It would appear, then, that women identified in the clinical setting of recurrent early pregnancy loss, particularly recurrent pre-embryonic and embryonic losses, without other important past medical history represent a different population from those identified because of thromboembolic disease, systemic lupus erythematosus, or adverse second or third trimester obstetric outcomes.

The relationship between antiphospholipid syndrome cases resulting in complications during the fetal period (fetal death or premature delivery due to obstetric complications) and those during the pre-embryonic and embryonic periods (identified by recurrent pregnancy loss) is seen as a continuum by some (Clark et al., 2001) and questioned by others (Branch and Khamashta, 2003; Branch, 2004). The former view would hold that the same underlying mechanism (e.g., aPL-mediated inflammation) can operate along the continuum of gestation to cause either predominantly first trimester or predominantly second and third trimester complications. Certainly, it is easy to envision a common mechanism for fetal death and preterm birth resulting from severe preeclampsia or placental insufficiency — defective utero-placental circulation and, in turn, diminished intervillous blood flow. But would the same mechanism also be responsible for recurrent pre-embryonic and embryonic losses and be associated with relatively low rates of second and third trimester complications? It is possible that widespread recognition of obstetric APS and treatment beginning early in pregnancy may decrease second and third trimester complications, making further study in this area difficult.

The 1999 preliminary criteria for APS (Wilson et al., 1999) recognized obstetric complications occurring in both the pre-embryonic–embryonic period and the fetal–neonatal periods, dividing them into three categories, one encompassing early pregnancy loss and the other two relating primarily to complications in second or third trimesters. Thus, the accepted obstetric clinical criteria are:

> One or more unexplained deaths of a morphologically normal fetus at or beyond the 10th week of gestation, or
>
> One or more premature births of a morphologically normal neonate at or before the 34th week of gestation, or
>
> Three or more unexplained consecutive spontaneous abortions before the 10th week of gestation.

The experts who authored the 1999 preliminary criteria strongly encouraged investigators to stratify groups of subjects according to the clinical and laboratory criteria.

4.2. Vascular occlusion and miscellaneous manifestations

The principal manifestations of APS are recurrent venous or arterial thromboses, pregnancy loss and morbidity, and catastrophic vascular occlusion. Many patients have livedo reticularis. Except for their severity, the youth of affected patients, and unusual anatomic locations (Budd-Chiari syndrome and sagittal sinus, and upper extremity thromboses), venous thromboses in APS do not clinically differ from thromboses attributable to other causes. Similarly, arterial thromboses differ from those not associated with aPL only because of their recurrent nature, unusual locations, and occurrence in young patients. Thrombosis of renal glomerular arterioles causes proteinuria without celluria or hypocomplementemia and may lead to renal failure (thrombotic microangiopathy) (Bhandari et al., 1998). Table 2 lists clinical and laboratory features that commonly occur in APS, but were not included in the 1999 International Criteria.

Valvular heart disease, a late manifestation, may necessitate valve replacement. Its pathogenesis in APS is unknown. Some patients develop non-focal neurologic symptoms such as lack of concentration, forgetfulness, and dizzy spells. Multiple small, hyper-intense lesions seen on magnetic resonance imaging (MRI), primarily in the periventricular white matter, do not correlate well with clinical symptoms.

4.3. Catastrophic vascular occlusion syndrome

The catastrophic vascular occlusion syndrome is a rare, abrupt, and life-threatening complication of

Table 2
Non-defining Clinical and Laboratory Features of the Antiphospholipid Antibody Syndrome. Components identified with an asterisk have been shown in formal studies to be statistically associated with the syndrome subsequent to publication of the criteria shown in Table 1

Type	Features
Clinical	Livedo reticularis*
	Thrombocytopenia (usually 50,000 to 100,000 platelets/mme)*
	Autoimmune hemolytic anemia
	Cardiac valve disease (late finding)*
	Multiple sclerosis-like syndrome and other myelopathy
	Nonfocal neurologic symptoms
	Chorea
	Catastrophic vascular occlusion syndrome*
	Pulmonary hypertension
	Uremia
Laboratory	IgA anticardiolipin antibody*
	Antibodies to phosphatidylserine, phosphatidylinositol, phosphatidylglycerol, phosphatidylethanolamine
	Antibody to β_2 glycoprotein I*
	Proteinuria
	False positive test for syphilis*
	Hyperintense lesions on brain MRI (T2 weighted)

APS. It consists of multiple thromboses of medium and small arteries occurring (despite apparently adequate anticoagulation) over a period of days, causing stroke, cardiac, hepatic, adrenal, renal, and intestinal infarction and peripheral gangrene (Asherson et al., 2002, 2003).

Acute adrenal failure may be the initial clinical event. Patients often have moderate thrombocytopenia, erythrocytes are less fragmented than in the hemolytic-uremic syndrome or thrombotic thrombocytopenic purpura, and fibrin split products are not strikingly elevated. Renal failure and pulmonary hemorrhage may occur. Tissue biopsies show non-inflammatory vascular occlusion (Asherson et al., 2001).

5. Diagnostic investigations

5.1. *Blood*

Patients with APS have persistent, moderate or high-titer anticardiolipin antibody (primarily IgG and IgM), lupus anticoagulant, or both. Antibodies to β_2GPI and prothrombin are commonly present. Because commercial laboratories vary in their consistency of measurement, tests should be repeated for verification. High antibody titer, IgG isotype, and IgG2 subclass impart poor prognoses (Sammaritano et al., 1997). Lupus anticoagulant is a more specific, but less sensitive predictor of thromboses than is anticardiolipin. Low titer, transient, or IgD and IgE antibody, and antibody to phosphatidylserine or phosphatidylethanolamine do not have a proven relationship to APS.

Antinuclear and anti-DNA antibodies occur in approximately 45% of patients clinically diagnosed as having PAPS (Lockshin et al., 2000); they do not mandate the additional diagnosis of systemic lupus erythematosus (SLE) if the patient has no clinical indicators of SLE. However, SLE should be sought in any patient with APS. Thrombocytopenia in APS is usually modest ($>50{,}000/mm^3$); proteinuria occurs in patients with thrombotic microangiopathy, which is diagnosable by renal biopsy. Hypocomplementemia, erythrocyte casts, and pyuria are not characteristic of thrombotic microangiopathy and imply lupus glomerulitis. Erythrocyte sedimentation rate, hemoglobin and leukocyte count are usually normal in patients with uncomplicated PAPS except during acute thrombosis. Prothrombin fragment 1 plus 2 and other markers of coagulation activation do not predict impending thrombosis.

5.2. Serologic tests

Initial diagnosis requires testing for anticardiolipin by ELISA and lupus anticoagulant with two sensitive phospholipid-dependent clotting assays; a positive screening test for lupus anticoagulant must be further investigated according to established criteria (see Table 1). Though lupus anticoagulant is interpreted as either present or absent, anticardiolipin must be abnormal in moderate to high titer. Positive results require a repeat test after several weeks to exclude transient, clinically unimportant antibody. Patients repeatedly negative in both tests who are still suspected of having APS should be tested for antibody to β_2GPI. Whether simultaneously to test persons with venous occlusive disease for protein C, protein S, and antithrombin deficiency or for the factor V Leiden or prothrombin mutations is a matter of economics and clinical likelihood; some genetic thrombophilias may cause fetal death (Paidas et al., 2004). Such testing is advisable when feasible.

Patients positive for aPL also should be tested for platelet count, antinuclear antibody, urinalysis, and erythrocyte sedimentation rate, with further evaluation for lupus if abnormalities are found. Patients tested as a part of pregnancy counseling also should be tested for anti-Ro/SSA and anti-La/SSB antibodies, because increased risk of neonatal lupus occurs in the same patient population.

5.3. Imaging studies

MRI studies show vascular occlusion and infarction consistent with clinical symptoms, without special characteristics, except that multiple otherwise unexplained cerebral infarctions in a young person suggest the syndrome. Multiple small hyper-intense white matter lesions are common and do not unequivocally imply brain infarction. Occlusions usually occur in vessels below the resolution limits of angiography; hence angiography or magnetic resonance angiography is not indicated unless clinical findings suggest medium or large vessel disease. Echocardiography or cardiac MRI may show severe Libman-Sacks endocarditis and intracardiac thrombi (Erel et al., 2002)

5.4. Biopsy

Skin, renal, and other tissue biopsies show non-inflammatory vascular occlusion. The finding of inflammatory necrotizing vasculitis suggests concomitant lupus or other connective tissue disease. There are no other diagnostic immunofluorescence or electron microscopic findings.

6. Differential diagnosis

6.1. Positive antiphospholipid antibody tests

Non-autoimmune causes for a positive aPL test are outlined in Table 3. High-titer β_2GPI-dependent aPL, repeatedly demonstrable over several months, in a patient with appropriate symptoms, confirms a diagnosis of APS. Infection-induced antibody is usually transient and is more commonly IgM than IgG (Levy et al., 1990). Transient and low-titer antibodies are inconclusive for diagnosis. In a patient who has lupus or lupus-like disease, livedo reticularis, or long-standing thrombocytopenia, and who has a strongly positive aPL test, it is usually unnecessary to exclude other diagnoses.

6.2. Pregnancy

Five to 21% of women with recurrent pregnancy losses, and 0.5–2% of normal pregnant women, have lupus anticoagulant or anticardiolipin antibodies in moderate to high titer. Heritable thrombophilias, such as deficiency of protein C, protein S, and antithrombin and presence of the factor V Leiden or the prothrombin mutation, may be other individually less common causes of fetal loss (Preston et al., 1996; Alfirevic et al.,

Table 3
Non-Autoimmune Causes for Positive Antiphospholipid Antibody Tests

Assay Type	Antibody Type	Causes
ELISA	β_2 –glycoprotein independent	Infection: syphilis, Lyme disease, leptospirosis, pinta, HIV
	β_2 –glycoprotein dependent	Advanced age
		Drugs
	Either	Lymphoproliferative disease
		Hyperimmunoglobulin M
Lupus anticoagulant	-	Infection; HIV, drugs

2002). The relationship between these inherited disorders and fetal loss is, however, a subject of current controversy (Rasmussen and Ravn, 2004). At least two prospective studies suggest that the mere presence of an inherited thrombophilia is not linked to fetal death (Vossen et al., 2004; Dizon-Townson et al., 2005). However, a randomized trial suggests that the presence of certain thrombophilias in women with a prior fetal death may be an indication for heparin treatment to improve pregnancy outcome (Gris et al., 2004).

Attribution of fetal death to APS is most certain when there is no coexisting, plausible alternative, when high-titer aPL is repeatedly positive before and after pregnancy, and when the placenta shows vasculopathy and infarction. Ideally, fetal deaths are evaluated with formal autopsy to search for anomalies, placental and fetal tissue culture for viral infection, fetal tissue culture for karyotype, and histologic examination of selected tissues to search for cytologic changes associated with specific causes of death. Maternal evaluations at the time of presentation with fetal death should include a test for possible fetal–maternal hemorrhage, and, in selected cases, assessment for diabetes. Women who have had a fetal death should have appropriate imaging studies for possible uterine abnormalities and laboratory tests for selected thrombophilias proven to be associated with fetal death and treatable using heparin [factor V Leiden, prothrombin A21210G mutation, and protein S deficiency, Gris et al., 2004)].

In addition to aPL, women presenting with recurrent early miscarriage (pre-embryonic or embryonic losses) should be evaluated for uterine anomalies and for parental karyotype abnormalities, both of which are widely accepted associations with recurrent miscarriage (ACOG, 2001). Less well-accepted evaluations include tests for thyroid abnormalities, luteal phase insufficiency, and cervical cultures for ureaplasma. Even in the absence of parental karyotype abnormalities, 25–60% abortuses in women with recurrent early miscarriage are chromosomally abnormal, usually with lethal triploidy or polyploidy (Stern et al., 1996; Sullivan et al., 2004). Thus, clinicians should employ appropriate caution before assigning a diagnosis of APS to a woman with recurrent early miscarriage.

7. Treatment

Anticoagulation is the treatment for APS. Warfarin, heparin, and low-molecular-weight heparin, often in association with low-dose aspirin, are all used. Anticoagulation is indicated for seropositive patients with thrombosis and at the diagnosis of pregnancy in a seropositive woman who has had prior pregnancy losses attributable to APS. A single strongly positive ELISA predicts an increased risk of thrombophlebitis or pulmonary embolus (Ginsburg et al., 1992), but the absolute risk is low. Thus, anticoagulation is not indicated for prophylactic treatment of asymptomatic seropositive persons. Because warfarin is teratogenic, only unfractionated or low-molecular-weight heparin is used for treatment of affected pregnancies in the United States; in other countries, converting to warfarin after the first trimester (prior to 6 weeks' gestation) is considered acceptable (Vilela et al., 2002; Branch and Khamashta, 2003).

Anticoagulation for thrombosis is initiated in a standard manner with heparin, followed by long-term maintenance with warfarin (Khamashta et al., 1995; Ruiz-Irastorza et al., 2002; Crowther et al., 2003). Some patients require larger than expected doses of both heparin and warfarin to achieve therapeutic anticoagulation. Although most physicians with special interest in this field now use low-molecular-weight heparin for pregnant patients and for patients unable or unwilling to take warfarin, no clinical trial has compared low-molecular-weight heparin to unfractionated heparin or warfarin. Many physicians add low-dose (81–325 mg/day) aspirin and/or hydroxychloroquine to heparin or warfarin; the justification for this practice rests primarily on retrospective data and association studies. Corticosteroids have no established role in the treatment of PAPS but are used for rheumatic symptoms in sAPS. However, high doses of corticosteroids are usually empirically given to patients with severe thrombocytopenia, hemolytic anemia, and the catastrophic syndrome.

In some patients, lupus anticoagulants cause the INR to be unreliable (Ortel and Moll, 1997). Such patients may be treated with warfarin monitored by special assays, or with unfractionated or low-molecular-weight heparin monitored by measurement of antifactor Xa activity or other appropriate assays. For well-anticoagulated patients who continue to have thromboses, aspirin, hydroxychloroquine, a statin drug, intravenous immunoglobulin, and plasmapheresis have theoretical bases for efficacy and have all been used. No published experience in APS patients exists for clopidogrel, pentoxifylline, Aggrenox, argatroban, hirudins, and other new anticoagulant agents. Clinical experience suggests that thrombolytic agents for acute thrombosis are unhelpful, because re-occlusion rapidly occurs.

Asymptomatic persons serendipitously found to have a weakly or *transiently positive* aPL test need no prophylactic therapy. For those with *moderate to high titer*, *persistent* aPL, education about the meaning of the abnormal test is appropriate, as is a discussion of warning signs to report. Pregnant women with low-titer antibody should be closely monitored and retested during pregnancy.

Some patients with positive aPL tests have clinical events of ambiguous meaning (dizzy or confusional episodes, non-specific visual disturbance, very early pregnancy loss). There is no consensus for the treatment of such persons. Because full anticoagulation carries high risk, many physicians prescribe low-dose (81 mg) aspirin daily and/or hydroxychloroquine. No published data support or refute this recommendation.

Normalization of the lupus anticoagulant or anticardiolipin antibody tests is *not* an indication to discontinue anticoagulation, because patients remain at risk for new thrombosis regardless of the change in titer.

7.1. Pregnancy

The ideal treatment for APS during pregnancy would: (1) improve maternal and fetal-neonatal outcome by preventing pregnancy loss, preeclampsia, placental insufficiency, and preterm birth, and (2) reduce or eliminate the maternal thrombotic risk of APS during pregnancy. Two recent reviews (Branch and Khamashta, 2003; Derksen et al., 2004) have emphasized that case series and treatment trials each tend to include a majority of individuals whose APS diagnosis falls into one of the two groups:

1. *Those with recurrent early pregnancy loss or (at least) one fetal loss in absence of SLE or a thrombotic history*. In terms of pregnancy outcome, these women appear to respond favorably to fairly low doses of heparin and have relatively few obstetric complications, such as preeclampsia and fetal growth restriction, and are apparently at lower risk for thrombosis.
2. *Those with high frequencies of fetal loss, SLE, a thrombotic history, or combinations of these.* Women in this subcategory of APS patients are at relatively higher risk for obstetric complications, recurrent fetal death, and maternal thrombosis.

The need for treatment, as well as the nature of that treatment, in women who fall into the first of these two groups is currently a subject of debate among experts (Branch and Khamashta, 2003). For now, however, clinicians are advised to strongly consider treatment with heparin for either group during pregnancy when APS is diagnosed with reasonable certainty.

The foregoing discussion notwithstanding, it is perhaps more pragmatic to discuss the specifics of pregnancy treatment in terms of whether or not the patient has suffered a previous thrombotic event. Management of women who have previously failed heparin treatment ('refractory cases') or who have a positive aPL test in the absence of clinical criteria for APS will also be discussed below.

7.1.1. APS with previous thrombosis

Most experts recommend full heparin anticoagulation for women with APS who have had a thrombotic event (ACOG, 2000a; Bates et al., 2004). Thus, any question about the dose of heparin required for obstetric outcome is essentially moot. Some commonly used full anticoagulation heparin regimens are shown in Table 4. Patients in most published series received low-dose aspirin as well as heparin, but the benefit of adding aspirin is unknown.

Non-pregnant women with APS and previous thrombosis are commonly treated long term with warfarin. This agent is a known teratogen and should be discontinued either prior to conception or by the 5th week of gestation (menstrual). Women with particularly egregious thrombotic histories, such as those with recurrent thrombotic events or cerebral thrombotic events and those who have had a recurrent thrombosis while on heparin, are viewed as being at very high risk for thrombosis during pregnancy. In selected such cases, some experts recommend the judicious use of warfarin anticoagulation, rather than heparin, during pregnancy (Branch and Khamashta, 2003).

Clopidogrel and newer antithrombotic agents are not cleared for use in pregnancy, but, together with intravenous immunoglobulin and hydroxychloroquine, may be considered in patients unable to use heparin. These approaches should be undertaken in consultation with a maternal–fetal medicine specialist.

The peripartum management of anticoagulation therapy rarely poses a significant problem, although concerns abound. There are three acceptable approaches, and the choice of one in particular will be influenced primarily by the degree of concern in a given individual, rather than scientific proof that one approach is superior to another. For most individuals, subcutaneous unfractionated heparin treatment may be discontinued with the onset of uterine contractions or 6–12 h prior to induction of labor or Cesarean section. A second approach, generally reserved for higher risk individuals, is to continue subcutaneous unfractionated heparin injections through labor at a low dose (e.g., 5000 IU every 12 h). A third approach, especially applicable to women with a recent thrombosis or those at very high risk, is to use intravenous unfractionated heparin treatment at a dose adjusted to maintain the aPTT 1.5 times the control mean, turning the infusion off as delivery becomes imminent.

Excessive bleeding with vaginal delivery is unusual, especially when heparin levels are less than 0.4 IU/mL. Unfractionated heparin treatment should be restarted 4–6 h following delivery when the individual is clinically stable. As with LMWH (see below), it is prudent to re-start unfractionated heparin no sooner than 2 h after epidural catheter removal.

The safety of LMWH with the use of regional anesthesia has generated considerable concern, largely from case series and case reports suggesting an increased risk for spinal or epidural-related hematomas (Yin et al., 1999; Hynson et al., 1996). Both the American Society of Regional Anesthesia and Pain Medicine and the American College of Obstetrics and Gynecology have made formal recommendations regarding neuraxial anesthesia and LMWH (ACOG, 2000a; Horlocker et al., 2003). Patients on preoperative LMWH thromboprophylaxis (e.g., 40 mg of enoxaparin once daily) should have needle placement no sooner than 10–12 h after the LMWH dose. Patients receiving higher (treatment) doses of LMWH, such as enoxaparin 1 mg/kg every 12 h, enoxaparin 1.5 mg/kg daily, dalteparin 120 U/kg every 12 h, or dalteparin 200 U/kg daily, require delays of at least 24 h to assure normal hemostasis at the time of needle insertion. LMWH may be restarted 46 h following delivery when the individual is clinically stable, but no sooner than 2 h after epidural catheter removal.

Table 4
Subcutaneous Heparin Regimens Used in the Treatment of Antiphospholipid Syndrome During Pregnancy

Prophylactic Regimens		
	Recommended in women with no history of thrombotic events - diagnosis because of recurrent pre-embryonic and embryonic loss or prior fetal death or early delivery because of severe preeclampsia or severe placental insufficiency	
	Standard heparin:	(1) 7,500 – 10,000 U every 12 hours in the first trimester, 10,000 U every 12 hours in the second and third trimesters
	Low molecular weight heparin:	(1) Enoxaparin 40 mg once daily or dalteparin 5,000 U once daily, OR (2) Enoxaparin 30 mg every 12 hours or dalteparin 5,000 U every 12 hours
Anticoagulation Regimens		
	Recommended in women with a history of thrombotic events	
	Standard heparin:	(1) ⩾7,500 U every 8–12 hours adjusted to maintain the mid-interval heparin levels in *the therapeutic range
	Low molecular weight heparin:	(1) Weight-adjusted (e.g., enoxaparin 1 mg/kg every 12 hours or dalteparin 200 U/kg every 12 hours) (2) Intermediate dose (e.g., enoxaparin 40 mg once daily or dalteparin 5,000 U once daily until 16 weeks' gestation and every 12 hours from 16 weeks' gestation onwards)

* Heparin levels = anti-Factor Xa levels. Women without a lupus anticoagulant in whom the activated partial thromboplastin time is normal can be followed using the activated partial thromboplastin time.

Women with a history of previous thrombosis should be re-started on warfarin after delivery, overlapping with heparin for several days until the International Normalized Ratio (INR) reaches the desired range. Breast-feeding is permissible with both heparin and warfarin.

7.1.2. APS without a history of thrombotic events

Treatment during pregnancy in women with obstetric APS is aimed at improving maternal and fetal-neonatal outcome by preventing pregnancy loss, preeclampsia, placental insufficiency, and preterm birth, while minimizing or eliminating maternal thrombotic risk. Maternally-administered heparin is widely considered the treatment of choice, usually initiated in the early first trimester after ultrasonographic demonstration of a live embryo. Some physicians recommend initiation of heparin prior to conception; no clinical trial supports this recommendation. The dose of heparin required for safe and effective treatment is debated, however. Suggested regimens are shown in Table 4. Patients in most published series received low-dose aspirin as well as heparin, but here again, the benefit of adding aspirin is unknown.

Even in the absence of prior thrombosis, most experts recommend postpartum thromboprophylaxis in women with obstetric APS (Branch and Khamashta, 2003). Warfarin is preferred by most patients, and thromboprophylactic coverage should extend for 6–8 weeks after delivery. The need for postpartum anticoagulation in women with primary APS diagnosed solely on the basis of recurrent pre-embryonic and embryonic losses is uncertain.

7.1.3. APS pregnancy in 'refractory' cases

In spite of treatment with heparin, recurrent pregnancy losses occur in 20–30% of APS patients in most case series and trials. The best approach to such cases in subsequent pregnancies is unknown, though clinicians and patients understandably feel as if they should try an alternative therapy or add another drug to their regimen in a next pregnancy attempt. In the early 1990s, experts were often inclined to use glucocorticoids, often in substantial doses, though this approach is untested in clinical trials. By the mid-1990s, intravenous immune globulin, usually used in conjunction with heparin and low-dose aspirin, was touted as beneficial based in selected cases. Two randomized trials have found that immune globulin is no more efficacious than heparin (Branch et al., 2000; Triolo et al., 2003). However, as with a combination of glucocorticoids and heparin, a properly designed trial of intravenous immune globulin in refractory APS has never been done.

Hydroxychloroquine has been shown to diminish the thrombogenic properties of antiphospholipid antibodies in a murine thrombosis model (Edwards et al., 1997). Past concerns about ocular damage or defects in exposed embryos and fetuses has been allayed to some degree by recent reports (Levy et al., 2001). There are few case reports and no trials of APS patients being treated during pregnancy with hydroxychloroquine.

In the absence of an evidence-based recommendation for refractory APS, clinicians can only offer speculative opinion as to promising and acceptable treatment alternatives. In women whose treated pregnancy failure occurred on a prophylactic regimen, full anticoagulation in the next pregnancy would seem rational. If the treated pregnancy failed while on full anticoagulation, some experts would be inclined to add an immunomodulatory agent, such as glucocorticoids, immune globulin, or hydroxychloroquine, to the anticoagulation regimen.

7.1.4. No APS, but persistently positive aPL

Occasionally, a woman without a clinical history compatible with APS will be identified as having aPL. Examples include SLE patients without thrombosis or pregnancy morbidity, women with false-positive serological tests for syphilis, and control women in research studies of aPL. Two prospective studies indicate a slightly increased risk of pregnancy loss in general obstetric patients who test positive for aPL (Lockwood et al., 1989; Lynch et al., 1994; Yasuda et al., 1995), but many aPL positive women in these studies had normal pregnancy outcomes. No data support treatment of such individuals during pregnancy, though it is common for them to be offered low-dose aspirin. Also, a biologic false-positive test for syphilis, in the absence of aPL, does not predict pregnancy loss (Koskela et al., 1998). Clinical judgment will be required in cases wherein other factors suggest an increased thrombotic risk, e.g., marked obesity, prolonged bedrest, or severe proteinuria.

7.2. Special situations

Although drugs that induce lupus (hydralazine, phenytoin) may also induce aPL, if alternatives are not available they may be prescribed for patients with aPL. Drugs that promote thrombosis (estrogen and estrogen-containing oral contraceptives) are not currently deemed safe, even for asymptomatic women serendipitously known to bear high-titer antibody. This advice does not translate to a recommendation to test all normal women prior to prescription of such medications, but it does suggest special attention to and further evaluation of those with family histories or clinical suggestions of rheumatic disease, livedo reticularis, biologic false-positive tests for syphilis, or borderline thrombocytopenia. Experts believe that progestin-only contraceptives do not increase the risk of thrombosis (ACOG, 2000b), and thus may be an appropriate choice to prevent pregnancy in women with APS. There is no reliable information regarding the safety of 'morning after' contraception, or use of raloxifene, bromocriptine, or leuprolide in APS patients. A small retrospective review of women undergoing artificial reproductive technology ('IVF') procedures demonstrated no thrombotic events (Guballa et al., 2000).

7.3. Complications and prognosis

The complications of APS pregnancy are primarily related to the increased risks of maternal thrombosis, preeclampsia, placental insufficiency, and indicated preterm birth. However, as noted above, women presenting with recurrent preembryonic and embryonic losses and no history of SLE or thrombosis are at considerably lower risk of these complications than women who have SLE, prior thrombosis, or prior fetal death associated with preeclampsia and placental insufficiency. As an important counseling point, studies from the later 1980s and early 1990s suggest that women in the latter group face an approximately 5–10% risk of thrombosis during pregnancy or the postpartum period (Branch et al., 1992; Lima et al., 1996). Importantly, clinicians must be aware of the increased risk of thrombosis in the postpartum period and manage patients accordingly. Long-term outcomes of children born of APS pregnancies are not known, though small studies indicate the risks are primarily those related to premature birth (Pollard et al., 1992; Botet et al., 1997) or intrauterine growth restriction (Brewster et al., 1999).

The potential complications of heparin treatment during pregnancy include hemorrhage, osteoporosis with fracture, and heparin-induced thrombocytopenia. Fortunately, the reported rate of osteoporosis and associated fracture is low, though cases have occurred, even with low-molecular weight heparin (Lima et al., 1996). It is likely, though, that the risk is higher in women with underlying autoimmune disease who have required glucocorticosteroid treatment. Heparin-induced thrombocytopenia, which may be lethal, is also fortunately infrequent in pregnant women (Fausett et al., 2001).

Long-term risks for women with APS include thrombosis and stroke. In studies of women with APS, including studies of women without prior thrombosis, half developed thromboses during 3–10 years follow-up and 10% developed SLE (Silver et al., 1994; Shah et al., 1998; Erkan et al., 2001). The studied populations were highly selected referral populations that may have been biased toward severe disease, but follow-up studies of obstetric patients with autoantibodies show similar results (Clark et al., 2002). In many patients with long-standing APS, development of severe cardiac valvular necessitates valve replacement. Atherosclerosis also occurs, as does progressive multi-infarct dementia. Recent studies suggest that APS does not add to the risk of atherosclerosis imparted by SLE (Roman et al., 2003; Maksimowicz et al., 2002).

Key points

The diagnosis of antiphospholipid syndrome requires that a patient have both a clinical event (thrombosis or pregnancy complication) and a repeatedly positive aPL documented by a solid phase serum assay (anticardiolipin) or by an inhibitor of phospholipid-dependent clotting (lupus anticoagulant).

The obstetric criteria for the diagnosis of antiphospholipid syndrome include complications occurring in both the pre-embryonic-embryonic period and the fetal–neonatal periods:

- one or more unexplained deaths of a morphologically normal fetus at or beyond the 10th week of gestation,
- one or more premature births of a morphologically normal neonate at or before the 34th week of gestation, or
- three or more unexplained consecutive spontaneous abortions before the 10th week of gestation.

The exact mechanism(s) of adverse pregnancy outcomes associated with antiphospholipid antibodies is unknown, but current candidates include both thrombogenic and inflammatory events at the maternal–fetal interface.

Women diagnosed with antiphospholipid syndrome on the basis of obstetric criteria (but without thrombosis) should be treated with heparin (standard or low molecular weight) during pregnancy. Low dose or 'thromboprophylactic' doses are adequate.

Women diagnosed with antiphospholipid syndrome and who have had a previous thrombotic event should be anticoagulated with heparin (standard or low molecular weight) during pregnancy.

Continuation of anticoagulant treatment in the postpartum period is important to decrease the risk of maternal thrombosis.

References

Alfirevic, Z., Roberts, D., Martlew, V. 2002. How strong is the association between maternal thrombophilia and adverse pregnancy outcome? A systematic review. Eur. J. Obstet. Gynecol. Reprod. Biol. 101, 6–14.

American College of Obstetricians and Gynecologists (ACOG). 2000a. Thromboembolism in pregnancy. ACOG Practice Bulletin 19. ACOG, Washington, DC.

American College of Obstetricians and Gynecologists (ACOG). 2000b. The use of hormonal contraception in women with coexisting medical conditions. ACOG Practice Bulletin 18. ACOG, Washington, DC.

American College of Obstetricians and Gynecologists (ACOG). 2001. Management of Recurrent Early Pregnancy Loss. American College of Obstetrics Gynecologists Practice Bulletin 24. ACOG, Washington, DC.

Arbuckle, M.R., James, J.A., Kohlhase, K.F., Rubertone, M.V., Dennis, G.J., Harley, J.B. 2001. Development of anti-dsDNA autoantibodies prior to clinical diagnosis of systemic lupus erythematosus. Scand. J. Immunol. 54, 211.

Asherson, R.A., Cervera, R., de Groot, P.G., Erkan, D., Boffa, M.C., Piette, J.C., Khamashta, M.A., Shoenfeld, Y. 2003. Catastrophic Antiphospholipid Syndrome Registry Project Group. Catastrophic antiphospholipid syndrome: international consensus statement on classification criteria and treatment guidelines. Lupus 12, 530–534.

Asherson, R.A., Cervera, R., Piette, J.-C., Espinosa, G., Garcia-Carrasco, M., Ramos-Casals, M., Font, J. 2002. CAPS Registry: a review of 150 cases from the international registry of patients with catastrophic antiphospholipid syndrome (CAPS) [abstract]. Arthritis Rheum. 46, s218.

Asherson, R.A., Cervera, R., Piette, J.C., Shoenfeld, Y., Espinosa, G., Petri, M.A., Lim, E., Lau, T.C., Gurjal, A., Jedryka-Goral, A., Chwalinska-Sadowska, H., Dibner, R.J., Rojas-Rodriguez, J., Garcia-Carrasco, M., Grandone, J.T., Parke, A.L., Barbosa, P., Vasconcelos, C., Ramos-Casals, M., Font, J., Ingelmo, M. 2001. Catastrophic antiphospholipid syndrome: clues to the pathogenesis from a series of 80 patients. Medicine (Baltimore) 80, 355.

Bates, S.M., Greer, I.A., Hirsh, J., Ginsberg, J.S. 2004. Use of antithrombotic agents during pregnancy: the Seventh ACCP Conference on Antithrombotic and Thrombolytic Therapy. Chest 126 (Suppl.), 627S–644S.

Bhandari, S., Harnden, P., Brownjohn, A.M., Turney, J.H. 1998. Association of anticardiolipin antibodies with intraglomerular thrombi and renal dysfunction in lupus nephritis. QJM 91, 401.

Blank, M., Krause, I., Fridkin, M., Keller, N., Kopolovic, J., Goldberg, I., Tobar, A., Shoenfeld, Y. 2002. Bacterial induction of autoantibodies to beta2-glycoprotein-I accounts for the infectious etiology of antiphospholipid syndrome. J. Clin. Invest. 109, 797.

Bordron, A., Dueymes, M., Levy, Y., Jamin, C., Ziporen, L., Piette, J.C., Shoenfeld, Y., Youinou, P. 1998. Anti-endothelial cell antibody binding makes negatively charged phospholipids accessible to antiphospholipid antibodies. Arthritis Rheum. 41, 1738.

Botet, F., Romera, G., Montagut, P., Figueras, J., Carmona, F., Balasch, J. 1997. Neonatal outcome in women treated for the antiphospholipid syndrome during pregnancy. J. Perinat. Med. 25, 192–196.

Branch, D.W. 1987. Immunologic disease and fetal death. Clin. Obstet. Gynecol. 30, 295–311.

Branch, D.W. 2004. Antiphospholipid antibodies and fetal compromise. Thromb. Res. 114, 415–418.

Branch, D.W., Dudley, D.J., Mitchell, M.D., Creighton, K.A., Abbott, T.M., Hammond, E.H., Daynes, R.A. 1990. Immunoglobulin G fractions from patients with antiphospholipid antibodies cause fetal death in BALB/c misb: a model for autoimmune fetal loss. Am. J. Obstet. Gynecol. 163, 210–216.

Branch, D.W., Khamashta, M.A. 2003. Antiphospholipid syndrome: obstetric diagnosis, management, and controversies. Obstet. Gynecol. 101, 1333–1344.

Branch, D.W., Peaceman, A.M., Druzin, M., Silver, R.K., El-Sayed, Y., Silver, R.M., Esplin, M.S., Spinnato, J., Harger, J. 2000. A multicenter, placebo-controlled pilot study of intravenous immune globulin treatment of antiphospholipid syndrome during pregnancy. The Pregnancy Loss Study Group. Am. J. Obstet. Gynecol. 182, 122–127.

Branch, D.W., Silver, R.M., Blackwell, J.L., Reading, J.C., Scott, J.R. 1992. Outcome of treated pregnancies in women with antiphospholipid syndrome: an update of the Utah experience. Obstet. Gynecol. 80, 614–620.

Brewster, J.A., Shaw, N.J., Farquharson, R.G. 1999. Neonatal and pediatric outcome of infants born to mothers with antiphospholipid syndrome. J. Perinat. Med. 27, 183–187.

Clark, C.A., Spitzer, K.A., Goldberg, A.S., Laskin, A.S., Laskin, C.A. 2002. Long-term follow-up of women with autoantibodies and recurrent pregnancy loss (RPL) [abstract]. Arthritis Rheum. 46, s45.

Clark, C.A., Spitzer, K.A., Laskin, C.A. 2001. The spectrum of the antiphospholipid syndrome: a matter of perspective. J. Rheumatol. 28, 1939–1941.

Cowchock, F.S., Reece, E.A., Balaban, D., Branch, D.W., Plouffe, L. 1992. Repeated fetal losses associated with antiphospholipid antibodies: a collaborative randomized trial comparing prednisone with low-dose heparin treatment. Am. J. Obstet. Gynecol. 166, 1318–1323.

Crowther, M.A., Ginsberg, J.S., Julian, J., Denburg, J., Hirsh, J., Douketis, J., Laskin, C., Fortin, P., Anderson, D., Kearon, C., Clarke, A., Geerts, W., Forgie, M., Green, D., Costantini, L., Yacura, W., Wilson, S., Gent, M., Kovacs, M.J. 2003. A comparison of two intensities of warfarin for the prevention of recurrent thrombosis in patients with the antiphospholipid antibody syndrome. N. Engl. J. Med. 349, 1133–1138.

Day, H.M., Thiagarajan, P., Ahn, C., Reveille, J.D., Tinker, K.F., Arnett, F.C. 1998. Autoantibodies to β2-glycoprotein I in systemic lupus erythematosus and primary antiphospholipid syndrome—clinical correlations in comparison with other antiphospholipid antibody tests. J. Rheumatol. 25, 667.

Derksen, R.H., Khamashta, M.A., Branch, D.W. 2004. Management of the obstetric antiphospholipid syndrome. Arthritis Rheum. 50, 1028–1039.

Dizon-Townson, D., Miller, C., Sibai, B., Spong, C.Y., Thom, E., Wendel, G., Jr., Wenstrom, K., Samuels, P., Cotroneo, M.A., Moawad, A., Sorokin, Y., Meis, P., Miodovnik, M., O'sullivan, M.J., Conway, D., Wapner, R.J., Gabbe, S.G. 2005. The relationship of the factor V Leiden mutation and pregnancy outcomes for mother and fetus. Obstet. Gynecol. 106 (3), 517–524.

Edwards, M.H., Pierangeli, S., Liu, X., Barker, J.H., Anderson, G., Harris, E.N. 1997. Hydroxychloroquine reverses thrombogenic properties of antiphospholipid antibodies in mice. Circulation 96, 4380–4384.

Erel, H., Erkan, D., Lehman, T.J., Prince, M.R. 2002. Diagnostic usefulness of 3 dimensional gadolinium enhanced magnetic resonance venography in antiphospholipid syndrome. J. Rheumatol. 29, 1338.

Erkan, D., Merrill, J.T., Yazici, Y., Sammaritano, L., Buyon, J.P., Lockshin, M.D. 2001. High thrombosis rate after fetal loss in antiphospholipid syndrome: effective prophylaxis with aspirin. Arthritis Rheum. 44, 1466–1467.

Farquharson, R.G., Quency, S., Greaves, M. 2002. Antiphospholipid syndrome in pregnancy: a randomized, controlled trial of treatment. Obstet. Gynecol. 100, 408–413.

Fausett, M.B., Vogtlander, M., Lee, R.M., Esplin, M.S., Branch, D.W., Rodgers, G.M., Silver, R.M. 2001. Heparin-induced thrombocytopenia is rare in pregnancy. Am. J. Obstet. Gynecol. 185, 148–152.

Gharavi, A.E., Pierangeli, S.S., Harris, E.N. 2001. Origin of antiphospholipid antibodies. Rheum. Dis. Clin. North Am. 27, 551.

Gharavi, A.E., Sammaritano, L.R., Wen, J., Elkon, K.B. 1992. Induction of antiphospholipid antibodies by immunization with beta 2 glycoprotein I (apolipoprotein H). J. Clin. Invest. 90, 1105.

Ginsburg, K.S., Liang, M.H., Newcomer, L., Goldhaber, S.Z., Schur, P.H., Hennekens, C.H., Stampfer, M.J. 1992. Anticardiolipin antibodies and the risk for ischemic stroke and venous thrombosis. Ann. Intern. Med. 117, 997.

Girardi, G., Berman, J., Redecha, P., Spruce, L., Thurman, J.M., Kraus, D., Hollmann, T.J., Casali, P., Caroll, M.C., Wetsel, R.A., Lambris, J.D., Holers, V.M., Salmon, J.E. 2003. Complement C5a receptors and neutrophils mediate fetal injury in the antiphospholipid syndrome. J. Clin. Invest. 112, 1644–1654.

Gris, J.C., Mercier, E., Quere, I., Lavigne-Lissalde, G., Cochery-Nouvellon, E., Hoffet, M., Ripart-Neveu, S., Tailland, M.L., Dauzat, M., Mares, P. 2004. Low-molecular-weight heparin versus low-dose aspirin in women with one fetal loss and a constitutional thrombophilic disorder. Blood 103, 3695–3699.

Guballa, N., Sammaritano, L., Schwartzman, S., Buyon, J., Lockshin, M.D. 2000. Ovulation induction and in vitro fertilization in systemic lupus erythematosus and antiphospholipid syndrome. Arthritis Rheum. 43, 550.

Harris, E.N. 1987. Syndrome of the black swan. Br. J. Rheumatol. 26, 324–326.

Holers, V.M., Girardi, G., Mo, L., Guthridge, J.M., Molina, H., Pierangeli, S.S., Espinola, R., Xiaowei, L.E., Mao, D., Vialpando, C.G., Salmon, J.E. 2002. Complement C3 activation is required for antiphospholipid antibody-induced fetal loss. J. Exp. Med. 195, 211–220.

Horbach, D.A., van Oort, E., Derksen, R.H., de Groot, P.G. 1998. The contribution of anti-prothrombin-antibodies to lupus anticoagulant activity—discrimination between functional and non-functional anti-prothrombin antibodies. Thromb. Haemost. 79, 790–795.

Horlocker, T.T., Wedel, D.J., Benzon, H., Brown, D.L., Enneking, K.F., Heit, J.A., Mulroy, M.F., Rosenquist, R.W., Rowlingson, J., Tryba, M., Yuan, C.S. 2003. American Society of Regional Anesthesia and Pain Medicine. Regional anesthesia in the anticoagulated patient: defining the risks (the second ASRA consensus conference on neuraxial anesthesia and anticoagulation). Region. Anesth. Pain Med. 28, 172–197.

Hynson, J.M., Katz, J.A., Bueff, H.U. 1996. Epidural hematoma associated with enoxaparin. Anesth. Analg. 82, 1072–1075.

Jankowski, M., Vreys, I., Wittevrongel, C., Boon, D., Vermylen, J., Hoylaerts, M.F., Arnout, J. 2002. Thrombogenicity of β2-glycoprotein I-dependent antiphospholipid antibodies in a photochemically-induced thrombosis model in the hamster. Blood 2003; 101: 157–162. Epub 2002 Sep 5.

Khamashta, M.A., Cuadrado, M.J., Mujic, F., Taub, N.A., Hunt, B.J., Hughes, G.R.V. 1995. The management of thrombosis in the antiphospholipid–antibody syndrome. N. Eng. J. Med. 332, 993–997.

Koskela, P., Vaarala, O., Makitalo, R., Palosuo, T., Aho, K. 1998. Significance of false positive syphilis reactions and anticardiolipin antibodies in a nationwide series of pregnant women. J. Rheumatol. 15, 70.

Kutteh, W.H. 1996. Antiphospholipid antibody-associated recurrent pregnancy loss: treatment with heparin and low-dose aspirin is superior to low-dose aspirin alone. Am. J. Obstet. Gynecol. 174, 1584–1589.

Levine, S.R., Brey, R.L., Sawaya, K.L., Salowich-Palm, L., Kokkinos, J., Kostrzema, B., Perry, M., Havstad, S., Carey, J. 1995. Recurrent stroke and thrombo-occlusive events in the antiphospholipid syndrome. Ann. Neurol. 38, 119.

Levy, R.A., Gharavi, A.E., Sammaritano, L.R., Habina, L., Qamar, T., Lockshin, M.D. 1990. Characteristics of IgG antiphospholipid antibodies in patients with systemic lupus erythematosus and syphilis. J. Rheum. 17, 1036.

Levy, R.A., Vilela, V.S., Cataldo, M.J., Ramos, R.C., Duarte, J.L., Tura, B.R., Albuquerque, E.M., Jesus, N.R. 2001. Hydroxychloroquine (HCQ) in lupus pregnancy: double-blind and placebo-controlled study. Lupus 10, 401–404.

Lima, F., Khamashta, M.A., Buchanan, N.M., Kerslake, S., Hunt, B.J., Hughes, G.R. 1996. A study of sixty pregnancies in patients with the antiphospholipid syndrome. Clin. Exp. Rheumatol. 14, 131–136.

Lockshin, M.D., Druzin, M.L., Goei, S., Qamar, T., Magid, M.S., Jovanovic, L., Ferenc, M. 1985. Antibody to cardiolipin as a predictor of fetal distress or death in pregnant patients with systemic lupus erythematosus. N. Engl. J. Med. 313, 152–156.

Lockshin, M.D., Sammaritano, L.R., Schwartzman, S. 2000. Brief report: validation of the Sapporo Criteria for antiphospholipid antibody syndrome. Arthritis Rheum. 43, 440.

Lockwood, C.J., Romero, R., Feinberg, R.F., Clyne, L.P., Coster, B., Hobbins, J.C. 1989. The prevalence and biologic significance of lupus anticoagulant and anticardiolipin antibodies in a general obstetric population. Am. J. Obstet. Gynecol. 161 (2), 369–373.

Lutters, B.C., Derksen, R.H., Tekelenburg, W.L., Lenting, P.J., Arnout, J., de Groot, P.G. 2003. Dimers of beta 2-glycoprotein I increase platelet deposition to collagen via interaction with phospholipids and the apolipoprotein E receptor 2′. J. Biol. Chem. 278 (36), 33831–33838. Epub 2003 June 13.

Lynch, A., Marlar, R., Murphy, J., Davila, G., Santos, M., Rutledge, J., Emlen, W. 1994. Antiphospholipid antibodies in predicting adverse pregnancy outcome. A prospective study. Ann. Intern. Med. 120, 470.

Mak, I.Y., Brosens, J.J., Christian, M., Hills, F.A., Chamley, L., Regan, L., White, J.O. 2002. Regulated expression of signal transducer and activator of transcription, Stat5, and its enhancement of PRL expression in human endometrial stromal cells in vitro. J. Clin. Endocrinol. Metab. 87, 2581.

Maksimowicz, K., Petri, M., Magder, L. 2002. Predictors of carotid atherosclerosis in systemic lupus erythematosus[abstract]. Arthritis Rheum. 46, s54.

Ortel, T.L., Moll, S. 1997. Monitoring warfarin therapy in patients with lupus anticoagulants. Ann. Intern. Med. 127, 177.

Oshiro, B.T., Silver, R.M., Scott, J.R., Yu, H., Branch, D.W. 1996. Antiphospholipid antibodies and fetal death. Obstet. Gynecol. 87, 489–493.

Paidas, M.J., Ku, D.H., Arkel, Y.S. 2004. Screening and management of inherited thrombophilias in the setting of adverse pregnancy outcome. Clin. Perinatol. 31 (4), 783–805. vii.

Pattison, N.S., Chamley, L.W., Birdsall, M., Zanderigo, A.M., Liddell, H.S., McDougall, J. 2000. Does aspirin have a role in improving pregnancy outcome for women with the antiphospholipid syndrome? A randomized controlled trial. Am. J. Obstet. Gynecol. 183, 1008–1012.

Pierangeli, S.S., Liu, X.W., Barker, J.H., Anderson, G., Harris, E.N. 1995. Induction of thrombosis in a mouse model by IgG, IgM, and IgA immunoglobulins from patients with the antiphospholipid syndrome. Thromb. Haemost. 74, 1361.

Pierangeli, S.S., Vega-Ostertag, M., Harris, E.N. 2004. Intracellular signaling triggered by antiphospholipid antibodies in platelets and endothelial cells: a pathway to targeted therapies. Thromb. Res. 114, 467–476.

Pollard, J.K., Scott, J.R., Branch, D.W. 1992. Outcome of children born to women treated during pregnancy for the antiphospholipid syndrome. Obstet. Gynecol. 80, 365–368.

Preston, F.E., Rosendaal, F.R., Walker, I.D., Briet, E., Berntorp, E., Conard, J., Fontcuberta, J., Makris, M., Mariani, G., Noteboom, W., Pabinger, I., Legnani, C., Scharrer, I., Schulman, S., van der Meer, F.J. 1996. Increased fetal loss in women with heritable thrombophilia. Lancet 348, 913–916.

Rai, R., Cohen, H., Dave, M., Regan, L. 1997. Randomised controlled trial of aspirin and aspirin plus heparin in pregnant women with recurrent miscarriage associated with phospholipid antibodies. Br. Med. J. 314, 253–257.

Rai, R.S., Regan, L., Clifford, K., Pickering, W., Dave, M., Mackie, I., McNally, T., Cohen, H. 1995. Antiphospholipid antibodies and beta 2-glycoprotein-I in 500 women with recurrent miscarriage: results of a comprehensive screening approach. Hum. Reprod. 10, 2001–2005.

Rand, J.H. 2002. Molecular pathogenesis of the antiphospholipid syndrome. Circ. Res. 90, 29.

Rand, J.H., Wu, S., Andree, H.A.M., Lockwood, C.J., Guller, S., Scher, J., Harpel, P.C. 1997. Pregnancy loss in the antiphospholipid antibody syndrome — a possible thrombogenic mechanism. N. Engl. J. Med. 337, 154–160.

Rasmussen, A., Ravn, P. 2004. High frequency of congenital thrombophilia in women with pathological pregnancies?. Acta Obstet. Gynecol. Scand. 83, 808–817.

Roman, M.J., Shankar, B.A., Davis, A., Lockshin, M.D., Sammaritano, L., Simantov, R., Crow, M.K., Schwartz, J.E., Paget, S.A., Devereux, R.B., Salmon, J.E. 2003. Prevalence and correlates of accelerated atherosclerosis in systemic lupus erythematosus. N. Engl. J. Med. 349 (25), 2399–2406.

Ruiz-Irastorza, G., Khamashta, M.A., Hunt, B.J., Escudero, A., Cuadrado, M.J., Hughes, G.R. 2002. Bleeding and recurrent thrombosis in definite antiphospholipid syndrome: analysis of a series of 66 patients treated with oral anticoagulation to a target international normalized ratio of 3.5. Arch. Intern. Med. 162, 1164.

Sammaritano, L.R., Gharavi, A.E., Soberano, C., Levy, R.A., Lockshin, M.D. 1992. Phospholipid binding of antiphospholipid antibodies and placental anticoagulant protein. J. Clin. Immunol. 12, 27.

Sammaritano, L.R., Ng, S., Sobel, R., Lo, S.K., Simantov, R., Furie, R., Kaell, A., Silverstein, R., Salmon, J.E. 1997. Anticardiolipin IgG subclasses. Association of IgG2 with arterial and/or venous thrombosis. Arthritis Rheum. 40, 1998.

Shah, N.M., Khamashta, M.A., Atsumi, T., Hughes, G.R. 1998. Outcome of patients with anticardiolipin antibodies: a 10 year follow-up of 52 patients. Lupus 7, 3.

Silver, R.K., MacGregor, S.N., Sholl, J.S., Hobart, J.M., Neerhof, M.G., Ragin, A. 1993. Comparative trial of prednisone plus aspirin versus aspirin alone in the treatment of anticardiolipin antibody-positive obstetric patients. Am. J. Obstet. Gynecol. 169, 1411–1417.

Silver, R.M., Draper, M.L., Scott, J.R., Lyon, J.L., Reading, J., Branch, D.W. 1994. Clinical consequences of antiphospholipid antibodies: an historic cohort study. Obstet. Gynecol. 83, 372.

Simantov, R., Lo, S.K., Salmon, J.E., Sammaritano, L.R., Silverstein, R.L. 1996. Factor V Leiden increases the risk of thrombosis in patients with antiphospholipid antibodies. Thromb. Res. 84, 361–365.

Spitzer, K.A., Clark, C.A., Laskin, A.S., Goldberg, A.S., Laskin, C.A. 2002. Prevalence of inherited thrombophilias in women with unexplained recurrent pregnancy loss [abstract]. Arthritis Rheum. 46, s231.

Stephenson, M.D. 1996. Frequency of factors associated with habitual abortion in 197 couples. Fertil. Steril. 66, 24.

Stern, J.J., Dorfmann, A.D., Gutierrez-Najar, A.J., Cerrillo, M., Coulam, C.B. 1996. Frequency of abnormal karyotypes among abortuses from women with and without a history of recurrent spontaneous abortion. Fertil. Steril. 65, 250–253.

Sullivan, A.E., Silver, R.M., LaCoursiere, D.Y., Porter, T.F., Branch, D.W. 2004. Recurrent fetal aneuploidy and recurrent miscarriage. Obstet. Gynecol. 104, 784–788.

The Antiphospholipid Antibody Stroke Study (APASS) Group. 1993. Anticardiolipin antibodies are an independent risk factor for first ischemic stroke. Neurology 43, 2069.

Triolo, G., Ferrante, A., Ciccia, F., Accardo-Palumbo, A., Perino, A., Castelli, A., Giarratano, A., Licata, G. 2003. Randomized study of subcutaneous low molecular weight heparin plus aspirin versus intravenous immunoglobulin in the treatment of recurrent fetal loss associated with antiphospholipid antibodies. Arthritis Rheum. 48, 728–731.

Vilela, V.S., de Jesus, N.R., Levy, R.A. 2002. Prevention of thrombosis during pregnancy. Isr. Med. Assoc. J. 4 (10), 794–797.

Vossen, C.Y., Preston, F.E., Conard, J., Fontcuberta, J., Makris, M., van der Meer, F.J., Pabinger, I., Palareti, G., Scharrer, I., Souto, J.C., Svensson, P., Walker, I.D., Rosendaal, F.R. 2004. Hereditary thrombophilia and fetal loss: a prospective follow-up study. J. Thromb. Haemost. 2, 592–596.

Wilson, W.A., Gharavi, A.E., Koike, T., Lockshin, M.D., Branch, D.W., Piette, J-C., Brey, R., Derksen, R., Harris, E.N., Hughes, G.R.V., Triplett, D.A., Khamashta, M.A. 1999. International consensus statement on preliminary classification criteria for definite antiphospholipid syndrome. Report of an international workshop. Arthritis Rheum. 42, 1309–1311.

Yasuda, M., Takakuwa, K., Tokunaga, A., Tanaka, K. 1995. Prospective studies of the association between anticardiolipin antibody and outcome of pregnancy. Obstet. Gynecol. 86, 555–559.

Yetman, D.L., Kutteh, W.H. 1996. Antiphospholipid antibody panels and recurrent pregnancy loss: prevalence of anticardiolipin antibodies compared with other antiphospholipid antibodies. Fertil. Steril. 66, 540–546.

Yin, B., Barratt, S.M., Power, I., Percy, J. 1999. Epidural haematoma after removal of an epidural catheter in a patient receiving high-dose enoxaparin. Br. J. Anaesth. 82, 288–290.

Handbook of Systemic Autoimmune Diseases, Volume 4
Reproductive and Hormonal Aspects of Systemic Autoimmune Diseases
Michael Lockshin and D. Ware Branch, editors

CHAPTER 7

Pregnancy in Rheumatoid Arthritis, Sjögren Syndrome and Other Rare Autoimmune Rheumatic Diseases

Andrea Doria[a,*], Luca Iaccarino[a], Anna Ghirardello[a], Chiara Briani[b], Sandra Zampieri[a], Angela Tincani[c], Pier Franca Gambari[a]

[a]*Division of Rheumatology, Department of Clinical and Experimental Sciences, University of Padova, Italy*
[b]*Department of Neurosciences, University of Padova, Italy*
[c]*Rheumatology Unit, General Hospital and University of Brescia, Italy*

1. Introduction

Autoimmune rheumatic diseases (ARD) affect young females in their childbearing age. Over the last decades, the improvement of survival rate as well as quality of life in patients affected with ARD have led to more pregnancies observed during these diseases.

Pregnancy is a condition in which profound immune and endocrine changes occur. The physiological increase of cortisol, progesterone, estradiol and testosterone during the 3rd trimester of pregnancy seems to lead to Th-2 cytokine polarization both at the systemic level and at the feto–maternal interface (Munoz-Valle et al., 2003).

It has been suggested that some autoimmune diseases, such as systemic lupus erythematosus (SLE), which are mediated mainly by Th-2 cytokines, tend to occur or relapse during pregnancy (Doria et al., 2002, 2004), whereas Th-1 mediated diseases, such as rheumatoid arthritis (RA), tend to improve. In either case a flare or onset of disease occur during post-partum, when the anti-inflammatory Th-2 cytokines collapse.

SLE is the most frequently observed ARD during pregnancy. However, pregnancy occurs in patients with RA, Sjögren Syndrome (SS) and undifferentiated connective tissue diseases (UCTD) and is instead rare in patients with rare ARD, namely systemic sclerosis (SSc), mixed connective tissue diseases (MCTD), polymyositis–dermatomyositis (PM–DM), systemic vasculitis including Wegener's granulomatosis (WG), Churg–Strauss syndrome (CSS), polyarteritis nodosa (PAN), microscopic polyangitis (MPA), Takayasu arteritis (TA) and Behçet disease (BD). The onset of most of these latter diseases occurs in patients after the age of 40 (Table 1).

This chapter focuses on the relationship between pregnancy and the above-mentioned ARD.

Guidelines for the management of these conditions during pregnancy are provided. Data on pregnancy outcome of some of these ARD are very limited.

2. Rheumatoid arthritis

Rheumatoid arthritis (RA) is an articular and systemic chronic inflammatory disease capable of damaging joints leading to severe anatomic and functional alterations.

2.1. Effect of the oral contraceptive and parity in the development of RA

Exogenous hormonal influences are implicated in disease risk. The risk factor most widely studied is

*Corresponding author.
Tel.: +39-49-8212190; fax: +39-49-8212191.
E-mail address: adoria@unipd.it (A. Doria).

DOI: 10.1016/S1571-5078(05)04007-9

Table 1
Epidemiology of pregnancy in rheumatoid arthritis, Sjögren syndrome and other rare autoimmune rheumatic diseases

Disease	Incidence (× 10.6)	F/M ratio	Peak onset (years)	Pregnancy occurrence
Rheumatoid arthritis	200–400	4/1	>40	Relatively common
S. Sjögren	Common	10/1	>40	Relatively commnon
Systemic sclerosis	10–20	3–9/1	>40	Rare
UCTD	Not known	9/1	<40	Relatively common
MCTD	30	7–8/1	>40	Rare
PM–DM	1–12	1.5–2/1	>40	Rare
Takayasu arteritis	2.6	8–9/1	<40	Rare
Wegener's granulomatosis	4	M>F	>40	Rare
Churg–Strauss syndrome	0.5–2.7	1	>40	Rare
Polyarteritis nodosa	4.6–9	0.5	>40	Rare
Microscopic polyangitis	2.7–8	0.8	>40	Rare
Behçet disease	Variable[a]	M>F	<40	Relatively common[a]

[a] The incidence changes depending on geographical areas: Turkey and Japan 1/1000 and North America/North Europe 1/500,000; pregnancy is common in Japan, Middle East and Mediterranean countries.

exposure to oral contraceptives following an observation made over 20 years ago (Anonymous, 1978). Since then, several studies suggested that women who take oral contraceptive are at reduced risk of developing RA (Brennan et al., 1997; Silman and Hichberg, 2001). Although this association has not been clearly explained, it seems to be independent of oral contraceptive formulations used between populations and over time (Silman, 2002). The explanatory hypotheses include a direct hormonal effect of the pill, delayed pregnancy, or delayed breast-feeding (Gordon, 2004).

The influence of pregnancy in the development of RA is still a matter of debate. In the past, nulliparity was considered to be a risk for developing RA (Silman and Hichberg, 2001); although, increased risk was not observed in single women (Silman, 1994). It has also been suggested that subfertility highlights a group at higher risk. More recent studies do not support this view and suggest that parity, particularly having more than three children, increases the risk of developing RA (Gordon, 2004).

2.2. *Effects of pregnancy on the disease*

Joint involvement tends to improve during pregnancy in patients with RA. The improvement generally starts during the 1st trimester and continues during the 2nd and 3rd trimesters.

The improvement of arthritis seems to be related to cytokine profiles during pregnancy, with increased Th-2 type and reduced Th-1 type responses. An alternative hypothesis, not mutually exclusive, is that peptides derived from class II major histocompatibility complex (MHC) antigens of the foetus might compete with maternal self-antigens and divert the immune response away from an autoimmune response. Finally, pregnancy may promote the development of regulatory T cell that suppress T cells responses associated with the disease. At present, there is evidence only for the first of these three hypotheses (Brennan et al., 2000; Østensen and Villiger, 2002).

Philip Hench (1938) first observed that 90% of patients with RA improved during pregnancy. Some decades later, a retrospective study including a total of 345 pregnancies indicated that arthritis improved in about 75% of patients with RA (Neely and Persellin, 1977) and prospective studies comprising 177 pregnancies found improvement or remission in about two-third of the cases (Østensen and Husby 1983; Unger et al., 1983; Nelson et al., 1993; Quinn et al., 1993).

Recently, Barrett et al. (1999) evaluated 140 pregnancies and observed that arthritis improves in 66% and goes into remission in 16% of the cases. In the same study, the authors reported a worsening of arthritis in 20% of cases during pregnancy.

Using validated clinical instruments to assess disease activity, Østensen et al. (2004) prospectively evaluated 10 pregnancies in RA patients and noted a complete disease remission in three cases (30%), improvement of joint inflammation in four (40%), worsening in three (30%), and no changes in one (10%).

Regarding the post-partum period, old studies showed that arthritis worsened in more than 80–90% of cases 3–4 months after delivery (Fiddler, 1997; Nelson and Østensen, 1997). More recently, Barrett et al. (1999) and Østensen et al. (2004) observed a relapse of arthritis after 1 month in 54% and 60% of cases, respectively. Moreover, Barrett et al. (1999) observed a relapse in 77% of cases after 6 months from delivery.

In addition it has been shown that the post-partum period, particularly after the first pregnancy, imparts a higher risk for disease development (Silman et al., 1992). A subsequent investigation showed that much of this increased risk might be due to exposure to breast-feeding (Brennan and Silman, 1994).

Barrett et al. (2000) studied three groups of patients with RA after delivery: 49 non-breast-feeders, 38 first-time breast-feeders, and 50 repeat breast-feeders. After adjustment for possible confounders, including treatment, first-time breast-feeders had the highest disease activity at 6 months post-partum, based on self-reported symptoms, joint counts and C-reactive protein levels. The authors concluded that breast-feeding for the first time has an adverse effect on 6-month post-partum outcome in women with RA, and underlined the importance of breast-feeding in influencing inflammatory processes. A possible explanation is that post-partum flare in RA patients could be related to proinflammatory effects of the increased prolactin level associated with breast-feeding, as in lupus patients (Gordon, 2004).

2.3. Effects of the disease on pregnancy

Obstetric complications, such as spontaneous abortion, premature birth or intrauterine growth restriction (IUGR) are not increased in RA patients compared to normal population (Fiddler, 1997). However, vaginal delivery can be difficult in patients with severe coxo-femoral joint damage or in those with coxo-femoral prosthesis. In the case of the subluxation of the atlanto-axial joint, particular attention has to be taken when the intubation of the patient is required; if necessary, naso-tracheal intubation is considered safer.

2.4. Disease treatment during pregnancy

Sulfasalazine, cyclosporine and hydroxychloroquine seem to be safe enough to take during pregnancy. Among the other disease modifying anti-rheumatic drugs (DMARDs) commonly used in the treatment of RA, methotrexate (MTX) is toxic for the foetus. The congenital anomalies observed in animals and human exposed to MTX in the 1st trimester most often involve the central nervous system, cranial ossification and the palate; however, other anomalies have also been reported.

MTX should be stopped 3–6 months before conception (Lloyd et al., 1999; Jansen and Genta, 2000). Adequate contraception is necessary in females using MTX in the fertile age range. Therapeutic abortion is suggested if pregnancy occurs in patients taking MTX, which is also an abortifacient.

Leflunomide induces skeletal and central nervous system malformations in rats and rabbits. A safety update of the manufacturer in 2003 reported 310 pregnancies exposed to this drug with known outcome in 164. Therapeutic abortion was performed in 43 cases, spontaneous abortion occurred in 36 cases and 85 pregnancies went to term. Congenital malformations occurred in seven children. Thus, leflunomide is contraindicated during pregnancy; women with childbearing potential should be started on the drug only under safe contraception. Due to its long half-life and protracted elimination from plasma, leflunomide must be withdrawn before a planned conception, and residual leflunomide should be eliminated using cholestyramine or active charcoal (Brent, 2001).

Data on TNF alpha antagonists are very limited. Animal studies reported no teratogenic or fetotoxic effects (Goroir et al., 1992); in addition, limited studies on human pregnancy in patients taking TNF alpha antagonists have not shown an increase in birth defects or adverse pregnancy outcomes (Antoni et al., 2001). Further studies are necessary to establish if these drugs are safe during pregnancy.

3. Sjögren syndrome

Sjögren syndrome (SS) is an autoimmune exocrinopathy, which mainly involves salivary and lacrimal glands. Its primary form (SSp) is characterized by sicca syndrome either with or without systemic involvement; its secondary form is associated with other ARD. Since the disease onset is after 40 years of age, pregnant SSp patients are infrequent.

3.1. Effects of pregnancy on the disease and vice versa

Only some data have been published on SS clinical course during pregnancy; the available data regard mainly foetal and neonatal complications.

Takaya et al. (1991) analyzed 117 pregnancies in 40 patients with SS, 13 of whom had SSp. The frequency of spontaneous abortion was similar in pregnancies of SS patients compared to the 129 pregnancies of healthy controls. Nevertheless, in patients with SS secondary to SLE, the frequency of spontaneous abortion and premature delivery was significantly higher when compared to SSp patients. Anti-Ro/SSA and anti-La/SSB autoantibodies were not associated with obstetric complications. Moreover, spontaneous abortion was more frequent in patients with secondary SS or in those with thrombocytopenia, anti-erythrocyte antibodies, prolongation of activated partial thromboplastin time (aPTT) or syphilis false positivity. The conclusion was that SS does not influence pregnancy outcome, except for patients with SS secondary to SLE or with serological and haematological abnormalities, such as antiphospholipid antibodies (aPL) or lupus anticoagulant (LAC).

In 1995, a Finnish group carried out a case–control retrospective study on foetal prognosis of pregnancies in SSp patients. In particular, the study aimed to evaluate the possible association between foetal loss and anti-cardiolipin (aCL), anti-Ro/SSA and anti-La/SSB autoantibodies (Julkunen et al., 1995). Fifty-five pregnancies in 21 SSp patients were included, along with 100 pregnancies in 42 SLE patients and 94 pregnancies in 42 healthy women. Of the 55 SSp pregnancies, 8 (15%) occurred after disease onset. The percentage of foetal loss was 20%, with a relative risk of 2.7 that went down to 2.0 after the exclusion of one patient with four spontaneous abortions. By comparison, the relative risk of foetal loss in the SLE pregnancies was 2.2. Foetal loss in SSp patients was not associated with high levels of aCL or with anti-Ro/SSA or anti-La/SSB antibodies. No significant differences were found in premature birth or IUGR in babies from SSp patients in comparison to healthy subjects. The birth weight of babies from SLE patients was significantly lower compared to that of healthy controls. The study concluded that the majority of the pregnancies in SSp patients occur before disease onset and that these patients have a higher risk of foetal loss, which is not associated with high serum levels of aCL, anti-Ro/SSA and anti-La/SSB antibodies.

Recently, we prospectively followed 16 pregnancies in 15 SSp patients with regular clinical and laboratory evaluation, including specific questionnaire and Schirmer and Saxon tests. We did not observe variations in glandular or extra-glandular manifestations during either gestation or post-partum.

3.2. Disease treatment during pregnancy

Administration of drugs during pregnancy in SSp patients is not necessary except for patients with systemic manifestations such as fever or arthralgia. In these cases, treatment with low-to-medium doses of corticosteroids can be of benefit.

4. Systemic sclerosis

Systemic sclerosis or scleroderma (SSc) is a systemic connective tissue disease characterized by a widespread fibrotic process, primarily involving skin and selected viscera.

4.1. Effects of parity in the development of SSc

Recently, Lambe et al. (2004) used the Swedish Multi-Generation register to study the association between childbearing and the risk of developing SSc. Pregnancy history was restricted to birth before the first scleroderma-related hospitalization for cases and the corresponding age for their matched controls. Nulliparity was found to be associated with an increased risk of SSc. The risk decreased with increasing number of births. The association between lower parity and increased risk of SSc could be due to subfecundity caused by SSc before disease become clinically evident, a possible common aetiology of both infertility and SSc, or a protective effect of pregnancy through an unknown mechanism.

4.2. Effects of pregnancy on the disease

The effect of pregnancy on SSc disease course is less known than that on RA, SSp or UCTD because it is not common to observe pregnancies in SSc patients due to the peak onset after the age of 40 and/or severe disease complications. The analysis of the first case reports published, summarized by Black and Stevens (1989) and Steen (1997), showed a frequent worsening of the disease during pregnancy and a high mortality rate (33.3%). More recent studies, both retrospective (Steen et al., 1989) and prospective (Steen, 1999), show that in a high percentage of cases (60–88%) the disease remains clinically stable; it rarely tends to get worse or improve, and does so with a similar frequency (5–20%).

As it concerns clinical manifestations, cutaneous involvement seems to remain stable during pregnancy and Raynaud's phenomenon tends to improve. Gastro-esophageal reflux tends to worsen, during pregnancy, in part because the tone of the inferior oesophageal sphincter is physiologically reduced (Steen, 1997). Mallory-Weiss tears have occurred in women with SSc with oesophageal disease who vomit in early or late pregnancy (Cho et al., 2003). This can be associated with life-threatening bleeding; recurrent vomiting in these patients may require prompt inpatient treatment.

The cardiopulmonary manifestations, when they lead to organ failure, are associated with a high risk of maternal complications during pregnancy (Steen, 1997), as in patients with the similar clinical manifestations due to other causes.

Renal crisis, with the acute-onset of severe hypertension, represents the most severe risk for both the mother and the foetus. Renal crisis can be difficult to differentiate from pre-eclampsia and HELLP (haemolysis, elevated liver enzymes, and low platelet count) syndrome. A daily increase in serum creatinine level and the lack of proteinuria in the early stage favour the diagnosis of renal crisis, whereas elevated liver function tests and proteinuria with oedema are more suggestive of pre-eclampsia and HELLP syndrome (Gordon, 2004).

As described in the early literature (Black and Stevens, 1989; Steen, 1997), renal crisis often led to maternal death. In more recent studies (Steen et al., 1989; Steen, 1999), the frequency of renal crisis was lower, similar to that observed in non-pregnant SSc patients. This manifestation occurs with higher frequency in SSc patients with diffuse form and recent onset of disease. A previous renal crisis is not a contraindication for a future pregnancy provided that the disease has been stable for several years prior to conception.

4.3. Effects of the disease on pregnancy

Only a few studies on obstetric complications during pregnancy in SSc patients are available. Preliminary studies showed an increased risk of foetal loss (Slate and Graham 1968; Silman and Black, 1988). A retrospective study of patients in which pregnancy occurred after disease onset (Steen et al., 1989) reported a foetal loss rate of 9% in SSc patients and 7.5% in healthy controls. The same study reported a higher risk of premature delivery and low birth weight in SSc patients compared to controls. Finally, a high frequency of neonatal death has also been observed (Black and Stevens, 1989; Steen, 1997).

More recently, a prospective study on 91 pregnancies in 59 SSc patients (Steen, 1999) demonstrated that frequency of spontaneous abortion is similar in SSc patients compared to controls. However, the frequency of spontaneous abortion was higher in patients with diffuse SSc (20%). Premature delivery was more common in SSc patients in comparison to controls (26% vs. 5%); this percentage rose to 28% only when patients with diffuse SSc were considered and to 65% in patients with diffuse SSc of recent onset. In this study, only one 25-week-old baby died immediately after birth. The risk of spontaneous abortion or premature birth seems to be more elevated in patients with diffuse SSc, especially of recent onset (Steen, 1999). Therefore, in counselling SSc patients it is important to consider disease duration and the extension of organ involvement. Patients with disease duration less than 4 years, with diffuse SSc and anti-topoisomerase antibodies have a higher risk of clinical disease worsening, including the occurrence of renal crisis, or obstetric complications in comparison to patients with long disease duration and anti-centromeric antibodies (Steen, 1998).

In the case of cardiomyopathy with ejection fraction <30%, restrictive respiratory insufficiency, vital capacity <50%, malabsorption or renal insufficiency, the opportunity to interrupt the pregnancy should be carefully evaluated, because of the elevated risk of maternal and foetal complications.

4.4. *Disease treatment during pregnancy*

The treatment of SSc consists of d-penicillamine (rarely used now), cyclosporine or other immunosuppressants alone or in combination.

For the treatment of the musculoskeletal manifestations non-steroidal anti-inflammatory drugs (NSAIDs) and/or paracetamol can be used. NSAID use should cease in the 3rd trimester because of risk of foetal pulmonary hypertension. It is better to avoid steroids because, some believe, they can induce a renal crisis.

The improvement of Raynaud's phenomenon often observed during pregnancy allows withdrawal of calcium channel blockers, if used. In order to control gastro-esophageal reflux, anti-H2 or proton pump drugs may be used cautiously when clinically necessary.

The treatment of renal crisis during pregnancy still remains a matter of debate. Angiotensin-converting enzyme (ACE)-inhibitors or receptor blockers (ARBs) are the only drugs effective in controlling hypertension and renal insufficiency, which leads to dialysis or death in untreated patients. Use of ACE-inhibitors during pregnancy is associated with IUGR, oligohydramnios, congenital malformations, renal failure and neonatal death (Rosa et al., 1989; Mehta and Modi, 1989). However, cases of SSc patients treated with ACE-inhibitors during pregnancy without complications have been described (Altieri and Cameron, 1988; Baethgep and Wolf, 1989).

5. Undifferentiated connective tissue diseases

Undifferentiated connective tissue diseases (UCTD) are paucisymptomatic conditions characterized by clinical manifestations suggestive of connective tissue diseases (CTDs), but in a number and/or combination insufficient to allow diagnosis of a definite CTD, i.e., SLE, SS, SSc or PM–DM. UCTD can indefinitely remain undifferentiated or evolve into a definite CTD after a variable period of time. The studies on UCTD published until now (Alarcon et al., 1991, 1996; Mosca et al., 1998; Williams et al., 1999; Danieli et al., 1999) have shown that UCTD evolve into 'definite' CTDs with a frequency ranging between 6% and 51%. This large variability is due to the different criteria for patient selection (Mosca et al., 1999), the most important being the time elapsed between the disease onset and the study entry. In fact, all the studies (Alarcon et al., 1996; Mosca et al., 1998; Williams et al., 1999; Danieli et al., 1999, Doria et al., 2005) showed that evolution is more common in the first 2–3 years after the onset of the symptoms; conversely, it is rare after 5 years.

The onset of UCTD usually occurs before the age of 40; it is therefore relatively common to observe pregnancies in patients affected with such diseases. In UCTD patients, it is important to consider the risks of foetal and maternal complications, including the possibility that UCTD may evolve into a definite CTD because of pregnancy.

5.1. The effects of pregnancy on the disease

5.1.1. Role of pregnancy in modifying the disease course

Mosca et al. (2002) retrospectively evaluated 25 pregnancies in 20 patients affected with UCTD, followed by a multidisciplinary team, consisting of a rheumatologist and an obstetrician–gynaecologist. The diagnosis was based on the following criteria: signs and symptoms of CTDs not fulfilling the existing classification criteria for a definite CTD, and presence of anti-nuclear antibody (ANA) determined on at last two different occasions (Mosca et al., 1999). The diagnosis was reassessed at every clinical observation during pregnancy.

The mean age of the patients was 30 years and the mean disease duration at the time of pregnancy onset was 7 years. In six patients (24%) a disease flare was observed during pregnancy or post-partum. One patient, who developed a severe flare with serositis and glomerulonephritis, was considered to have evolved into a clear SLE. In the other patients the manifestations during flares were mild: arthritis in four cases, fever in one case, skin rash in another one, all treated with low-dose methylprednisolone and hydroxychloroquine. Another patient developed an overt SLE 2 years after pregnancy.

5.1.2. Role of pregnancy in the evolution of UCTD into a definite CTD

Because of the low number of pregnancies considered in Mosca's study (Mosca et al., 2002), it was not possible to definitely establish the role of pregnancy as a factor triggering the evolution of UCTD into a definite CTD. However, since this possibility cannot be ruled out, it should be considered in the counselling of such patients before pregnancy. Since UCTD evolution mostly occurs in the first 3–5 years after disease onset, Mosca et al. (2002) suggested that patients with disease duration of less than 5 years have a higher risk of developing a definite CTD during or soon after pregnancy.

During the last 10 years, Doria et al. (unpublished observation) prospectively followed 20 pregnancies in patients with UCTD, and no cases relapsed or evolved into a definite CTD. All patients had disease duration longer than 3 years at the time of conception, which might explain the stability during pregnancy.

Taken all together, these data suggest that patients affected with UCTD generally have a good pregnancy outcome. However, due to the potential occurrence of a disease flare and/or an evolution into a definite CTD as well as obstetrical and neonatal complications, close clinical monitoring is always advisable.

5.2. Effects of the disease on pregnancy

In the study of Mosca et al. (2002), obstetrical complications occurred in 6 of the 22 pregnancies (27%) that ended in a live birth: one patient had transitory hypertension; four patients had a premature birth, in one case with a disseminated intravascular coagulation in the post-partum period, and one patient had an IUGR. Recently, it was suggested that anti-Ro/SSA-positive UCTD patients might have a slightly higher frequency of pregnancy loss than those anti-Ro/SSA-negative patients (Brucato et al., 2002). However, this hypothesis is still unproven.

In the study by Mosca et al. (2002) there were no neonatal complications; particularly, no cases of neonatal lupus in patients positive for anti-Ro/SSA and anti-La/SSB antibodies were observed. However, in a prospective study on congenital complete heart block (CCHB) in the offspring of anti-Ro/SSA-positive women affected with CTDs (Brucato et al., 2001), one out of two babies who developed CCHB was born to a mother with UCTD.

5.3. Disease treatment during pregnancy

For the treatment of patients with UCTD during pregnancy an approach similar to that adopted for patients with mild SLE (low-dose prednisone and/or hydroxychloroquine) should be considered.

6. Polymyositis—dermatomyositis

Polymyositis (PM) is an ARD characterized by inflammation of striated muscles. In dermatomyositis (DM) muscle inflammation is associated with characteristic skin manifestations. Since the two peaks of PM–DM onset are in childhood and over the age of 45 years, women in reproductive age group are uncommonly affected. Therefore, pregnancies in patients affected with PM–DM are rare.

6.1. The effects of pregnancy on the disease

The available data on pregnancy in PM-DM patients derive from the analysis of several case reports (Glickman, 1958; Massé, 1962; Tsai et al., 1973; Bauer et al., 1979; Katz, 1980; Barnes and Link, 1983; King and Chow, 1985; Emy et al., 1986; England et al., 1986; Houck et al., 1987; Ditzian-Kadanoff et al., 1988; Le Thi Huong et al., 1988; Rosenweig et al., 1989; Ishii et al., 1991; Ohno et al., 1992; Steiner et al., 1992; Suwa et al., 1992; Pinheiro et al., 1992; Satoh et al., 1994; Harris et al., 1995; Solomon and D'Alton, 1996; Papapetropoulos et al., 1998; Kofteridis et al., 1999; Kanoh et al., 1999; Messina et al., 2002; Juarez-Azpilcueta et al., 2003; Park et al., 2003; Silva et al., 2003) and one retrospective series (Gutierrez et al., 1984) which shows a rather high frequency of disease flare (40%) in pregnant patients with childhood onset of PM–DM, even if in long-term remission, and a low frequency (17%) in pregnant patients with adult onset of PM–DM, either inactive or active but controlled by prednisone therapy (Gutierrez et al., 1984; Mintz, 1989). Two cases of PM–DM-associated pregnancy resulting in maternal death have been reported (England et al., 1986; Rosenweig et al., 1989).

6.2. The effects of the disease on pregnancy

Pregnancy outcome in patients with PM–DM is summarized in Table 2; data are obtained from the case reports (Glickman, 1958; Massé, 1962; Tsai et al., 1973; Bauer et al., 1979; Katz, 1980; Barnes et al., 1983; King and Chow, 1985; Emy et al., 1986; England et al., 1986; Houck et al., 1987; Ditzian-Kadanoff et al., 1988; Le Thi Huong et al., 1988; Rosenweig et al., 1989; Ishii et al., 1991; Ohno et al., 1992; Steiner et al., 1992; Suwa et al., 1992; Pinheiro et al., 1992; Satoh et al., 1994; Harris et al., 1995; Solomon and D'Alton, 1996; Papapetropoulos et al., 1998; Kofteridis et al., 1999; Kanoh et al., 1999; Messina et al., 2002; Juarez-Azpilcueta et al., 2003; Park et al., 2003; Silva et al., 2003) and one retrospective series (Gutierrez et al., 1984). Foetal prognosis is influenced by the age of PM–DM onset, the timing of PM–DM onset in relation to the pregnancy, and the disease activity during pregnancy.

In patients with childhood onset the percentage of at-term births was approximately 70%, while in women with adult PM–DM onset before pregnancy this percentage decreased to 50% (Gutierrez et al., 1984).

When the disease was inactive during pregnancy the percentage of term births was 86%, and there was no increased rate of foetal loss. In patients with active disease the probability of delivering a live baby was 57% and the probability of foetal loss was 35%.

A few cases of PM–DM onset during pregnancy have been reported (Table 2). The majority of the cases diagnosed in the 1st trimester resulted in pregnancy loss or neonatal demise (Mintz, 1989; Kofteridis et al., 1999; Kanoh et al., 1999; Silva et al., 2003), whereas the majority of those diagnosed in the 2nd and 3rd trimester resulted in live infants,

Table 2
Pregnancy outcome in patients with PM–DM, data reported are from the analysis of case reports and one small retrospective series[a]

	Total	PM/DM[b]		Onset before pregnancy	Onset during pregnancy			Onset during post-partum
		Active	Inactive		Total	1st trim.	2nd 3rd trim.	
Number of pregnancies	56	28 (51%)	22 (39.3%)	32 (57.1%)	18 (33%)	6 (33%)	12 (66%)	6 (11%)
Live birth	40 (71.4%)	16 (57.1%)	19 (86.4%)	25 (80.6%)	10 (55.5%)	1 (16.6%)	9 (75%)	5 (83.3%)
Foetal loss	13 (28.5%)	10 (35.7%)	2 (9.1%)	6 (18.7%)	6 (33.3%)	3 (50%)	3 (25%)	1 (16.7%)
Stillbirth	4 (7.2%)	4 (14.3%)	—	2 (6.4%)	2 (11.1%)	2 (33%)		—
Abortion	7 (12.5%)	4 (14.3%)	2 (9.1%)	3 (10%)	3 (16.6%)	1 (16.6%)	3 (25%)	1 (16.7%)
Therapeutic abortion	2 (3.6%)	2 (7.1%)	—	1 (3.2%)	1 (5.5%)	—	1 (8.3%)	—
Neonatal death	3 (5.4%)	2 (7.1%)	1 (4.5%)	1 (3.2%)	2 (11.1%)	2 (33%)	—	—
IUGR	7 (12.5%)	3 (10.7%)	4 (18.2%)	6 (19.4%)	1 (5.5%)	—	1 (8.3%)	—
Pre-term delivery	9 (16.1%)	6 (21.4%)	3 (13.6%)	6 (19.4%)	3 (16.6%)	—	3 (25%)	—

[a] Glickman (1958); Massé (1962); Tsai et al. (1973); Bauer et al. (1979); Katz (1980); Barnes et al. (1983); King et al. (1985); Emy et al. (1986); England et al. (1986); Houck et al. (1987); Ditzian-Kadanoff et al. (1988); Le Thi Huong et al. (1988); Rosenweig et al. (1989); Ishii et al. (1991); Ohno et al. (1992); Steiner et al. (1992); Suwa et al. (1992); Pinheiro et al. (1992); Satoh et al. (1994); Harris et al. (1995); Solomon and D'Alton (1996); Papapetropoulos et al. (1998); Kofteridis et al. (1999); Kanoh et al. (1999); Messina et al. (2002); Juarez-Azpilcueta et al. (2003); Park et al. (2003); Silva et al. (2003); and one retrospective series (Gutierrez et al., 1984).

[b] Onset before and during pregnancy (50 pregnancies).

despite a high frequency of premature births (Mintz, 1989; Kofteridis et al., 1999; Kanoh et al., 1999; Silva et al., 2003). In patients who were diagnosed with PM–DM during pregnancy the percentage of living newborns was 55%.

High serum creatine kinase (CK) levels were reported in two babies born to mothers who were diagnosed with PM–DM during pregnancy (Messina et al., 2002). The CK levels of both, otherwise healthy, newborns remained elevated for a few months after birth. The authors hypothesized that an active factor capable of damaging skeletal muscle tissue may come from the mother across the placenta. However, the existence and the nature of this hypothetical maternal factor remains unknown.

6.3. *Disease treatment during pregnancy*

In the case of PM–DM flare during pregnancy, treatment has to be started as soon as possible, since foetal complications are more frequent in patients with active disease. Similarly, in the treatment used in non-pregnant women, prednisone should be started at the dosage of 1 mg/kg/day and maintained till the normalization of serum CK levels. If response to prednisone is insufficient, cyclosporine A or azathioprine can be added. Plasma-exchange or high-dose intravenous immunoglobulins (IVIG) are other therapeutic options acceptable during pregnancy. However, the efficacy of these two treatments in patients with PM–DM during pregnancy has not yet been demonstrated. Available evidence suggests that when PM–DM arises during pregnancy, the disease course is more severe and a more aggressive therapy is required.

7. Mixed connective tissue diseases

Mixed connective tissue disease (MCTD) is an ARD characterized by overlapping clinical features of CTDs including SLE, SSc and PM–DM, associated with anti-U1RNP antibody positivity, usually at high titre (Doria et al., 1992).

7.1. Effects of pregnancy on the disease and vice versa

Only a few old studies on pregnancy outcome in patients affected with MCTD are available and their results are contradictory (Table 3). The oldest studies (Bennett and O'Connell, 1980; Kaufman and Kitridou, 1982) showed a high rate of maternal and foetal complications. Ten years later, Lundberg and Hedfors (1991) retrospectively evaluated 40 pregnancies in 20 women with high-titre anti-U1RNP antibody; 18 pregnancies occurred after the disease onset. No cases of disease flares during pregnancy or post-partum were observed, and the authors concluded that the risk of foetal loss or damage, as well as of disease worsening was low in patients with high-titre anti-U1RNP antibody, even after MCTD onset.

7.2. Disease treatment during pregnancy

Since MCTD has a relatively good prognosis, no therapy changes are required during pregnancy, unless the patients are taking known teratogenic drugs which, of course, should be discontinued and replaced with safer ones. Disease flares, particularly with renal involvement, should instead be treated aggressively (Horita et al., 2001) with the same drugs and schemes as for patients with severe SLE.

8. Takayasu arteritis

Takayasu arteritis (TA) is a granulomatosus vasculitis which affects large vessels such as the aorta, its major branches and the pulmonary arteries. TA typically occurs in women during their childbearing age; therefore, it is more common to observe pregnancy in patients with TA than in those with other vasculitides (Table 1).

8.1. Effects of pregnancy on the disease and vice versa

Although the disease does not seem to relapse during pregnancy (Ishikawa and Matsuura, 1982; Wong et al., 1983; Matsumura et al., 1992; Sharma et al., 2000), maternal complications, particularly hypertension and pre-eclampsia, are commonly observed in TA patients (Table 4). Although less frequent, congestive heart failure and renal insufficiency have been reported (Sharma et al., 2000).

Spontaneous abortion was reported in 8–16% of cases (Ishikawa and Matsuura, 1982; Wong et al., 1983; Matsumura et al., 1992; Sharma et al., 2000) and intrauterine foetal death in 20% of cases studied by Sharma et al. (2000), but this complication was not observed in other studies (Ishikawa and Matsuura, 1982; Wong et al., 1983; Matsumura et al., 1992). IUGR and premature delivery were found in approximately 40% of cases (Ishikawa and Matsuura, 1982; Wong et al., 1983; Matsumura et al., 1992; Sharma et al., 2000) and occurred more frequently in infants born to patients with more severe disease.

Severe aortic valvular disease and aortic aneurysm are risk factors for severe maternal morbidity and fatality, therefore patients with these complications should be discouraged from pregnancy

Table 3
Pregnancy outcome in patients with MCTD: main retrospective studies

	Kaufman et al. (1982)	Lundberg et al. (1991)
Group of patients	MCTD	High-titre anti-U1RNP
No. of pregnancies	17	18
No. of patients	10	9
Foetal loss	13 (76%)	3 (16%)
Spontaneous abortion	6 (35%)	3 (16%)
Stillbirth	3 (18%)	0
Therapeutic abortion	4 (24%)	0
Pre-eclampsia	n.r.	2 (11%)
Disease flares	8 (47%)	0

Table 4
Effects of pregnancy on the course of systemic vasculitis and maternal/foetal complications

Disease	Status of the disease at conception: Disease worsening/flare — Active	Disease worsening/flare — Inactive	Maternal/foetal risk — Active	Maternal/foetal risk — Inactive
Takayasu arteritis	Rare	Rare	Frequent	Frequent
Wegener's granulomatosis	Frequent flares	Rare flares (25%)	Frequent	Rare
Churg–Strauss syndrome	Frequent flares	Frequent flares (50%)	Frequent	Frequent
Polyarteritis nodosa	Frequent flares	Rare flares	Frequent	Rare
Microscopic polyangitis	Frequent flares	Rare flares	Frequent	Rare
Behçet disease	Frequent improvement (50%), rare flares (25%)		Rare	Rare

The frequencies of maternal morbidity and fatality are higher in patients with disease onset during pregnancy.

and, if pregnancy unexpectedly occurs, therapeutic abortion should be considered.

8.2. *Disease treatment during pregnancy*

In the case of disease relapse during pregnancy, treatment consists of prednisone 1 mg/kg/day until disease control is obtained, thereafter prednisone can be tapered to the lowest effective dose. In refractory cases the use of azathioprine is recommended. Hypertension has to be managed very aggressively with α-methyldopa, calcium channel blockers or hydralazine. ACE-inhibitors are contraindicated because of their foetal toxicity. It may be difficult to judge core blood pressure, since radial pressure may not reflect renal, uterine or cerebral pressure.

9. Wegener's granulomatosis

Wegener's granulomatosis (WG) is an uncommon, small-vessel, necrotizing vasculitis that usually affects the upper respiratory tract, the lungs and the kidney. The disease peaks after the age of 40, thus pregnancies in women with WG are not commonly observed (Table 1).

9.1. *Effects of pregnancy on the disease and vice versa*

Few data on pregnancy in patients with WG are available and they are based on case reports: twenty-six pregnancies in 20 patients with WG have been described since 1970 (Cooper et al., 1970; Talbot et al., 1984; Milford and Bellini 1986; Harrison, 1989; M'Rad et al., 1989; Palit and Clague, 1990; Biesenbach et al., 1991; Fields et al., 1991; Pauzner et al., 1994; Lima et al., 1995; Parnham and Thatcher, 1996; Habib et al., 1996; Luisiri et al., 1997; Koldingsnes, 1998; Kumar et al., 1998; Dayoan et al., 1998; Harber et al., 1999; Auzary et al., 2000; Masterson et al., 2004). A review of these cases finds that patients with active disease at conception are at high risk of poor outcome because of foetal and maternal death.

The foetal prognosis is also poor in patients with onset of WG during pregnancy. Seven cases are reported; these resulted in three premature births, two therapeutic abortions, one maternal death and one term-delivery of a healthy baby (Talbot et al., 1984; Luisiri et al., 1997; Dayoan et al., 1998; Masterson et al., 2004).

In patients who conceived when the disease was in remission, relapse occurred in 25% of cases (Table 4). However, it is not known if this figure is higher than that expected in non-pregnant WG patients. The relapse or worsening of renal disease in the late pregnancy can be difficult to differentiate from pre-eclampsia. Very few parameters are useful in this regard, among them active urine sediment, which is indicative of WG nephritis, and hypertension, which is more commonly observed in pre-eclampsia, seem to be the most reliable. Moreover, as in SLE patients, the possibility that both features coexist at the same time cannot be ruled out. Premature delivery is a common complication of pregnancy in patients with WG, particularly in those with active disease during gestation.

9.2. Disease treatment during pregnancy

The treatment of disease relapse during pregnancy largely depends on the type and extension of the disease manifestations. For symptoms limited to the upper airways local antibiotic treatment and, if necessary, low-dose oral prednisone are recommended. Systemic manifestations require more aggressive treatment with high-dose oral prednisone (1 mg/kg/day). In case of insufficient response to corticosteroids, azathioprine should be started.

If life-threatening manifestations occur during the 2nd or 3rd trimester of pregnancy, cyclophosphamide should also be considered. Although conventional treatment with steroids and cyclophosphamide is able to control disease activity in 90% of patients, the potential adverse effects of cyclophosphamide must be weighed against the potential benefits and the patient should be involved in the decision-making process.

Recently, Masterson et al. (2004) described a successful remission with the combined use of intravenous immunoglobulin and steroids in a woman diagnosed with WG during the 1st trimester of pregnancy.

10. Churg–Strauss syndrome

Churg–Strauss syndrome (CSS) is a disorder characterized by pulmonary and systemic small-vessel vasculitis, extravascular granulomas and hypereosinophilia occurring in patients with asthma and allergic rhinitis.

10.1. Effects of pregnancy on the disease and vice versa

CSS relapse was reported in 50% of women who conceive while the disease is in remission, as shown in Table 4 (Debby et al., 1993; Lima et al., 1995; Hiyama et al., 2000). During relapse, the prevalent manifestations were worsening of asthma, mononeuritis multiplex and skin rash. Although prematurity is commonly observed, the majority of these patients delivered normal but low-birth-weight infants.

Patients with disease onset during pregnancy had a very poor prognosis (Barry et al., 1997; Priori et al., 1998). In these cases pregnancy complications were very common, including foetal and maternal death.

10.2. Disease treatment during pregnancy

Treatment of CSS relapses during pregnancy consists of prednisone, dosage of which has to be adjusted according to the severity of manifestations. In CSS patients, special care should be taken in monitoring bronchospasm during pregnancy and post-partum.

11. Polyarteritis nodosa

Polyarteritis nodosa (PAN) is a disorder characterized by necrotizing inflammation of medium size or small arteries. In patients with PAN prevalent features are fever, weight loss, myalagia, musculoskeletal, skin, gastrointestinal manifestations and peripheral neuropathy, especially mononeuritis multiplex.

11.1. Effects of pregnancy on the disease and vice versa

A few case reports on pregnancy in PAN patients are available (Reed and Smith, 1980; Pitkin, 1983; Fernandes et al., 1996). Patients who conceive during disease remission seem to have a favourable outcome with no maternal death, rare disease relapse and, in the majority of cases, delivery of healthy—although premature and low-birth-weight—babies. Conversely, the pregnancy outcome is poor when PAN is diagnosed during pregnancy.

11.2. Disease treatment during pregnancy

Patients with active disease during pregnancy are at high risk of death; therefore, therapeutic abortion should be considered in the early phase of pregnancy, whereas high-dose corticosteroid and cyclophosphamide are indicated in late pregnancy.

12. Microscopic polyangiitis

Microscopic polyangiitis (MPA) is a systemic, pauci-immune, necrotizing, small-vessel vasculitis. MPA is initially recognized as a subset of PAN from which it may be difficult to distinguish. It is also possible that in many series reported in literature MPA patients had been grouped with PAN. However, unlike PAN, most patients with MPA developed severe renal disease and pulmonary haemorrhage.

Only a few case reports on pregnancy in patients with MPA are available in the literature. Cetinkaya et al. (2002) described a patient who developed MPA at 16th week of gestation. Treatment with high-dose methylprednisolone (1 g/day for 3 days) and one pulse of cyclophosphamide (0.5 g) was given, but unfortunately the patient died due to pulmonary infection.

Milne et al. (2004) reported another case where MPA occurred at 24th week of gestation and was successfully treated with plasma-exchange, 1 g i.v. cyclophosphamide and 1 g daily iv. methylprednisolone, switched to 60 mg oral prednisone after 3 days. To reduce the risk of infections, prophylactic treatment with co-trimoxazole and oral anti-fungal agents was introduced.

It is possible that, as for PAN or other vasculitis, patients with MPA diagnosed and treated prior to pregnancy have a more favourable outcome with no need of aggressive treatment, which may increase the risk of maternal and foetal mortality.

13. Behçet disease

Behçet disease (BD) is a chronic, relapsing, multisystemic, inflammatory process characterized by recurrent oral and genital ulcers, ocular, gastrointestinal, neurological manifestations and thrombosis, occurring primarily in the Mediterranean basin, Middle East, South Asia and Japan. Most reports of large series come from Turkey or Japan. It predominantly affects young women during childbearing age; therefore, in endemic areas it is not rare to observe pregnancy in patients with BD (Table 1). In fact, a number of case reports as well as retrospective series of pregnancies in BD patients are available (Hamza et al., 1988; Bang et al., 1997; Marsal et al., 1997; Gul, 2000; Uzun et al., 2003).

13.1. Effects of pregnancy on the disease and vice versa

Pregnancy outcome appears favourable in patients with BD. The disease tends to improve during pregnancy in approximately half of the cases, and relapse occurs in 25% of cases (Table 4). During relapses, disease manifestations consist of oral or genital ulcers, arthritis and eye inflammation. Foetal and neonatal complications do not occur at an increased rate during pregnancy in patients with BD (Uzun et al., 2003).

13.2. Disease treatment during pregnancy

Nevertheless, the patients should be strictly monitored during pregnancy and post-partum, since relapses could occur and an early diagnosis and prompt treatment can guarantee the most favourable pregnancy outcome.

Key points

- The physiological adaptation of the immune system to pregnancy can potentially affect the course of all autoimmune rheumatic diseases (ARD). Conversely, the autoimmune processes characteristic of these conditions may compromise the foetal outcome.
- Pregnancy is not rare in patients with RA, SS and UCTD; it is rare in patients with systemic vasculitis.

- Some general guidelines seem to be valid for all ARD including those more rare:
  (1) Patients should be correctly informed about the risk of becoming pregnant,
  (2) Pregnancies should be planned when the disease is in remission in order to increase the probability of successful maternal and foetal outcome,
  (3) Patients should be regularly monitored during gestation and post-partum by a multidisciplinary team including rheumatologist, obstetrician, and neonatologist,
  (4) In case of disease relapse on adequate treatment, aggressive therapy should be recommended since active disease can be more detrimental to the foetus than drugs,
  (5) Pregnancies complicated by the onset of ARD have a particularly severe prognosis.

References

Alarcon, G.S., Williams, G.V., Singer, J.Z., et al. 1991. Early undifferentiated connective tissue disease. I. Early clinical manifestation in a large cohort of patients with undifferentiated connective tissue diseases compared with cohorts of well established connective tissue disease. J. Rheumatol. 18, 1332.

Alarcon, G.S., Willkens, R.F., Ward, J.R., et al. 1996. Early undifferentiated connective tissue disease. IV. Musculoskeletal manifestations in a large cohort of patients with undifferentiated connective tissue diseases compared with cohorts of patients with well-established connective tissue diseases: follow up analyses in patients with unexplained polyarthritis and patients with rheumatoid arthritis at baseline. Arthritis Rheum. 39, 403.

Altieri, P., Cameron, J.S. 1988. Scleroderma renal crisis in a pregnant woman with late partial recovery of renal function. Nephrol. Dial. Transplant. 3, 677.

Anonymous 1978. Reduction in incidence of rheumatoid arthritis associated with oral contraceptive. Royal College of General Practoiners' oral contraceptive study. Lancet 1, 569.

Antoni, C.E., Furst, D., Manger, B., et al. 2001. Outcome of pregnancy in women receiving remicade (Infliximab) for the treatment of Chron's disease or rheumatois arthritis. Arthritis Rheum. 44, S84.

Auzary, C., Huong, D.T., Wechsler, B., et al. 2000. Pregnancy in patients with Wegener's granulomatosis: report of five cases in three women. Ann. Rheum. Dis. 59, 800.

Baethgep, B.A., Wolf, R.E. 1989. Successful pregnancy with scleroderma renal disease and pulmonary hypertension in a patient using angiotensin converting enzyme inhibitors. Ann. Rheum. Dis. 48, 776.

Bang, D., Chun, Y.S., Haam, I.B., et al. 1997. The influence of pregnancy on Behçet's disease. Yonsei Med. J. 38, 437.

Barnes, A.B., Link, D.A. 1983. Childhood dermatomyositis and pregnancy. Am. J. Obstet. Gynecol. 146, 335.

Barrett, J.H., Brennan, P., Fiddler, M., et al. 2000. Breast-feeding and post partum relapse in women with rheumatoid and inflammatory arthritis. Arthritis Rheum. 43, 1010.

Barrett, J.H., Brennan, P., Fiddler, M.A., et al., 1999. Does rheumatoid arthritis remit during pregnancy and relapse post-partum? Arthritis Rheum. 42, 1219.
This is the largest study on the influence of pregnancy on RA activity. The authors prospectively studied 140 pregnancies in patients with RA during the last trimester and one and 6 month post-partum. Main measure of disease activity was Health Assessment Questionnaire (HAQ) for disability and assessment of joint symptoms by examination of inflamed joints.

Barry, C., Davis, S., Garrard, P., et al. 1997. Churg–Strauss disease: deterioration in a twin pregnancy. Successful outcome following treatment with corticosteroids and cyclophosphamide. Br. J. Obstet. Gynaecol. 104, 746.

Bauer, K.A., Siegler, M., Lindheimer, M.A. 1979. Polymyositis complicating pregnancy. Arch. Intern. Med. 139, 449.

Bennett, R.M., O'Connell, D.J. 1980. Mixed connective tissue disease: a clinicopathologic study of 20 cases. Semin. Arthritis Rheum. 10, 25.

Biesenbach, G., Stöger, H., Zazgornik, J. 1991. Successful pregnancy of twin in a renal transplant patient with Wegener's granulomatosis. Nephrol. Dial. Transplant 6, 139.

Black, C., Stevens, W.M. 1989. Scleroderma Rheum. Dis. Clin. North Am. 15, 193.

Brennan, P., Bankhead, C., Silman, A.J., et al. 1997. Oral contraceptive and rheumatoid arthritis: results from primary care-based incident case control study. Semin. Arthritis Rheum. 26, 817.

Brennan, P., Barrett, J., Fiddler, M., et al. 2000. Maternal–fetal HLA incompatibility and the course of inflammatory arthritis during pregnancy. J. Rheumatol. 27, 2843.

Brennan, P., Silman, A.J. 1994. Breast-feeding and the onset of rheumatoid arthritis. Arthritis Rheum. 37, 808.

Brent, R.L. 2001. Teratogen update: reproductive risks of leflunomide (Arava), o pirimidine syntesis inhibitor: counseling women taking leflunomide before or during pregnancy and men taking leflunomide who are contemplating fathering a child. Teratology 63, 106.

Brucato, A., Doria, A., Frassi, M., et al. 2002. Pregnancy outcome in 100 women with autoimmune diseases and anti-Ro/SSA antibodies: a prospective controlled study. Lupus 11, 716.

Brucato, A., Frassi, M., Franceschini, F., et al. 2001. Risk of congenital complete heart block in newborns of mothers with anti-Ro/SSA antibodies detected by counter-immunoelectrophoresis: a prospective study of 100 women. Arthritis Rheum. 44, 1832.

Cetinkaya, R., Odabas, A.R., Gursan, N., et al. 2002. Microscopic polyangiitis in a pregnant woman. South. Med. J. 95, 1441.

Cho, K.H., Heo, S.W., Chung, S.H., et al. 2003. A case of Mallory–Weiss syndrome complicating pregnancy in a patient with scleroderma. Korean J. Intern. Med. 18, 238.

Cooper, K., Stafford, J., Warwick, M.T. 1970. Wegener's granulomatosis complicating pregnancy. J. Obstet. Gynaecol. 77, 1028.

Danieli, M.G., Fraticelli, P., Franceschini, F., et al. 1999. Five-year follow up of 165 Italian patients with undifferentiated connective tissue disease. Clin. Exp. Rheumatol. 17, 585.

Dayoan, E.S., Dimen, L.L., Boylen, C.T. 1998. Successful treatment of Wegener's granulomatosis during pregnancy: a case report and review of the medical literature. Chest 113, 836.

Debby, A., Tanay, A., Zakut, H. 1993. Allergic granulomatosis and angiitis (Churg-Strauss vasculitis) in pregnancy. Int. Arch. Allergy Immunol. 102, 307.

Ditzian-Kadanoff, R., Reinhard, J.D., Thomas, C., et al. 1988. Polymyositis with myoglobinuria in pregnancy: a report and review of the literature. J. Rheumatol. 15, 513.

Doria, A., Cutolo, M., Ghirardello, A., et al. 2002. Steroid hormones and disease activity during pregnancy in systemic lupus erythematosus. Arthritis Rheum. 47, 202.

Doria, A., Ghirardello, A., de Zambiasi, P., et al. 1992. Japanese diagnostic criteria for mixed connective tissue disease in Caucasian patients. J. Rheumatol. 19, 259.

Doria, A., Ghirardello, A., Iaccarino, L., et al., 2004. Pregnancy, cytokines and disease activity in systemic lupus erythematosus. Arthritis Rheum. 51, 989.
The authors prospectively studied levels of some cytokine and soluble receptors involved in the humoral immune response in 17 consecutive patients with systemic lupus erythematosus and 8 matched healthy controls during pregnancy.

Doria, A., Mosca, M., Gambari, P.F., et al. 2005. Defining unclassifiable connective tissue diseases: incomplete, undifferentiated or both?. J. Rheumatol. 32, 213.

Emy, P., Lenormand, V., Maitre, F., et al. 1986. Polymyositis, dermatomyositis and pregnancy: high-risk pregnancy. A further case report and review of the literature. J. Gynecol. Obstet. Biol. Reprod. 15, 785.

England, M.J., Perlmann, T., Veriava, Y. 1986. Dermatomyositis in pregnancy. A case report. J. Reprod. Med. 31, 633.

Fernandes, S.R., Cury, C.P., Samara, A.M. 1996. Pregnancy with a history of treated polyarteritis nodosa. J. Rheumatol. 23, 1119.

Fiddler, M.A. 1997. Rheumatoid arthritis and pregnancy: issues for consideration in clinical management. Arthrit. Care Res. 10, 264.

Fields, C.L., Ossario, M.A., Roy, T.M., et al. 1991. Wegener's granulomatosis complicated by pregnancy. A case report. J. Reprod. Med. 36, 463.

Glickman, F.S. 1958. Dermatomyositis associated with pregnancy. US Armed Forces Med. J. 9, 417.

Gordon, C. 2004. Pregnancy and autoimmune diseases. Best Pract. Res. Clin. Rheumatol. 18, 359.
This is a recent review which covers the maternal and foetal aspects of pregnancy in systemic lupus erythematosus, antiphospholipid syndrome, inflammatory arthritis especially RA, vasculitis and systemic sclerosis. The author also discussed the management of analgesic, anti-rheumatic and immunosuppressive therapy during pregnancy and breast-feeding period.

Goroir, B.P., Peppel, K., Silva, M., et al. 1992. The biosynthesis of tumor necrosis factor during pregnancy: studies with CAT reporter transgene and TNF inhibitors. Eur. Cytokine Netw. 3, 533.

Gul, U. 2000. Pregnancy and Behçet disease. Arch. Dermatol. 136, 1063.

Gutierrez, G., Dagnino, R., Mintz, G. 1984. Polymyositis–dermatomyositis and pregnancy. Arthritis Rheum. 27, 291.

Habib, A., MacKay, K., Abrons, H.L. 1996. Wegener's granulomatosis complicating pregnancy: presentation of two patients and review of the literature. Clin. Nephrol. 46, 332.

Hamza, M., Elleuch, M., Zribi, A. 1988. Behçet's disease and pregnancy. Ann. Rheum. Dis. 47, 350.

Harber, M.A., Tso, A., Taheri, S., et al. 1999. Wegener's granulomatosis in pregnancy: the therapeutic dilemma. Nephrol. Dial. Transplant. 14, 1789.

Harris, A., Webley, M., Usherwood, M., et al. 1995. Dermatomyositis presenting in pregnancy. Br. J. Dermatol. 133, 783.

Harrison, D.F.N. 1989. Ear, nose and throat symptoms in subacute Wegener's granulomatosis (letter). BMJ 299, 791.

Hench, P.S. 1938. The ameliorating effect of pregnancy on chronic atrophic (infectious rheumatoid) arthritis, fibrosistis, and intermittent hydrartrosis. Mayo Clinic. Proc. 13, 161.

Hiyama, J., Shiota, Y., Marukawa, M., et al. 2000. Churg–Strauss syndrome associated with pregnancy. Intern. Med. 39, 985.

Horita, Y., Tsunoda, S., Inenaga, T., et al. 2001. Pregnancy in nephrotic syndrome with mixed connective tissue disease. Nephron 89, 354.

Houck, W., Melnyk, C., Gast, M.J. 1987. Polymyositis in pregnancy. A case report and literature review. J. Reprod. Med. 32, 208.

Ishii, N., Ono, H., Kawaguchi, T., et al. 1991. Dermatomyositis and pregnancy. Case report and review of the literature. Dermatologica 183, 146.

Ishikawa, K., Matsuura, S. 1982. Occlusive thromboaortopathy (Takayasu's disease) and pregnancy. Clinical course and management of 33 pregnancies and deliveries. Am. J. Cardiol. 50, 1293.

Jansen, N.M., Genta, M.S. 2000. The effects of immunosoppressive and anti-inflammatory medications on fertility, pregnancy, and lactation. Arch. Inten. Med. 160, 610.

Juarez-Azpilcueta, A., Pol-Kipes, G., Olivo-Arroyo, G., et al. 2003. Dermatomyositis and pregnancy. Gac. Med. Mex. 139, 509.

Julkunen, H., Kaaja, R., Kurki, P., et al. 1995. Fetal outcome in women with primary Sjögren's Syndrome. A retrospective case–control study. Clin. Exp. Rheumatol. 13, 65.

Kanoh, H., Izumi, T., Seishima, M., et al. 1999. A case of dermatomyositis that developed after delivery: the involvement of pregnancy in the induction of dermatomyositis. Br. J. Dermatol. 141, 897.

Katz, A.L. 1980. Another case of polymyositis in pregnancy. Arch. Intern. Med. 140, 1123.

Kaufman, R.L., Kitridou, R.C. 1982. Pregnancy in mixed connective tissue disease: comparison with systemic lupus erythematosus. J. Rheumatol. 9, 549.

King, C.R., Chow, S. 1985. Dermatomyositis and pregnancy. Obstet. Gynecol. 66, 589.

Kofteridis, D.P., Malliotakis, P.I., Sotsiou, F., et al. 1999. Acute onset of dermatomyositis presenting in pregnancy with rhabdomyolysis and fetal loss. Scand. J. Rheumatol. 28, 192.

Koldingsnes, W. 1998. Pregnancy in Wegener's granulomatosis: a case report (abstract). Scand. J. Rheumatol. 27 (Suppl. 107), 85.

Kumar, A., Mohan, A., Gupta, R., et al. 1998. Relapse of Wegener's granulomatosis in the first trimester of pregnancy: a case report. Br. J. Rheumatol. 37, 331.

Lambe, M., Björnådal, L., Neregård, P., et al. 2004. Childbearing and the risk of scleroderma: a population-based study in Sweden. Am. J. Epidemiol. 159, 162.

Le Thi Huong, D., Wechsler, B., Combes, R., et al. 1988. Twin pregnancy in polymyositis. Ann. Med. Interne 139, 286.

Lima, F., Buchanan, N., Froes, L., et al. 1995. Pregnancy in granulomatosus vasculitis. Ann. Rheum. Dis. 54, 604.

Lloyd, M.E., Carr, M., McElhatton, P., et al. 1999. The effects of methotrexate on pregnancy, fertility and lactation. Q. J. Med. 92, 551.

Luisiri, P., Lance, N.J., Curan, J.J. 1997. Wegener's granulomatosis in pregnancy. Arthritis Rheum. 40, 1354.

Lundberg, I., Hedfors, E. 1991. Pregnancy outcome in patients with high titre anti-RNP antibodies. A retrospective study of 40 pregnancies. J. Rheumatol. 18, 359.
The authors retrospectively studied 40 pregnancies in 20 women with high titer of anti-RNP antibodies. They studied the obstetric complications and maternal disease during pregnancy and post-partum period.

Marsal, S., Falga, C., Simeon, C.P., et al. 1997. Behçet's disease and pregnancy relationship study. Br. J. Rheumatol. 36, 234.

Massé, M.R. 1962. Pregnancies and dermatomyositis. Bull. Soc. Fr. Dermatol. Syphiligr. 69, 921.

Masterson, R., Pellicano, R., Bleasel, K., et al. 2004. Wegener's granulomatosis in pregnancy: a novel approach to management. Am. J. Kidney Dis. 44, 86.

Matsumura, A., Moriwaki, R., Numano, F. 1992. Pregnancy in Takayasu arteritis from the view of internal medicine. Heart Vessels Suppl. 7, 120.

Mehta, N., Modi, N. 1989. ACE inhibitors in pregnancy. Lancet 2 (8654), 96.

Messina, S., Fagiolari, G., Lamperti, C., et al. 2002. Women with pregnancy-related polymyositis and high serum CK levels in the newborn. Neurology 58, 482.

Milford, C.A., Bellini, M. 1986. Wegener's granulomatosis arising in pregnancy. J. Laringol. Otol. 100, 475.

Milne, K.L., Stanley, K.P., Temple, R.C., et al. 2004. Microscopic polyangiitis: first report of a case with onset during pregnancy. Nephrol. Dial. Transplant. 19, 234.

Mintz, G. 1989. Dermatomyositis. Rheum. Dis. Clin. North Am. 15, 375.

Mosca, M., Neri, R., Bombardieri, S. 1999. Undifferentiated connective tissue diseases (UCTD): a review of the literature and a proposal for preliminary classification criteria. Clin. Exp. Rheumatol. 17, 615.

Mosca, M., Neri, R., Strigini, F., et al., 2002. Pregnancy outcome in patients with undifferentiated connective tissue disease: a preliminary study on 25 pregnancies. Lupus 11, 304.
The authors studied 25 pregnancies in patients with undifferentiated connective tissue disease (UCTD) in order to evaluate: (1) pregnancy outcome; (2) whether pregnancy is associated with flares of disease activity; and (3) whether pregnancy may be a trigger for development of a defined connective disuse disease (CTD). This is the first study on pregnancy in patients with UCTD.

Mosca, M., Tavoni, A., Neri, R., et al. 1998. Undifferentiated connective tissue diseases: the clinical and serological profiles of 91 patients followed for at least 1 year. Lupus 7, 95.

M'Rad, S., Moalla, M., Ben Milled, K., et al. 1989. Granulomatose de Wegener et grossesse: une observation. Rev. Med. Interne 10, 69.

Munoz-Valle, J.F., Vazquez-Del Mercado, M., Garcia-Iglesias, T., et al. 2003. T(H)1/T(H)2 cytokine profile, metalloprotease-9 activity and hormonal status in pregnant rheumatoid arthritis and systemic lupus erythematosus patients. Clin. Exp. Immunol. 131, 377.

Neely, N.T., Persellin, R.H. 1977. Activity of rheumatoid arthritis during pregnancy. Texas Med. 73, 59.

Nelson, J.L., Hughes, K.A., Smith, A.G., et al. 1993. Maternal–fetal disparity in HLA class II alloantigenes and the pregnancy-induced amelioration of rheumatoid arthritis. N. Engl. J. Med. 329, 466.

Nelson, J.L., Østensen, M. 1997. Pregnancy and rheumatoid arthritis. Rheum. Dis. Clin. North Am. 23, 195.

Ohno, T., Imai, A., Tamaya, T. 1992. Successful outcomes of pregnancy complicated with dermatomyositis. Case reports. Gynecol. Obstet. Invest. 33, 187.

Østensen, M., Fuher, L., Mathieu, R., et al., 2004. A prospective study of pregnant patients with rheumatoid arthritis and ankylosing spondylits using validated clinical instruments. Ann. Rheum. Dis. 63, 1212.
The authors prospectively evaluated 10 pregnancies in patients with RA and analyzed the disease course before conception, during each trimester of pregnancy, and at weeks 6, 12 and 24 post-partum by means of some validated clinical instruments for measurement of disease activity namely the Rheumatoid Arthritis Disease Activity Index (RADAI), the 44 joint count, and the Health Assessment Questionnaire (HAQ).

Østensen, M., Husby, G. 1983. A prospective clinical study of the effect of pregnancy on rheumatoid arthritis and ankylosing spondylitis. Arthritis Rheum. 26, 1155.

Østensen, M., Villiger, P.M. 2002. Immunology of pregnancy as a remission inducing agent in rheumatoid arthritis. Transpl Immunol. 9, 155.

Palit, J., Clague, B. 1990. Wegener granulomatoisis presenting during first trimester of pregnancy. Br. J. Rheumatol. 29, 389.

Papapetropoulos, T., Kanellakopoulou, N., Tsibri, E., et al. 1998. Polymyositis and pregnancy: report of a case with three pregnancies. J. Neurol. Neurosurg. Psychiatry 64, 406.

Park, I.W., Suh, Y.J., Han, J.H., et al. 2003. Dermatomyositis developing in the first trimester of pregnancy. Korean J. Intern. Med. 18, 196.

Parnham, A.P., Thatcher, G.N. 1996. Pregnancy and active Wegener granulomatosis. Aust. N.Z. J. Obstet. Gynaecol. 36, 361.

Pauzner, R., Mayan, H., Hershko, E., et al. 1994. Exacerbation of Wegener's granulomatosis during pregnancy: report of a case with tracheal stenosis and literature review. J. Rheumatol. 21, 1153.

Pinheiro, G.R., Goldenberg, J., Atra, E., et al. 1992. Juvenile dermatomyositis and pregnancy: report and literature review. J. Rheumatol. 19, 1798.

Pitkin, R.M. 1983. Polyarteritis nodosa. Clin. Obstet. Gynecol. 26, 579.

Priori, R., Tommassini, M., Magrini, L., et al. 1998. Churg-Strauss syndrome during pregnancy after steroid withdrawal. Lancet 352, 1599.

Quinn, C., Mulpeter, K., Casey, E.B., et al. 1993. Changes in levels of IgM RF and alpha2 PAG correlate with increased disease activity in rheumatoid during puerperium. Scand. J. Rheumatol. 22, 273.

Reed, N.R., Smith, M.T. 1980. Periarteritis nodosa in pregnancy: report of a case and review of the literature. Obstet. Gynecol. 55, 381.

Rosa, F.W., Bosco, L.A., Graham, C.F., et al. 1989. Neonatal anuria with maternal angiotensis-converting enzyme inhibition. Obstet. Gynecol. 74, 371.

Rosenweig, B.A., Rotmensch, S., Binette, S., et al. 1989. Primary idiopathic polymiositis and dermatomyositis complications in pregnancy: diagnosis and treatment. Obstet. Gynecol. Surv. 44, 162.

Satoh, M., Ajmani, A.K., Hirakata, M., et al. 1994. Onset of polymyositis with autoantibodies to threonyl-tRNA synthetase during pregnancy. J. Rheumatol. 21, 1564.

Sharma, B.K., Jain, S., Vasishta, K. 2000. Outcome of pregnancy in Takayasu arteritis. Int. J. Cardiol. 75 (Suppl. 1), S159.

Silman, A.J. 2002. Contraceptives, pregnancy, and RA. Ann. Rheum. Dis. 61, 383.

Silman, A.J. 1994. Epidemiology of rheumatoid arthritis. APMIS 102, 721.

Silman, A.J., Black, C.M. 1988. Increased incidence of spontaneous abortion and infertility in women with scleroderma before disease onset: a controlled study. Ann. Rheum. Dis. 47, 6441.

Silman, A.J., Hichberg, M.C. 2001. Rheumatoid arthritis. In: A.J. Silman, M.C. Hochberg (Eds.), Epidemiology of the Rheumatic Disease. Oxford University Press, Oxford, p. 31.

Silman, A.J., Kay, A., Brennan, P. 1992. Timing of pregnancy in relation to the onset of rheumatoid arthritis. Arthritis Rheum. 35, 152.

Silva, C.A., Sultan, S.M., Isenberg, D.A. 2003. Pregnancy outcome in adult-onset idiopathic inflammatory myopathy. Rheumatology 42, 1168.

Slate, W.G., Graham, A.R. 1968. Scleroderma and pregnancy. Am. J. Obstet. Gynecol. 101, 335.

Solomon, J.E., D'Alton, M.E. 1996. Dermatomyositis in pregnancy. Curr. Opin. Obstet. Gynecol. 8, 83.

Steen, V.D., Conte, C., Day, N. 1989. Pregnancy in women with systemic sclerosis. Arthritis Rheum. 32, 151.

Steen, V.D. 1998. Pregnancy in systemic sclerosis. Scand. J. Rheumatol. 107, 72.
This is a comprehensive review of the available information on fertility and pregnancy outcomes in women with systemic sclerosis.

Steen, V.D. 1999. Pregnancy in women with systemic sclerosis. Obstet. Gynecol. 94, 15.

Steen, V.D. 1997. Scleroderma and pregnancy. Rheum. Dis. Clin. North Am. 23, 133.

Steiner, I., Averbuch-Heller, L., Abramsky, O., et al. 1992. Postpartum idiopathic polymyositis. Lancet 339, 256.

Suwa, A., Hirakata, M., Tsuzaka, K., et al. 1992. Spontaneous remission of dermatomyositis which developed one month after normal delivery. Ryumachi 32, 73.

Takaya, M., Ichikawa, Y., Shimizu, H., et al. 1991. Sjögren syndrome and pregnancy. Tokai Exp. Clin. Med. 16, 83.

Talbot, S.F., Main, D.M., Levinson, A.I. 1984. Wegener's granulomatosis: first report of a case with onset during pregnancy. Arthritis Rheum. 27, 109.

Tsai, A., Lindheimer, M.D., Lamberg, S.I. 1973. Dermatomyositis complicating pregnancy. Obstet. Gynecol. 41, 570.

Unger, A., Kay, A., Griffin, A.J., et al. 1983. Disease activity and pregnancy associated alpha2-glycoprotein in rheumatoid arthritis during pregnancy. BMJ 286, 750.

Uzun, S., Alpsoy, E., Durdu, M., et al. 2003. The clinical course of Behçet's disease in pregnancy: a retrospective analysis and review of the literature. J. Dermatol. 30, 499.

Williams, H.J., Alarcon, G.S., Joks, R., et al. 1999. Early undifferentiated tissue disease (CTD). VI. An inception cohort after 10 years: disease remission and changes in diagnoses in well established and undifferentiated CTD. J. Rheumatol. 26, 816.

Wong, V.C.W., Yang, R.Y.C., Tse, T.F. 1983. Pregnancy and Takayasu's arteritis. Am. J. Med. 75, 597.

Handbook of Systemic Autoimmune Diseases, Volume 4
Reproductive and Hormonal Aspects of Systemic Autoimmune Diseases
Michael Lockshin and D. Ware Branch, editors

CHAPTER 8

A Bedside Perspective of Neonatal Lupus

Jill P. Buyon[a,*]

[a]*Division of Rheumatology, Hospital for Joint Diseases, New York University School of Medicine, New York, NY, USA*

1. Introduction

Detection of isolated congenital heart block (CHB) in the latter half of the 2nd trimester predicts with high certainty, the presence of maternal autoantibodies to the intracellular ribonucleoproteins SSA/Ro and SSB/La (Buyon, 2004; Lee, 1993). CHB is considered a passively acquired autoimmune disease, in which maternal autoantibodies cross the placenta and injure an otherwise normally developing heart. Other neonatal abnormalities, including cutaneous manifestations, cholestasis and cytopenias, are also associated with anti-SSA/Ro-SSB/La antibodies in the maternal and fetal circulation and are now grouped under the heading of neonatal lupus (NL) syndromes. This term–derived from the resemblance of the neonatal rash to the subacute cutaneous rash of systemic lupus erythematosus (SLE) in adults–is clearly a misnomer, as the newborn does not have a systemic autoimmune disease and the mother may be completely asymptomatic. The noncardiac manifestations of NL are generally transient, resolving at about 6 months of life coincident with the disappearance of maternal autoantibodies from the neonatal circulation. To date, however, complete (3rd degree) heart block is irreversible.

*Corresponding author.
Hospital for Joint Diseases, 301 East 17th Street, New York 10003. NY, USA.
Tel.: +1-212-598-6522.
E-mail address: Jill.Buyon@NYUMC.org (J.P. Buyon).

DOI: 10.1016/S1571-5078(05)04008-0

The relative rarity of autoimmune-associated CHB has posed a challenge to clinical and epidemiologic researchers. The establishment in 1994 of the Research Registry for Neonatal Lupus (Registry) (Buyon et al., 1998), a rare disease registry funded by the U.S. National Institutes of Health, has enabled the acquisition of larger and thus more statistically reliable series, data from which are reported here. As of March 1, 2005, the Registry follows 345 mothers (309 with verified anti-SSA/Ro and/or SSB-La antibodies) and their children with NL syndromes, including 214 with CHB only, 107 with NL rash only, 29 with CHB and rash, 3 with isolated cardiomyopathy (CM), and 7 with hepatic and/or hematologic manifestations.

2. Clinical presentation

The classic description of NL is one of a fetus or newborn discovered to be bradycardic due to a conduction defect in the absence of causative structural abnormalities, for which laboratory investigation reveals antibodies to SSA/Ro and/or SSB/La in the maternal serum. Although the mother may have SLE, Sjögren's syndrome (SS) or an undifferentiated autoimmune syndrome (UAS), over a third are entirely asymptomatic.

Many cases are discovered *in utero*, most commonly between 18 and 24 wk of gestation. The degree of heart block includes all levels from 1st degree, discovered only incidentally on electrocardiogram (i.e., after birth) or in utero by a prolonged

PR interval detected on echocardiogram, through 3rd degree (complete) heart block. Mortality (including fetal demise) is ~20%; most often in utero or the 1st few months of life (Buyon et al., 1998). Approximately, two-thirds of all recognized cases receive pacemaker insertion before reaching adulthood (Buyon et al., 1998), and current practice suggests that virtually all patients with complete heart block will have a pacemaker at some point in their lives. Risk factors for permanent pacing include very slow heart rates (below 55 bpm), symptoms such as poor exercise tolerance, cardiomegaly, long QRS or QT durations, ectopy, syncope, or structural or functional heart disease (Kertesz et al., 1997).

Unfortunately, cardiac injury may extend beyond the conduction system. There is a 10% incidence of late CM leading to low output congestive heart failure, death or transplant, even after successful pacemaker implantation for the associated heart block (Buyon et al., 1998; Moak et al., 2001). CM can be seen in the absence of heart block; three children of antibody-positive mothers from the Registry series had CM with no apparent block, and CM associated with 1st degree block/prolonged PR interval was seen in another Registry child. Nield et al. (2002) have reported isolated endocardial fibroelastosis in three cases (one fetus and two infants) exposed to maternal anti-SSA/Ro antibodies. The authors concluded that autoantibody-mediated EFE may be an etiological factor in cases of fetal and neonatal "idiopathic" dilated cardiomyopathy. A minority of offspring (23 of 128 currently in the Registry with sufficient records, or 18%) exhibit congenital structural abnormalities that do not in themselves account for CHB, including atrial septal defect and patent ductus arteriosus.

Other organ systems may be transiently involved in the newborn, in the presence or absence of CHB. The characteristic NL rash usually affects the scalp and face, particularly the periorbital region, and is typically photosensitive. In some instances the rash is present in other locations and can cover virtually the entire body. The lesions are superficial inflammatory plaques, typically annular or elliptic with erythema and scaling. The rash most often appears within a few weeks of life (most commonly at 6 wk) and resolves by 6–8 months of life, usually with minimal scarring (Neiman et al., 2000). Occasionally, newborns of mothers with anti-SSA/Ro-SSB/La antibodies may present with various cytopenias (Buyon et al., 1998, 2004; Watson et al., 1988) and/or liver enzyme abnormalities (Kanagasegar et al., 2002; Laxer et al., 1990; Lee et al., 2002; Schoenlebe et al., 1993).

The incidence of CHB in an offspring of a mother with anti-SSA/Ro antibodies is ~2% (Lee, 1993; Ramsey-Goldman et al., 1986; Lockshin et al., 1988; Brucato et al., 2001). When an anti-SSA/Ro-positive mother has previously given birth to a child with NL, the risk of CHB in a subsequent pregnancy rises to ~18% (Buyon et al., 1998; Julkunen and Eronen, 2001). In our Registry, of 95 subsequent pregnancies after having a child with CHB, 18 (19%) resulted in CHB and 7 (7%) in a child with NL rash. Importantly, a mother who has given birth to a child with cutaneous manifestations can subsequently give birth to a child with CHB. Of 41 pregnancies subsequent to the birth of a child with NL rash, 11 (28%) resulted in CHB and 15 (38%) in a 2nd child with rash. This latter observation was remarkable and may represent some bias in the data collection in that many mothers entered the Registry because of a child with CHB. The history of a previous child with rash was obtained by questionnaire and verified by photographs, doctors' notes, and/or biopsy. What is not known is the universe of women who may have had children with NL rash but remained undiagnosed. Of 15 pregnancies in mothers already enrolled because of a child with rash, two resulted in a subsequent child with CHB. Even if these latter numbers are more accurate it is clear that a previous child with any manifestation of NL puts the mother at greater risk for having a child with CHB than if she were a primigravida or only had healthy children. As previously reported, there is no gender-based difference in the frequency of either CHB or NL rash (Buyon et al., 1998; Neiman et al., 2000).

3. Diagnostic considerations

The identification of fetal bradycardia by either auscultation or routine obstetric ultrasound should prompt two immediate responses. The first is to obtain a two-dimensional and M-mode fetal echocardiographic and Doppler ultrasound to document whether there is an atrial arrhythmia or AV block, and to what degree. Only 2nd or 3rd degree block will be clinically manifest as bradycardia. These studies will also ascertain whether there are any major structural abnormalities of the heart such as AV septal defects, left atrial isomerism or abnormalities of the great arteries, which can themselves cause heart block independent of maternal autoantibodies. An associated myocarditis is supported by the finding of decreased contractility in addition to secondary changes such as an increase of cardiac size, pericardial effusions and tricuspid regurgitation.

The second response is to evaluate the mother's serum for the presence of anti-SSA/Ro and anti-SSA/La antibodies. The enzyme-linked immunosorbent assay (ELISA) is the most common and probably the most sensitive method for detection of these antibodies. In our laboratory at the Hospital for Joint Diseases which employs a commercial ELISA (Diamedix, Miami, FL), the titer of anti-SSA/Ro antibodies in the mothers of children with CHB is characteristically over 100 EU with most being well into the thousands. Titers less than 100 (19 is cutoff for normal controls) were only seen in 6 of over 200 CHB-sera evaluated. Gordon et al. recently evaluated sera from 125 CHB mothers using a commercially available line immunoassay, which employs a natural 60 kDa Ro protein (INNO-LIA^{TM} ANA Update, Innogenetics NV, Ghent, Belgium) (Gordon et al., 2004). By this method, 96% of the sera had antibodies to 60 kDa Ro, 86% to 52 kDa Ro and 78% to 48 kDa La. Sensitivity of the three antibodies was assessed in the symptomatic mothers of children with CHB (78 women) and disease-matched controls with unaffected children (65 women). There was no significant difference between the groups for 60 kDa Ro or for anti-52 kDa Ro antibody. However, there was a significant difference for the anti-SSB/La antibody ($P = 0.001$) with an odds ratio of 3.59. This translates to an increase in risk from a published 2% for CHB in an anti-SSA/Ro positive mother to 3.1% if the woman is also anti-SSB/La positive and to a decrease in risk to 0.9% if anti-SSB/La negative.

4. Therapeutic options

Because CHB is most often identified between 18 and 24 wk of gestation, intrauterine therapy should be possible. The clinical approach includes obstetric and rheumatologic management of both the fetus identified with CHB and the fetus with a normal heart rate but at high risk of developing CHB. In either situation, the critical decision is whether any treatment is necessary. Guidelines are not well established and are based empirically on anecdotal evidence. For the fetus identified with CHB, the clinician needs to know if the presence of bradycardia represents an irreversible fibrotic process and if continued autoimmune tissue injury will cause progressive damage. The rationale for treatment of identified heart block is to diminish a generalized inflammatory insult and lower the titer of maternal autoantibodies. Several intrauterine therapeutic regimens have been tried, including dexamethasone (Nield et al., 2002; Saleeb et al., 1999), which is not metabolized by the placenta and is available to the fetus in an active form, and plasmapheresis (Buyon et al., 1987). Maternal risks of dexamethasone are similar to those of any glucocorticoid and include infection, osteoporosis, osteonecrosis, diabetes, hypertension and preeclampsia. Fetal risks include oligohydramnios, intrauterine growth retardation and adrenal suppression. Recently in the United States, an NIH-funded multicenter open-label prospective trial has been initiated to evaluate the efficacy of 4 mg/day of dexamethasone (taken orally by the mother) in the treatment of newly identified 1st, 2nd or 3rd degree block [the PRIDE (PR interval and dexamethasone evaluation) in CHB Trial]. Results should be available within the next year.

With regard to prophylactic therapy of the highest-risk mother (previous child with CHB) there is little support for initiation of either prednisone or dexamethasone. Maternal prednisone (at least in low and moderate doses) early in pregnancy does not prevent the development of CHB (Waltuck and Buyon, 1994). This might be anticipated since prednisone given to the mother is not active in the fetus (Blanford and Murphy, 1977) and levels of anti-SSA/Ro -SSB/La antibodies remain relatively constant during corticosteroid therapy. Shinohara et al. (Shinohara et al., 1999) reported CHB in 15 of 61 infants born to 40 mothers with anti-SSA/Ro antibodies who did not receive glucocorticoids. This unexpectedly high prevalence may be explained by the retrospective nature of the study and potential referral bias. Conversely, CHB did not occur in any of 26 fetuses whose anti-SSA/Ro positive-mothers were given steroids prior to the 16th wk of gestation, Given published risks of ~2% (first)–18% (recurrence) (Lee, 1993; Ramsey-Goldman et al., 1986; Lockshin et al., 1988), the authors may have needed to follow more than 26 pregnancies to find an infant with CHB. In our group, we have noted that in 5 of 61 pregnancies in which CHB developed, the mothers had been taking prednisone prior to the fetal diagnosis (Waltuck and Murphy, 1994).

We recommend that the fetuses of all women with anti-SSA/Ro antibodies be evaluated by serial echocardiography (Friedman, 1992) preferably every week from 16 to 26 wk and perhaps less frequently thereafter. Justification for such close surveillance is based on cases in the Registry in which bradycardia attributable to AV nodal block was observed 1–2 wk after a normal heart beat. A recent major advance in echocardiography has made possible by the *in utero* detection of 1st degree block. The development of a non-invasive Doppler technique to measure the mechanical PR interval may allow earlier diagnosis and treatment possibilities. Normative data have been published (Glickstein et al., 2000), and the technique validated in two cases (Rosenthal et al., 2002; Copel, 2004). To explore related immune CM, a new Doppler index of fetal cardiac function, the Tei myocardial performance index, has been established *in utero* (Friedman et al., 2003). A U.S.-based multicenter NIH-funded trial is currently underway to assess the frequency of 1st degree block in mothers with anti-SSA/Ro antibodies, and whether it is a marker for more advanced block (PRIDE in CHB, discussed above). Echocardiograms are done weekly from 16 to 26 wk and every other week until 32 wk; all echocardiographers are trained to perform the novel measurement of the mechanical PR interval. The rationale is to evaluate the fetal heart with the most sensitive tools during the period of presumed vulnerability. Data should be forthcoming in the next year.

Fetuses with very slow heart rates and hydrops have been treated with sympathomimetics via the maternal circulation (Groves et al., 1995), or even digoxin or fetal pacing (Jaeggi, 2001). In the absence of controlled studies (which may never be feasible given the rarity of CHB), plasmapheresis, digoxin, diuretics and/or fetal pacing should be considered highly experimental and only reserved for those cases where the fetus is in a life-threatening situation with hydrops and deteriorating cardiac function.

After birth, treatment of the symptomatic infant often involves pacemaker therapy, and supportive treatment for low output or congestive heart failure. Despite the presence of intact antibody against SSA/Ro and SSB/La in breast milk, breastfeeding appears to confer no risk in the child's disease when compared with formula, although caution should prompt cessation of breastfeeding in a case of worsening CM or rash (Askanase et al., 2002).

All neonates (both healthy infants and those with CHB) whose mothers have anti-SSA/Ro or -SSB/La antibodies should be protected from excessive exposure to the sun, since they may develop skin lesions up to 6 months of age while the maternal antibodies persist. Treatment is generally conservative, and in many cases no intervention is required. Topical corticosteroids, preferably non-fluorinated, may be used. High-potency topical corticosteroids can produce systemic effects. Since the lesions are transient and generally benign, systemic therapies such as antimalarials are not recommended in young children, in whom the therapeutic dose approaches the toxic dose (Neiman et al., 2000). In most cases the other, rarer manifestations of NL such as liver enzyme abnormalities and cytopenias, are self-limited (Watson et al., 1988; Kanagasegar et al., 2002; Laxer et al., 1990; Lee et al., 2002).

Mothers who have had children with NL need to be aware of several important points to guide future management. If the mother has no signs or symptoms of a rheumatic disease, she should be reassured that she does not have SLE. Approximately half of these mothers develop rheumatological symptoms; however, severe life-threatening SLE is rare. Of 152 Registry mothers evaluated, 52 (34%) were asymptomatic, 28 (18%) had UAS, 29 (18%) had SLE, 31

(20%) had SS, 11 (7%) had SLE/SS and 1 (<1%) had rheumatoid arthritis (RA)/SS at the time NL was identified (prior to or at birth). Mean follow-up was 7.5 year. Twenty-one (40%) of the 52 initially asymptomatic mothers developed symptoms of a rheumatic disease: 3 (6%) developed UAS, 9 (17%) SS and 9 (17%) SLE. Of the 28 mothers initially categorized as having UAS, 3 (11%) developed SLE and 4 (14%) SS. 4 (13%) of 31 mothers with SS progressed to SLE. Notably, the majority of patients with SLE at the time of the affected pregnancy have not experienced disease progression.

A longitudinal study comparing 94 children of anti-SSA/Ro-SSB/La-positive mothers (including 49 born with NL and 45 unaffected siblings) with age- and ethnicity-matched controls whose mothers were antibody-negative, found that joint stiffness was the single rheumatological symptom reported significantly more often in the children of antibody-positive mothers than in the control group (Martin et al., 2002). Six (12%) of the 49 children born with NL developed a definable autoimmune disease (2 juvenile RA, 1 Hashimoto's thyroiditis, 1 psoriasis/iritis, 1 psoriasis/Type I diabetes, and 1 congenital hyothyroidism/nephrotic syndrome) by age 13 yr, compared with none of the unaffected siblings and none of the controls. Of the 6 mothers whose children subsequently developed a rheumatic/autoimmune disease, 5 (83%) had or developed symptoms or signs of SS, either alone or in association with SLE. A contribution of maternal health status to the development of disease in the children was suggestive, but restricted by the observation that of the mothers who consented to participate in the study, only six remained asymptomatic during the follow-up period. While the small sample size precludes definitive determinations of risk, children who have had NL and whose mothers have an autoimmune disease should be closely followed with regard to autoimmune symptoms in childhood.

Key points

- Approximately 2% of all mothers with anti -SSA/Ro antibodies have a baby with CHB, independent of whether the mother has a rheumatic disease or is totally asymptomatic.
- Mothers who have given birth to a child with NL, be it CHB or rash, face a nearly 20% risk that their next child will have CHB.
- All women with SLE, SS, RA or only the history of a positive ANA who are planning a pregnancy should be screened for anti-SSA/Ro and -SSB/La antibodies by ELISA. If these antibodies are present, prophylactic therapy is not indicated but serial echocardiographic analysis (preferably with assessment of the mechanical PR interval) is suggested.
- Treatment of CHB identified *in utero* is not established but guidelines are provided.

Acknowledgement

This work was supported in part by data and materials from the Research Registry for Neonatal Lupus (NIAMS contract AR4—2271).

References

Askanase, A.D., Miranda-Carus, M.E., Tang, X., Katholi, M., Buyon, J.P. 2002. The presence of IgG antibodies reactive with components of the ScSA/Ro–SSB/La complex in human breast milk: implications in neonatal lupus. Arthritis Rheum. 46, 269–271.

Blanford, A.T., Murphy, B.E.P. 1977. In vitro metabolism of prednisolone, dexamethasone, betamethasone, and cortisol by the human placenta. Am. J. Obstet. Gynecol. 127, 264–267.

Brucato, A., Frassi, M., Franceschini, F., Cimaz, R., Faden, D., Pisoni, M.P., Muscara, M., Vignati, G., Stramba-Badiale, M., Catelli, L., Lojacono, A., Cavazzana, I., Ghirardello, A., Vescovi, F., Gambari, P.F., Doria, A., Meroni, P.L., Tincani, A. 2001. Risk of congenital complete heart block in newborns of mothers with anti-Ro/SSA antibodies detected by counterimmunoelectrophoresis: a prospective study of 100 women. Arthritis Rheum. 44, 1832–1835.

Buyon, J.P. 2004. Neonatal lupus syndromes. In: R. Lahita (Ed.), Systemic Lupus Erythematosus, 4th ed., Elsevier Academic Press, San Diego, pp. 449–484.

Buyon, J.P., Hiebert, R., Copel, J., Craft, J., Friedman, D., Katholi, M., Lee, L., Marston, K., Provost, T., Reichlin, M., Rider, L., Rupel, A., Saleeb, S., Weston, W., Skovron,

M.L. 1998. Autoimmune-associated congenital heart block: mortality, morbidity, and recurrence rates obtained from a national neonatal lupus registry. J. Am. Coll. Cardiol. 31, 1658–1666.

Buyon, J.P., Swersky, S.H., Fox, H.E., Bierman, F.Z., Winchester, R.J. 1987. Intrauterine therapy for presumptive fetal myocarditis with acquired heart block due to systemic lupus erythematosus. Experience in a mother with a predominance of SS-B (La) antibodies. Arthritis Rheum. 30, 44–49.

Copel, J. 2004. Personal communication. Yale University Hospital, New Haven, CT.

Friedman, D.M. 1992. Fetal echocardiography in the assessment of lupus pregnancies. Am. J. Reprod. Immunol. 28, 164–167.

Friedman, D., Buyon, J., Kim, M., Glickstein, J.S. 2003. Fetal cardiac function assessed by Doppler myocardial performance index (Tei index). Ultrasound Obstet. Gynecol. 21, 33–36.

Glickstein, J.S., Buyon, J.P., Friedman, D. 2000. Pulsed Doppler echocardiographic assessment of the fetal PR interval. Am. J. Cardiol. 86, 236–239.

Gordon, P., Rosenthal, E., Simpson, J.M., Sharland, G., Brucato, A., Franceschini, F., De Bosschere, K., Meheus, L., Meroni, P.L., Hughesz, G.R., Buyon, J. 2004. Anti-52 kDa Ro, anti-60 kDa Ro, and anti-La antibody profiles in neonatal lupus. J. Rheumatol. 31, 2480–2487.

Groves, A.M.M., Allan, L.D., Rosenthal, E. 1995. Therapeutic trial of sympathomimetics in three cases of complete heart block in the fetus. Circulation 92, 3394–3396.

Jaeggi, E.T. 2001. Diagnosis, management and outcome of congenital atrio-ventricular block. Frontiers Fetal Health 3, 177–182.

Julkunen, H., Eronen, M. 2001. The rate of recurrence of isolated congenital heart block: a population-based study. Arthritis Rheum. 44, 487–488.

Kanagasegar, S., Cimaz, R., Kurien, B.T., Brucato, A., Scofield, R.H. 2002. Neonatal lupus manifests as isolated neutropenia and mildly abnormal liver functions. J. Rheumatol. 29, 187–191.

Kertesz, N.J., Fenrich, A.L., Friedman, R.A. 1997. Congenital complete atrioventricular block. Tex. Heart Inst J. 24, 301–307.

Laxer, R.M., Roberts, E.A., Gross, K.R., Britton, J.R., Cutz, E., Dimmick, J., Petty, R.E., Silverman, E.D. 1990. Liver disease in neonatal lupus erythematosus. J. Pediatr. 116, 238–242.

Lee, L.A. 1993. Neonatal lupus erythematosus. J. Invest Dermatol. 100, 9s–13s.

Lee, L.A., Sokol, R.J., Buyon, J.P. 2002. Hepatobiliary disease in neonatal lupus: prevalence and clinical characteristics in cases enrolled in a national registry. J. Pediatr. 109, E11.

Lockshin, M.D., Bonfa, E., Elkon, K., Druzin, M.L. 1988. Neonatal risk to newborns of mothers with systemic lupus erythematosus. Arthritis Rheum. 31, 697–701.

Martin, V., Lee, L.A., Askanase, A.D., Katholi, M., Buyon, J.P. 2002. Long term follow-up of children with neonatal lupus and their unaffected siblings. Arthritis Rheum. 46, 2377–2383.

Moak, J.P., Barron, K.S., Hougen, T.J., Cohen, M.H., Nordenberg, A., Van Hare, G.F., Perez, M., Cecchin, F., Schneider, D.S., Nehgme, R.A., Buyon, J.P. 2001. Congenital heart block: development of late-onset cardiomyopathy, a previously underappreciated sequela. J. Am. Coll. Cardiol. 37, 238–242.

Neiman, A.R., Lee, L.A., Weston, W.L., Buyon, J.P. 2000. Cutaneous manifestations of neonatal lupus without heart block: characteristics of mothers and children enrolled in a national registry. J. Pediatr. 37, 674–680.

Nield, L.E., Silverman, E.D., Smallhorn, J.F., Taylor, G.P., Mullen, J.B., Benson, L.N., Hornberger, L.K. 2002. Endocardial fibroelastosis associated with maternal anti-Ro and anti-La antibodies in the absence of atrioventricular block. J. Am. Coll. Cardiol. 40, 796–802.

Ramsey-Goldman, R., Hom, D., Deng, J.S., Ziegler, G.C., Kahl, L.E., Steen, V.D., LaPorte, R.E., Medsger, T.A., Jr. 1986. Anti-SS-A antibodies and fetal outcome in maternal systemic lupus erythematosus. Arthritis Rheum. 29, 1269–1273.

Rosenthal, D., Friedman, D.M., Buyon, J., Dubin, A. 2002. Validation of the Doppler PR interval in the fetus. J. Am. Soc. Echocardiogr. 15, 1029–1030.

Saleeb, S., Copel, J., Friedman, D., Buyon, J.P. 1999. Comparison of treatment with fluorinated glucocorticoids to the natural history of autoantibody–associated congenital heart block: retrospective review of the Research Registry for Neonatal Lupus. Arthritis Rheum. 42, 2335–2345.

Schoenlebe, J., Buyon, J.P., Zitelli, B.J., Friedman, D., Greco, M.A., Knisely, A.S. 1993. Neonatal hemochromatosis associated with maternal autoantibodies against Ro/SS-A and La/SS-B ribonucleoproteins. Am. J. Dis. Child. 147, 1072–1075.

Shinohara, K., Miyagawa, S., Fujita, T., Aono, T., Kidoguchi, K. 1999. Neonatal lupus erythematosus: results of maternal corticosteroid therapy. Obstet. Gynecol. 93, 952–957.

Waltuck, J., Buyon, J. 1994. Autoantibody-associated congenital heart block: outcome in mothers and children. Ann. Int. Med. 120, 544–551.

Watson, R., Kang, J.E., May, M., Hudak, M., Kickler, T., Provost, T.T. 1988. Thrombocytopenia in the neonatal lupus syndrome. Arch. Dermatol. 124, 560–563.

Handbook of Systemic Autoimmune Diseases, Volume 4
Reproductive and Hormonal Aspects of Systemic Autoimmune Diseases
Michael Lockshin and D. Ware Branch, editors

CHAPTER 9

Use of Anti-Rheumatic Drugs in Pregnancy

Roger A. Levy*

Disciplina de Reumatologia, Faculdade de Ciências Médicas, Universidade do Estado do Rio de Janeiro, RJ, Brasil

1. Introduction

Rheumatic diseases management in women of childbearing years involves counseling about contraception and pregnancy. It is crucial for the practicing internist, rheumatologist and obstetrician to be aware of the indications, limitations and risks of the increasingly expanding therapeutic armamentarium currently used in rheumatology. Judicious decisions have to be made according to each case, and issues related to a pregnancy are of particular concern because of the fetus. Some drugs classified as being of higher risk based on animal studies, are used during pregnancy in order to control maternal disease activity (Briggs et al., 2002). The recognition that in utero exposure to diethyl-stilbesterol could result in adenocarcinoma of the vagina 20 years later should serve to remind us that the long-term effects of some agents may only be known in the future.

Until the 1980s, the common advice to women with autoimmune rheumatic diseases, especially systemic lupus erythematosus (SLE), systemic sclerosis and vasculitic syndromes, was to avoid pregnancy because of the perception that maternal or fetal risks were of an unacceptable magnitude. Currently, there seems to be an agreement that pregnancy should be postponed until major disease activity is treated and certain appropriate medications (such as hydroxychloroquine for lupus) should be continued to reduce the chances of disease flare during pregnancy. Most of the data on pregnancy and autoimmune rheumatic conditions derived from retrospective analyses, but some prospective studies involving the use of *anti-rheumatic drugs* have been performed in the past two decades. The field remains, however, with very few randomized clinical trials (Gordon, 2004).

Women who take cytotoxic drugs should be informed of the risks of impaired fertility and congenital malformations, and must use effective methods of contraception. During pregnancy, nonsteroidal anti-inflammatory drugs (NSAID) may be used until the last 6 weeks, and low to moderate doses of corticosteroids are relatively safe throughout pregnancy. Among the disease-modifying agents, sulfasalazine and hydroxychloroquine treatment may be continued in pregnancy. Cytotoxic drugs may be used after the first trimester to treat life-threatening disease. During lactation, prednisone, sulfasalazine and hydroxychloroquine may be used cautiously. Women using heparin for treatment of anti-phospholipid antibody syndrome like those taking corticosteroids should take measures to prevent bone loss (Janssen and Genta, 2000).

The survey conducted by Ostensen in 2004 reviewed the maternal and fetal side effects of nonsteroidal anti-inflammatory drugs and immunosuppressive agents in pregnant patients. She concluded that the classic NSAID are not teratogenic, but if given in late pregnancy can induce renal and cardiac fetal deleterious effects. Similar effects may be

*Corresponding author.
Tel./fax: 55-21-2567-7530.
E-mail address: rlevy@uerj.br (R.A. Levy).

DOI: 10.1016/S1571-5078(05)04009-2

expected of the new, selective COX2-inhibitors. NSAID, when used, should therefore be stopped by gestational week 32.

Corticosteroids are frequently necessary to control rheumatic disease flares and for prevention of serious organic damage. Among disease-modifying drugs, sulfasalazine and anti-malarials have the safest record. Cyclosporine and azathioprine can be given throughout pregnancy if disease control requires it. There are insufficient data to conclude anything about mycophenolate mofetil usage in pregnancy. Animal studies suggest teratogenicity, and at least one report of human teratogenicity exists. In the United States, mycophenolate mofetil cannot be recommended in pregnancy. Monoclonal antibodies, although antibodies, may not be able to cross the placenta. The severity of the disease under treatment decides if continuation of one of these drugs is justified. Prophylactic withdrawal of drugs before pregnancy is mandatory for leflunomide and the cytotoxic agents methotrexate and cyclophosphamide, known teratogens (Ostensen, 2004).

The anti-rheumatic drug use during pregnancy should take into account their effect on disease activity and maternal side effects, as well as fetal development, teratogenic potential, nursing and potential late effects on the offspring. In the following pages, the recommendations for the indications and limitations of the most commonly used drugs in rheumatology during pregnancy will be reviewed. We will follow the order of the risk factor classification proposed by the Food and Drug Administration in 1980 adapted in 2002 (Briggs et al., 2002), outlined in Table 1. These ratings are indicated for drugs discussed below with the designations A–D, and X, with indications of * or $_M$ as indicated in Table 1.

2. Risk factor B drugs

Risk factor B drugs are those that either animal studies with no fetal risk have been published and no controlled human data or animal studies with defects were confirmed in humans in first trimester or later.

Table 1
Risk factors assigned based on the level of risk the drug poses to the fetus according to animal and human studies (Adapted from reference Briggs, Freeman and Yaffe, 2002)

Category	Justification	Example
A	Controlled studies without evidence of fetal harm in first trimester or later	Folic acid, vitamin D
B	Either animal studies with no fetal risk and no controlled human data or animal studies with defects were confirmed in humans in first trimester or later	Acetaminofen, low-dose ASA, sulfasalazine, anti-TNF, cyclobenzaprine
C	Either animal studies revealed teratogenic effects and there are no controlled studies in humans, or studies in animals and humans are not available. Used only if potential benefits justifies the potential risk to the fetus	Certain NSAIDs/D, COXIBs/D, prednisone, prednisolone*/D, gold salts, hydroxychloroquine, mycophenolate, cyclosporine, IVIG, cevimeline, pilocarpine, amitriptyline, tramadol, gabapentin
D	Positive evidence of human fetal risk, but the benefits may be acceptable despite the risk (life-threatening)	Azathioprine, d-Penicillamine, NSAIDs (third trimester), cyclophosphamide, colchicine, warfarin (second and third trimesters)
X	Fetal abnormalities in animal and human studies. The use clearly outweighs any possible benefit. Contraindicated in women who may become pregnant	Thalidomide, methotrexate, leflunomide, misoprostol, bosentan
M	Product rated by the manufacturer in its professional literature	
*	Divergence of rating between manufacturer and independent authors	Azathioprine

Acetaminophen (B) has been safely used in all stages of pregnancy; continuous high doses should be avoided due to liver toxicity. It is the most commonly used anti-pyretic agent just before delivery in cases of chorioamnionitis. A study evaluated the prevalence of congenital abnormalities and fetal growth in 123 women exposed to acetaminophen during pregnancy. The control group was composed of 13,329 pregnant women who did not receive any prescription. The authors found no excess risk of malformation [OR = 0.7 (95% CI 0.1–5.5)], and no evidence that acetaminophen influenced fetal growth (Thulstrup et al., 1999). Breast-feeding when taking acetaminophen appears safe (Committee on Drugs American Academy of Pediatrics, 1994).

Low-dose ASA (aspirin)—81–100 mg/day, is widely used as an anti-platelet agent, to prevent pre-eclampsia and thrombotic complications of anti-phospholipid syndrome. Low-dose ASA use during pregnancy does not increase the risk of neonatal or maternal bleeding and has been adopted as the current therapy by many referral centers (Tincani et al., 2003). It possesses no increased risk of fetal teratogenicity. Some practitioners suggest withdrawing low-dose ASA 1 or 2 weeks before delivery to decrease the possibility of bleeding from vaginal or cervical lacerations or the uterus. Aspirin taken in anti-inflammatory doses is classified as (C).

Sulfasalazine (B_M*) data in pregnant women are mostly derived from studies and reports in patients with inflammatory bowel diseases. It is well known that its use near term is related to prolonged neonatal jaundice and therefore should be avoided; thus its use in the late third trimester is classified as risk (D). The maximum dose recommended is 2 g/day and concomitant folic acid usage is advised. Because it acts as a folate inhibitor, sulfasalazine potentially could be teratogenic. Norgard et al. performed a case-control study within the Hungarian Case Control Surveillance of Congenital Abnormalities, 1980–1996, based on 22,865 newborn infants or fetuses with congenital abnormalities, and 38,151 babies without any detected congenital abnormalities (control group). They found that 17 pregnant women (0.07%) were treated with sulfasalazine in the case group, and 26 (0.07%) in the control group. The overall adjusted odds ratio of congenital abnormalities after sulfasalazine treatment was 1.2 (95% CI: 0.6–2.1). None of the analyses indicated any significant increased prevalence of selected congenital abnormalities among the exposed compared with the not exposed (Norgard et al., 2001). Breast-feeding is permitted when sulfasalazine is used (Committee on Drugs American Academy of Pediatrics 1994).

Cyclobenzaprine **(B_M*)** and sertraline **(B_M*)** are thought to be the safest therapeutic options for the treatment of fibromyalgia during pregnancy, although data are scarce.

Low molecular weight heparins (LMWH) **(B_M*)** such as enoxaparin and dalteparin have been widely used for thrombosis prophylaxis and treatment in pregnancy and in patients with anti-phospholipid syndrome. Though they have an excellent therapeutic index and a lower risk of heparin-induced thrombocytopenia compared to unfractionated heparins (UFH) (C_M), the long-term use of LMWH (as well as of unfractionated heparin) may be associated with increased bone mass loss during pregnancy. For that reason daily doses of 500 mg of calcium and 400 IU of vitamin D(A*) are recommended. Breast-feeding is not contraindicated in women using LMWH taken orally by the neonate is digested in the infants' gastrointestinal tract. UFH is not excreted in the human milk.

Limited human data suggest that biologic agents such as the **anti-TNF agents** [infliximab (B), etanercept (B_M) and adalimumab] and the **anti-CD20** agent rituximab are not teratogenic. These large proteins do not cross the placenta well, if at all, and do not appear to reach the fetal circulation. The best available information comes from reports of infliximab use in pregnancy. One case series described 96 women with Crohn's disease or rheumatoid arthritis who took infliximab during pregnancy, including some with first trimester exposure cases. The authors concluded that infliximab was not associated with either an increased frequency of birth defects or adverse pregnancy outcomes (Katz et al., 2004). There has been a report of unintentional use of rituximab during the first trimester of pregnancy in a patient with non-Hodgkin's lymphoma. The pregnancy was uncomplicated, and a healthy child was born at full term. Careful hematological and immunological monitoring revealed no adverse effects resulting from exposure to rituximab (Kimby et al., 2004).

At present very limited data suggest that TNF antagonists are neither embryotoxic nor teratogenic (Khanna et al., 2004).

Sills et al. described the first case of ovulation induction, intrauterine insemination, normal pregnancy and singleton delivery of a healthy infant following chronic (> 1 year) pre-ovulatory TNF-inhibitor therapy for rheumatoid arthritis (Sills et al., 2001). Reasonable proof of safety in pregnancy is, however, lacking for TNF antagonists.

Although TNF inhibitors, as well as other monoclonal antibody therapies, do not seem to cause fetal harm, and although rheumatologists generally concur that they should not be withdrawn when pregnancy is planned or diagnosed, it is not recommended that this kind of therapy be started during pregnancy due to lack of experience.

The monoclonal antibodies are excreted in the milk but digested by the infants' gastric juice.

3. Risk factor C drugs

Risk factor C drugs are those for which animal studies revealed teratogenic effects and there are no controlled studies in humans, or studies in animals and humans are not available. These drugs should be used only if potential benefits justify the potential risk to the fetus.

Most of the *non-steroidal anti-inflammatory drugs (NSAIDs)* are classified as (C), but they should not be used during the third trimester (when they are classified as risk factor D), because NSAIDs cause constriction of the fetal *ductus arteriosus* that can lead to pulmonary artery hypertension, and, later, in prolonged labor. Less frequently fetal loss, low birth weight and clotting and glomerular disorders have been reported. Nonetheless, some arthritic patients require such treatment (prednisone is preferred, if possible). Indomethacin (B*) is widely used to prevent premature labor, but its use has been linked to enterocolitis (Parilla et al., 2000). Ibuprofen (B_M*) use has been linked to glomerular defects leading to renal insufficiency or failure (Briggs 2002). The use of NSAIDs and conception was addressed on the Danish birth registry cohort study involving 1462 pregnant women who had taken up prescriptions for NSAIDs (excluding indomethacin users) in the period from 30 days before conception to birth compared to 17,259 pregnant women who were not prescribed any drugs during pregnancy. Analysis of the data was performed to estimate the risk of adverse birth outcome. A case-control study was carried on 4268 women who had miscarriages, of who 63 had taken NSAIDs, and 29,750 primiparous controls that had live births. The authors concluded that the use of NSAIDs during pregnancy does not seem to increase the risk of adverse birth outcome but is associated with increased risk of miscarriage (Nielsen et al., 2001).

A population-based cohort study on prenatal use of NSAIDs, aspirin and acetaminophen ascertained by in-person interviewing of the Kaiser Permanente Medical Care Program, in the San Francisco area, involved 1055 women. The pregnancy outcomes up to 20 weeks of gestation were evaluated. Fifty-three women (5%) reported prenatal NSAID use around conception or during pregnancy. After adjustment for potential confounders, prenatal NSAIDs use was associated with an 80% increased risk of miscarriage [adjusted hazard ratio 1.8 (95% CI 1.0–3.2)]. The association was stronger if the initial NSAIDs use was around the time of conception or if NSAIDs use lasted more than a week. Prenatal aspirin use was similarly associated with an increased risk of miscarriage. However, prenatal use of acetaminophen, was not associated with increased risk of miscarriage regardless of timing and duration of use (Li et al., 2003).

According to Ostensen up to 80% of patients with SLE are treated with NSAIDs for musculoskeletal symptoms, serositis and headache. Her survey reviewed the literature on non-selective and selective inhibitors of cyclooxygenases (COX) with an emphasis on the efficacy and safety profile reported in SLE patients. As ovulation is concerned, it can be adversely affected by non-selective and selective inhibitors of COX-inhibitors (Ostensen and Villiger, 2001).

NSAID safe use once pregnancy is under way is supported by a small and limited prospective study involving 88 pregnant patients with inflammatory rheumatic disease divided into 2 groups, 45 who were treated and 43 not treated with NSAIDs during pregnancy. Possible long-term effects of NSAIDs on offspring development were evaluated by telephone interview. There were no differences with regard to demographic data. Forty-nine pregnancies had been exposed to standard doses of NSAIDs for a mean duration of 15.3 weeks. The comparison of pregnancies exposed with those not exposed to NSAIDs had no differences in all of the parameters studied. No significant differences were found between the groups with respect to health and development of offspring at follow-up (Ostensen and Ostensen, 1996). The authors' personal experience is that short courses of low-dose steroids are safer to use in SLE pregnancy when indicated. Breast-feeding on NSAIDs is possible although they may be excreted in low concentrations in the milk, no toxicity has been reported (Committee on Drugs American Academy of Pediatrics, 1994).

The COX-2 selective inhibitors *celecoxib* (C_M*) and *lumiracoxib* have been introduced in the market more recently than the other NSAIDs and fewer data on pregnancy exposure are available. Pre- and post-implantation losses were evident with celecoxib the same way it was with the use of indomethacin in rats. The anti-implantation effect of the classical NSAIDs, as well as selective COX-2 inhibitors, may be due to decidualization defects. Thus COX-2 inhibitors should be used with caution in childbearing age women who either could or intend to become pregnant. Indeed, it has been suggested that specific COX-2 inhibitors with their good gastric safety profile may have a potential role in non-hormonal postcoital contraception (Sookvanichsilp and Pulbutr, 2002). Both celecoxib and lumiracoxib are indicated for the treatment of primary dysmenorrhea, and may be effective in postoperative pain, including hysterectomy, and pain associated with endometriosis. These substances have been studied and found to be effective tocolytic agents without the fetal risks seen with conventional NSAIDs (Hayes and Rock, 2002). The awareness of conception inhibition with specific COX-2 inhibitors should be the same as with the classical NSAIDs (Chan, 2004).

As with classic NSAIDs, COX-2 inhibitor use during the third trimester (D) is also associated with constriction or premature closure of *ductus arteriosus* (Stika et al., 2002). Breast-feeding should be avoided if celecoxib or lumiracoxib are used.

Unlike the fluorinated corticosteroids, *prednisone* (C*) and *prednisolone* (C*–D in the first trimester) are inactivated in the placenta, with less than 10% of the active drug appearing in the fetal circulation. However, the use of glucocorticoids during pregnancy is related in a dose-dependent fashion to several important maternal adverse effects, including diabetes, edema, aggravation of hypertension, preeclampsia, premature rupture of the membranes, immune suppression, osteopenia and osteonecrosis (Cortés-Hernández et al., 2002). Prednisone or prednisolone is indicated during SLE pregnancy in order to treat difficult to control arthritis, as well as alveolitis, pericarditis and myositis. Calcium and vitamin D supplementation is advised when more then 2 weeks use is planned.

The Israeli Teratogen Information Service studied prospectively 311 pregnancies counseled regarding systemic use of different corticosteroids in the first trimester and compared the rate of major congenital anomalies to that of 790 controls that were counseled for non-teratogenic exposure. The results of the study support that corticosteroids do not represent a major teratogenic risk in humans (Gur et al., 2004), though concern remains about the possibility of increased risk of cleft palate. Judicious use of prednisone or prednisolone is recommended in patients with SLE and dermatomyositis during pregnancy, when long-term moderate to high dosages are required and concomitant hydroxychloroquine is already prescribed, azathioprine use has to be considered.

There are several adopted protocols for adrenal protection during interventions such a labor or cesarean section for patients who are currently on or have been used steroids in the previous 2 years. We use intravenous hydrocortisone 100 mg TID for 3 days. Breast-feeding is permitted in patients using up to 40 mg/day of prednisone or prednisolone.

Fluorinated steroids such as dexamethasone and *betamethasone (C*)* are used in pregnancy to enhance fetal lung maturity in pregnancies at high risk for preterm birth. They also used in cases of newly identified congenital heart block associated with neonatal lupus syndrome (Buyon et al., 2004). Current clinical data indicate that betamethasone is the drug of choice for antenatal treatment for lung maturation when preterm delivery is highly likely (Jobe and Soll, 2004).

Gold salts (C_M) use during pregnancy has not been related to human teratogenicity, although abdominal wall and growth defects have been reported in rodents. Though infrequently used today, gold salts may be continued during pregnancy but should not be started during pregnancy. Breast-feeding is permitted for patients on gold therapy (Rayburn, 1998). Gold salts are excreted in the milk but the American Academy of Pediatrics considers gold salts to be compatible with breast-feeding (Committee on Drugs American Academy of Pediatrics, 1994).

Past concerns about potential adverse fetal effects due to the use of **anti-malarials** during pregnancy (Parke and Rothfield, 1996; Parke and West, 1996) have been allayed by recent analyses. Currently, *hydroxychloroquine* (C) should not be discontinued during lupus pregnancy. Not only is the elimination half-life 1–2 months, but stopping anti-malarial drugs can precipitate disease flares of SLE, which in turn may be detrimental to pregnancy (Buchanan et al., 1996; Borden and Parke, 2001).

In adults, chronic treatment with chloroquine or hydroxychloroquine carries a small risk of sight-threatening pigmentary retinopathy. To obtain safety data for its use in pregnancy, Klinger et al. did ophthalmic examinations in 21 children born to women who took anti-malarials during pregnancy. Average daily maternal doses were 317 mg hydroxychloroquine and 332 mg chloroquine, and the mean duration of gestational exposure was 7.2 months. No ophthalmic abnormality was detected in any infant. The authors concluded that the use of these drugs during pregnancy may not pose a significant risk of ocular toxicity to offspring (Klinger et al., 2001).

Additional recent studies in SLE patients treated with hydroxychloroquine or chloroquine also have shown no adverse effect, either on the pregnancy or on the fetus, suggesting that anti-malarials are safe during pregnancy (Cortés-Hernández, 2002). A randomized, controlled study designed to evaluate the need for hydroxychloroquine during lupus pregnancy and to assess safety included 20 consecutive pregnant patients with SLE or discoid lupus erythematosus (DLE). None of the patients on hydroxychloroquine group had a lupus exacerbation, and at conclusion the placebo group had significantly higher scores. Preeclampsia was diagnosed in three patients in the placebo group (one fetal death). Comparing prednisone dosage change, we noted a decrease in the hydroxychloroquine and an increase in the placebo group. Delivery age and Apgar scores were higher in the hydroxychloroquine group. Neonatal examination did not reveal congenital abnormalities, nor did a neuro-ophthalmological and auditory evaluation at 1.5–3 years of age (Levy et al., 2001).

Seventy-eight lupus experts from North America and UK answered a survey elaborated by Al-Herz et al. regarding their experience using anti-malarials in pregnancy and lactation. Of the 67% that responded, none reported having seen any fetal toxicity with anti-malarials use, and pregnancy was never terminated because of drug use, unless the patient insisted ($n = 1$). Postpartum, 63% continued anti-malarials and advised breast-feeding. The majority of lupus experts continue anti-malarials during pregnancy. This was particularly true for those who treated a larger number of pregnant lupus patients per year, and the majority recommended breast-feeding and continuation of anti-malarials postpartum. These practices are supported by the limited literature available (Al-Herz et al., 2002).

A large series of 133 pregnancies in women treated with hydroxychloroquine, resulting in 117 live births has been reported by Costedoat-Chalumeau et al. and the results were compared with a control group of 53 women with similar disorders who did not receive hydroxychloroquine. The authors performed electrocardiography in 47 children of mothers treated with hydroxychloroquine and in 45 children in the control group. Eighty-eight percent of pregnancies in the hydroxychloroquine group and 84% in the control group ended successfully. On the electrocardiograms, the PR interval and the corrected QT interval were not statistically different between groups. No visual, hearing, growth or developmental abnormalities were reported in any of the children at the last follow-up (ages 12–108 months; mean age 26 months). These findings support evidence for the safety of hydroxychloroquine therapy during pregnancy. The authors suggest that this treatment should be maintained throughout pregnancy in patients with SLE (Costedoat-Chalumeau et al., 2003). Breast-feeding is permitted for anti-malarial users and is well tolerated.

Mycophenolate Mofetil—MMF (C_M) induces fetal resorption and malformations in rats and rabbits at the recommended human dosage. It probably crosses the placenta and the recommendation is that the patient should wait 6 weeks before conception is attempted. Le Ray et al. reported multiple malformations in an infant born of a woman treated with MMF before conception and during the first trimester of pregnancy (Le Ray et al., 2004). On the other hand, Pergola et al. reported a successful pregnancy outcome on a patient exposed to MMF in the first trimester of pregnancy (Pergola et al., 2001). There is little evidence on safety of MMF in pregnancy it should only be used when the benefits are clearly outweighing the potential risks. Breast-feeding for patients on MMF is not advised due to the increased risks of infections and lymphoma.

Cyclosporine (C_M) is an immunosuppressive used for several clinical situations in rheumatology. It has been found to be embryotoxic in mice at 2.5-fold the maximum human recommended dose. In humans, cyclosporine has been linked to low birth weight, gestational diabetes and hypertension. Most of the data are derived from renal transplanted patients and the long-term immune effects are still unknown (Petri, 2003). Breast-feeding is not advised for patients on cyclosporine; transient leucopenia in the infant has been reported.

Intravenous immune globulin—IVIG (C_M) has been used for more then 20 years and is beneficial for patients with a variety of autoimmune disorders (Branch et al., 2004) including the antiphospholipid syndrome (Tincani et al., 2003).

There are no data concerning breast-feeding on patients on IVIG.

Cevimeline or **pilocarpine** (C_M) oral administration is indicated for improving the dryness symptoms of Sjögren's syndrome. Their use reduced implantation in rats at 5-fold the maximum human recommended dose and induced fetal death at 10-fold the maximum human recommended dose. Both substances have a low molecular weight and are capable of crossing the placenta. Milk excretion is expected for both cevimeline and pilocarpine and breast-feeding is not recommended.

4. Risk factor D drugs

Drugs ranked as risk D possess positive evidence of human fetal risk, but the benefits may be acceptable despite the risk (life-threatening disease conditions).

The use of *azathioprine* (D_M) in fertile women that are using intra uterine devices (IUD) contraceptives is associated with decreased IUD effectiveness. In human pregnancy it seems to be safe since the fetal liver is not capable of converting azathioprine into its active form. Preterm delivery and marrow toxicity have been reported and growth restriction may also occur. Large series have been performed in patients with inflammatory bowel disease (Moskovitz et al., 2004). In dosages of 1.5–2.0 mg/kg/day azathioprine has not been found to be teratogenic in humans (Rajapakse Korelitz, 2001).

The possible impact of azathioprine, as well as, cyclosporine, on the fetal immune system is a matter of debate. In neonates exposed to the drug, immunoglobulin levels and response to hepatitis B vaccine did not differ from that of controls. Limited data suggest that antenatal exposure to azathioprine or cyclosporine does not have a profound effect on the developing immune system (Cimaz, 2004). Breast-feeding is not advised for women using azathioprine, it has been related to delay in sexual development and impaired fertility in females (Committee on Drugs American Academy of Pediatrics, 1994).

Penicillamine (D_M) use during pregnancy is associated with a 5% risk of malformation. Systemic sclerosis patients considering pregnancy should be advised to discontinue *d*-penicillamine. Once the patient is pregnant, blood pressure, renal and pulmonary function should be checked regularly, and urinary sediment evaluation and creatinine clearance are mandatory during follow-up (Lyle, 1978). If penicillamine treatment must be continued, and this indication is questioned by many, lower doses (<500 mg/day) seem advisable. Breast-feeding is probably not safe.

First trimester exposure to *coumarin derivatives* (D*) is associated with an embryopathy syndrome known as "fetal warfarin syndrome". Exposure between the 6th and the 9th menstrual week of pregnancy results in a 10–25% chance of teratogenicity (Briggs et al., 2002). In selected cases, warfarin derivatives may be used during pregnancy in the second and third trimesters when the potential benefits appear to outweigh the risks (Tincani et al., 2003). A meta-analysis involving 208 pregnancies exposed during the second trimester found 84% of normal infants and no "fetal warfarin syndrome". Exposure near term may result in or neonatal bleeding and should be avoided. Warfarin is compatible with breast-feeding.

Cyclophosphamide (D_M) use in fertile females is related to diminished fertility due to premature ovarian failure. Cyclophosphamide use during the first trimester of pregnancy is related to multiple fetal abnormalities and frequently leads to abortion (Matalon et al., 2004). Use in the second or third trimesters should be limited to life threatening cases of lupus nephritis. Breast-feeding is not recommended, because cyclophosphamide is excreted into milk and has been linked to neonatal neutropenia, immune suppression and carcinogenesis.

5. Risk X Drugs

Risk X drugs are those that have been related to fetal abnormalities in animal and human studies. The use of such agents clearly outweighs any possible benefit, and they are formally contraindicated in women who may become pregnant. *Thalidomide* is the classical example of a drug of this group.

Methotrexate (MTX) and **leflunomide** (X) are folic acid inhibitors, they suppress lymphocyte proliferation, and are classified as a purine and pyrimidine inhibitors. Folic acid is essential for proper embryonic development. Both MTX- and leflunomide-induced congenital defects in human and in animal models. Leflunomide exhibits a dose-related teratogenicity and embryo/fetal toxicity in animals at doses equivalent to or lower than the used human doses. Even occupational exposure may present a risk to the fetus (Loyd et al., 1999).

Women recently or currently on leflunomide and who are considering pregnancy or are inadvertently pregnant should be treated with cholestyramine (B) (8 g TID for 11 days). If the plasma leflunomide level is >0.02 mg/mL on two occasions 14 days apart, cholestyramine should be continued (Brent, 2001). A pregnancy registry has been established to monitor fetal outcomes of leflunomide exposure. Health care providers are encouraged to call 1-877-311-8972 (USA) in order to register such patients. Both MTX and leflunomide are contraindicated if pregnancy is planned; because of their long half-life, leflunomide should be withdrawn 2 years before attempting conception. A recent survey replied by 175 rheumatologists inquiring about their perception of fetal risk, recommendations regarding the use of birth control in women of childbearing age taking DMARD, and the pregnancy outcomes of women with DMARD exposure, showed that pregnancy was contraindicated in women taking MTX (95%) or leflunomide (92.7%). The series reported 38 cases of pregnancy during MTX therapy and 10 on leflunomide, three of which in the MTX group had congenital malformations (Chakravarty et al., 2003). In case a patient on MTX is found to be pregnant, in the United States termination is recommended; if declined, folic acid 5 mg/day supplementation must be promptly instituted and close monitoring by ultrasonography is advised. In our experience, the cases with gross malformations are spontaneously aborted. The American Academy of Pediatrics recommends against breast-feeding while on MTX because of several potential problems, including immune suppression, neutropenia; as well as, adverse effects on growth and carcinogenesis. Breast-feeding is not recommended for women using leflunomide, its low molecular weight permits milk excretion (Committee on Drugs American Academy of Pediatrics, 1994).

6. Male Patients

Male patients taking cytotoxic agents like methotrexate, sulfasalazine, cyclosporine, azathioprine, or leflunomide should be apprised of the possibilities of infertility and *teratogenicity*. There is no evidence in the literature that MTX or leflunomide impair spermatogenesis or induce male infertility. There are no reports to date of adverse pregnancy outcomes among men exposed to MTX before conception. Several case reports and studies report no effect; others report reversible sterility. These studies were performed in oncology patients exposed to other agents. When used alone it apparently was not related to increased infertility (French and Koren, 2003, Rains et al., 1995). Men taking MTX or leflunomide, like those using cyclosporine and azathioprine seem to have normal sperm motility and count. On the other hand sulfasalazine use may induce oligospermia and more rarely azoospermia that can take up to 2 months to revert (Rains et al., 1995). A spermogram should be performed in patients on sulfasalazine intending to father a child (Janssen and Genta, 2000).

References

Al-Herz, A., Schulzer, M., Esdaile, J.M. 2002. Survey of antimalarial use in lupus pregnancy and lactation. J. Rheumatol. 29 (4), 700–706.

Borden, M.B., Parke, A.L. 2001. Antimalarial drugs in systemic lupus erythematosus: use in pregnancy. Drug Safety 24 (14), 1055–1063.

Branch, D.W., Peaceman, A.M., Druzin, M., Silver, R.K., El-Sayed, Y., Silver, R.M., Esplin, M.S., Spinnato, J., Harger, J. 2004. A multicenter, placebo-controlled pilot study of intravenous immune globulin treatment of antiphospholipid syndrome during pregnancy. The Pregnancy Loss Study Group. Am. J. Obstet. Gynecol. 182, 122–127.

Brent, R.L. 2001. Teratogen update: reproductive risks of leflunomide (Arava); a pyrimidine synthesis inhibitor: counseling women taking leflunomide before and during pregnancy and men taking leflunomide who are contemplating fathering a child. Teratology 63, 106–112.

Briggs, G.G., Freeman, R.K., Yaffe, S.J. 2002. Drugs in Pregnancy and Lactation. 6th ed., Lippincott Williams and Wilkins, Philadelphia, PA.

Buchanan, N.M., Toubi, E., Khamashta, M.A., Lima, F., Kerslake, S., Hughes, G.R. 1996. Hydroxychloroquine and lupus pregnancy: review of a series of 36 cases. Ann. Rheum. Dis. 55 (7), 486–488.

Buyon, J.P., Rupel, A., Clancy, R.M. 2004. Neonatal lupus syndromes. Lupus 13 (9), 705–712.

Chakravarty, E.F., Sanchez-Yamamoto, D., Bush, T.M. 2003. The use of disease modifying antirheumatic drugs in women with rheumatoid arthritis of childbearing age: a survey of practice patterns and pregnancy outcomes. J. Rheumatol. 30 (2), 241–246.

Chan, V.S. 2004. A mechanistic perspective on the specificity and extent of COX-2 inhibition in pregnancy. Drug Safety 27 (7), 421–426.

Cimaz, R., Meregalli, E., Biggioggero, M., Borghi, O., Tincani, A., Motta, M., Airo, P., Meroni, P.L. 2004. Alterations in the immune system of children from mothers treated with immunosuppressive agents during pregnancy. Toxicol. Lett. 149 (1–3), 155–162.

Committee on Drugs American Academy of Pediatrics. 1994. The transfer of drugs and other chemicals into human milk. Pediatrics 93, 137–150.

Cortés-Hernández, J., Ordi-Ros, J., Paredes, F., Casellas, M., Castillo, F., Vilardell-Tarres, M. 2002. Clinical predictors of fetal and maternal outcome in systemic lupus erythematosus: a prospective study of 103 pregnancies. Rheumatology 41, 643–650.

Costedoat-Chalumeau, N., Amoura, Z., Duhaut, P., Huong du, L.T., Sebbough, D., Wechsler, B., Vauthier, D., Denjoy, I., Lupoglazoff, J.M., Piette, J.C. 2003. Safety of hydroxychloroquine in pregnant patients with connective tissue diseases: a study of one hundred thirty-three cases compared with a control group. Arthritis Rheum. 48 (11), 3207–3211.

French, A.E., Koren, G. 2003. Effect of methotrexate on male fertility. Can. Fam. Physician 49, 577–578.

Gordon, C. 2004. Pregnancy and autoimmune diseases. Best Pract. Res. Clin. Rheumatol. 18 (3), 357–379.

Gur, C., Diav-Citrin, O., Shechtman, S., Arnon, J., Ornoy, A. 2004. Pregnancy outcome after first trimester exposure to corticosteroids: a prospective controlled study. Reprod. Toxicol. 18 (1), 93–101.

Hayes, E.C., Rock, J.A. 2002. COX-2 inhibitors and their role in gynecology. Obstet. Gynecol. Surv. 57 (11), 768–780.

Janssen, N.M., Genta, M.S. 2000. The effects of immunosuppressive and anti-inflammatory medications on fertility, pregnancy, and lactation. Arch. Intern. Med. 160 (5), 610–619.

Jobe, A.H., Soll, R.F. 2004. Choice and dose of corticosteroid for antenatal treatments. Am. J. Obstet. Gynecol. 190 (4), 878–881.

Katz, J.A., Antoni, C., Keenan, G.F., Smith, D.E., Jacobs, S.J., Lichtenstein, G.R. 2004. Outcome of pregnancy in women receiving infliximab for the treatment of Crohn's disease and rheumatoid arthritis. Am. J. Gastroenterol. 99 (12), 2385–2392.

Khanna, D., McMahon, M., Furst, D.E. 2004. Safety of tumour necrosis factor-alpha antagonists. Drug Safety 27 (5), 307–324.

Kimby, E., Sverrisdottir, A., Elinder, G. 2004. Safety of rituximab therapy during the first trimester of pregnancy: a case history. Eur. J. Haematol. 72 (4), 292–295.

Klinger, G., Morad, Y., Westall, C.A., Laskin, C., Spitzer, K.A., Koren, G., Ito, S., Buncic, R.J. 2001. Ocular toxicity and antenatal exposure to chloroquine or hydroxychloroquine for rheumatic diseases. Lancet 358 (9284), 813–814.

Le Ray, C., Coulomb, A., Elefant, E., Frydman, R., Audibert, F. 2004. Mycophenolate mofetil in pregnancy after renal transplantation: a case of major fetal malformations. Obstet. Gynecol. 103, 1091–1094.

Levy, R.A., Vilela, V.S., Cataldo, M.J., Ramos, R.C., Duarte, J.L., Tura, B.R., Albuquerque, E.M., Jesus, N.R. 2001. Hydroxychloroquine (HCQ) in lupus pregnancy: double-blind and placebo-controlled study. Lupus 10 (6), 401–404.

Li, D.K., Liu, L., Odouli, R. 2003. Exposure to non-steroidal anti-inflammatory drugs during pregnancy and risk of miscarriage: population based cohort study. BMJ 327 (7411), 368.

Loyd, M.E., Carr, M., Mcelhatton, P., Hall, G.M., Hughes, R.A. 1999. The effect of methotrexate on pregnancy, fertility and lactation. Q. J. Med. 92, 551–563.

Lyle, W.H. 1978. Penicillamine in pregnancy. Lancet 1, 606–607.

Matalon, S.T., Ornoy, A., Lishner, M. 2004. Review of the potential effects of three commonly used antineoplastic and immunosuppressive drugs (cyclophosphamide, azathioprine, doxorubicin on the embryo and placenta). Reprod. Toxicol. 18 (2), 219–230.

Moskovitz, D.N., Bodian, C., Chapman, M.L., Marion, J.F., Rubin, P.H., Scherl, E., Present, D.H. 2004. The effect on the fetus of medications used to treat pregnant inflammatory bowel-disease patients. Am. J. Gastroenterol. 99 (4), 656–661.

Nielsen, G.L., Sorensen, H.T., Larsen, H., Pedersen, L. 2001. Risk of adverse birth outcome and miscarriage in pregnant users of non-steroidal anti-inflammatory drugs: population based observational study and case-control study. BMJ 322, 266–270.

Norgard, B., Czeizel, A.E., Rockenbauer, M., Olsen, J., Sorensen, H.T. 2001. Population-based case control study of the safety of sulfasalazine use during pregnancy. Aliment. Pharmacol. Ther. 15 (4), 483–486.

Ostensen, M. 2004. Disease specific problems related to drug therapy in pregnancy. Lupus 13 (9), 746–750.

Ostensen, M., Ostensen, H. 1996. Safety of non-steroidal antiinflammatory drugs in pregnant patients with rheumatic disease. J. Rheumatol. 23 (6), 1045–1049.

Ostensen, M., Villiger, P.M. 2001. Nonsteroidal antiinflammatory drugs in systemic lupus erythematosus. Lupus 10 (3), 135–139.

Parilla, B.V., Grobman, W.A., Holtzman, R.B., Thomas, H.A., Dooley, S.L. 2000. Indomethacin tocolysis and risk of necrotizing enterocolitis. Obstet. Gynecol. 96 (1), 120–123.

Parke, A.L., Rothfield, N.F. 1996. Antimalarial drugs in pregnancy—the North American experience. Lupus 5 (Suppl. 1), S67–S69.

Parke, A., West, B. 1996. Hydroxychloroquine in pregnant patients with systemic lupus erythematosus. J. Rheumatol. 23 (10), 1715–1718.

Pergola, P.E., Kancharla, A., Riley, D.J. 2001. Kidney transplantation during the first trimester of pregnancy: immunosuppression with mycophenolate mofetil, tacrolimus, and prednisone. Transplantation 71 (7), 994–997.

Petri, M. 2003. Immunosuppressive drug use in pregnancy. Autoimmunity 36 (1), 51–56.

Rains, C.P., Noble, S., Faulds, D. 1995. Sulfasalazine. A review of its pharmacological properties and therapeutic efficacy in the treatment of rheumatoid arthritis. Drug 50 (1), 137–156.

Rajapakse, R., Korelitz, B.I. 2001. Inflammatory bowel disease during pregnancy. Curr. Treat. Options Gastroenterol. 4 (3), 245–251.

Rayburn, W.F. 1998. Connective tissue disorders and pregnancy. Recommendations for prescribing. J. Reprod. Med. 43 (4), 341–349.

Sills, E.S., Perloe, M., Tucker, M.J., Kaplan, C.R., Palermo, G.D. 2001. Successful ovulation induction, conception, and normal delivery after chronic therapy with etanercept: a recombinant fusion anti-cytokine treatment for rheumatoid arthritis. Am. J. Reprod. Immunol. 46 (5), 366–368.

Sookvanichsilp, N., Pulbutr, P. 2002. Anti-implantation effects of indomethacin and celecoxib in rats. Contraception 65 (5), 373–378.

Stika, C.S., Gross, G.A., Leguizamon, G., Gerber, S., Levy, R., Mathur, A., Bernhard, L.M., Nelson, D.M., Sadovsky, Y. 2002. A prospective randomized safety trial of celecoxib for treatment of preterm labor. Am. J. Obstet. Gynecol. 187 (3), 653–660.

Thulstrup, A.M., Sorensen, H.T., Nielsen, G.L., Andersen, L., Barrett, D., Vilstrup, H., Olsen, J. 1999. Fetal growth and adverse birth outcomes in women receiving prescriptions for acetaminophen during pregnancy. EuroMap Study Group. Am. J. Perinatol. 16 (7), 321–326.

Tincani, A., Branch, D.W., Levy, R.A., Piette, J.C., Carp, H., Rai, R.S., Khamashta, M., Shoenfeld, Y. 2003. Treatment of pregnant patients with antiphospholipid syndrome. Lupus 12 (7), 524–529.

Handbook of Systemic Autoimmune Diseases, Volume 4
Reproductive and Hormonal Aspects of Systemic Autoimmune Diseases
Michael Lockshin and D. Ware Branch, editors

CHAPTER 10

Offspring of Women with Systemic Autoimmune Diseases: Fetal and Neonatal Complications and Inheritance of Autoimmune Diseases

Chiara Biasini Rebaioli[a], Mario Motta[b], Micol Frassi[a], Antonio Brucato[c], Rolando Cimaz[d], Pierluigi Meroni[e], Andrea Doria[f], Andrea Lojacono[g], Sonia Zatti[g], David Faden[g], Angela Tincani[a,*]

[a]*Rheumatology and Clinical Immunology, General Hospital and University of Brescia, Brescia, Italy*
[b]*Neonatal Intensive Care Unit, General Hospital and University of Brescia, Brescia, Italy*
[c]*Department of Internal Medicine, Niguarda Hospital, Milano, Italy*
[d]*Istituti Clinici di Perfezionamento, Milano, Italy*
[e]*IRCCS Ist. Auxologico University of Milan, Milano, Italy*
[f]*Rheumatology, University Hospital Padua, Padova, Italy*
[g]*Department of Obstetrics and Gynecology, General Hospital and University of Brescia, Brescia, Italy*

1. Introduction

Pregnancy is a special period in every woman's life, especially in women affected by systemic autoimmune diseases.

Patients affected by systemic lupus erythematosus (SLE) were for a long time discouraged from becoming pregnant (Kitridou, 1997). It was in fact observed by some that the disease can worsen during gestation (Petri et al., 1991); high disease activity has profound implications on fetal outcome (see below).

Fortunately, owing to the increasing knowledge of pathophysiologic mechanisms and the development of clinics with combined obstetric and medical care, pregnancy is now a nearly normal event in women with SLE and other autoimmune diseases.

Normal does not mean uneventful, however. Pregnancies in this group of patients remain at high risk, even though now many women do not experience major complications. Potential adverse events include renal crisis in systemic sclerosis (SSc), thrombosis, miscarriage and preeclampsia in patients with anti-phospholipid antibodies (aPL) with or without SLE, neonatal lupus in babies born to mothers with anti-Ro/SSA antibodies, independently from maternal disease. In addition, some drugs used to care for the mothers can interfere with fetal outcome.

2. Obstetric complications in autoimmune disease

2.1. *Influence of maternal disease*

Maternal disease and the flare-ups occurring in pregnancy influence fetal/neonatal outcome.

The influence of pregnancy on SLE course is controversial, while some reports underline that the rate of flares, particularly in the renal and hematologic systems, is increased during pregnancy

*Corresponding author.
Reumatologia e Immunologia Clinica, Ospedale Civile, Piazza Spedali Civili 1, 25125 Brescia, Italy.
Fax: +39-030-3995085
E-mail address: tincani@bresciareumatologia.it (A. Tincani).

DOI: 10.1016/S1571-5078(05)04010-9

(Petri, 2004; Ruiz Irastorza et al., 1996), other studies (Tincani et al., 1992; Lockshin et al., 1984), including a very recent one (Tandon et al., 2004), show disease activity similar to that occurring in non-pregnant women. However, according to our experience, the majority of the flares occurring in pregnancy do not appear particularly severe and require only minor therapeutic adjustments (Doria et al., 2002).

Higher disease activity is associated with fewer live births, fewer full-term births and more pregnancy losses (Clowse et al., 2003); therefore, the pregnancy in lupus patients should be ideally planned in a period of complete disease remission.

In lupus pregnancies, fetal risks are often related to placental insufficiency, a condition often associated with gestational hypertension (Salafia and Parke, 1997; Lockshin and Sammaritano, 2003). Placental insufficiency can cause the restriction of nutrient and oxygen supply to the fetus and may include fetal growth restriction and respiratory insufficiency, leading to fetal distress and death. The consequences of placental insufficiency are more severe when it occurs before 25 weeks gestation, leading in this case to fetal death, and less severe near term when they tend to cause only mild growth restriction (Branch, 2004).

Infants born small for gestational age (SGA) have more frequent problems with perinatal depression ("asphyxia"), hypothermia, hypoglycemia, polycythemia, long-term deficits in growth, neurodevelopmental handicaps and higher rates of fetal and neonatal mortality. Recent literature suggests that adults who experienced severe growth restriction in utero have a significantly increased incidence of hypertension, insulin resistance and type 2 diabetes. Additionally, new evidence suggests that untoward metabolic events in utero that produce fetal growth restriction also may produce lifelong alterations in growth and development (Thureen et al., 2001).

In women with SSc, pregnancy outcome seems also related to disease activity and organ involvement. While pregnancy may be uneventful for both mother and fetus, SSc patients with moderate-to-severe cardiac or pulmonary involvement have an increased risk of morbidity or mortality (Branch, 2004). Patients with diffuse skin involvement, hypertension and renal disease face an increased risk of preeclampsia and perhaps of renal crisis, often dangerous both for mother and fetus (Traub et al., 1984; Brown and Bolster, 2003). Careful preconception evaluation is important to identify the patients for whom pregnancy is ill advised. Finally, there may be an increased risk of cardiopulmonary and renal complications in patients with early SSc (Steen et al., 1989, 1996); such patients should delay pregnancy until the disease is stabilized. Once pregnant, women with SSc and hypertension, as well as those with early diffuse disease, need to be closely monitored for evaluation of blood pressure.

SSc itself, independent of hypertension, may adversely affect pregnancy and requires close monitoring (Chin et al., 1998). Favorable outcome occurs in about 50% of cases, about 25% end in pre-term infants, particularly in women with early, diffuse disease (Steen, 1997). The overall rate of miscarriage among SSc patients may be only slightly increased (15–20%), but is significantly higher in patients severely ill, such as those with late diffuse SSc; finally fetal deaths occur in about 2–5% (Branch, 2004), confirming that these pregnancies should be regarded as high risk followed by a multidisciplinary experienced team.

2.2. *Influence of maternal autoantibodies*

Some autoantibodies can impair pregnancy outcome.

Women with aPL have an high rate of pregnancy losses within the fetal period (10 weeks or more of gestation), in the pre-embryonic period (less than 6 weeks of gestation) or the embryonic period (6–9 weeks of gestation) (Oshiro et al., 1996). Pregnancies in women with aPL can also be complicated by premature delivery due to utero-placental insufficiency (Branch et al., 1992).

These obstetric complications may arise from the pro-thrombotic or other effects of maternal aPL on placental function, related to endothelial cell activation, inhibition of protein C/S system and fibrinolysis (Meroni and Riboldi, 2001), or annexin V displacement (Rand et al., 1994). Direct antibody-mediated damage on the trophoblast has also been suggested (di Somone et al., 2000). During differentiation to syncytium, trophoblasts express cell membrane anionic phospholipids that can bind beta 2-glycoprotein I (β2GPI), the main cationic phospholipid-binding protein recognized by the aPL. Adherent β2GPI may be recognized by antibodies that, once bound, interfere with in vitro trophoblast cell maturation, resulting in a defective placentation and hormone production. These mechanisms may play a role in early fetal loss, while thrombosis may be responsible for losses occurring late in the pregnancy (Meroni et al., 2004). In addition pregnancy itself is a known risk factor for thromboembolism; women with aPL therefore bear two concomitant factors of enhanced vascular risk.

Thoughtful management of pregnancies (Tincani et al., 2003) with aPL can improve the rate of live births, now reaching 70% in most of the published reports (Branch and Khamashta, 2003). However the rate of pre-term delivery remains high, possibly with fewer severe consequences because of close obstetric monitoring, careful delivery timing, and progress recently achieved by neonatal intensive care units.

To investigate if aPL are associated with fetal damage other than prematurity, we compared the neonatal outcome of 71 babies from mothers with primary anti-phospholipid syndrome to that of 71 babies from healthy mothers (Tincani et al., 2002), matched for gestational age, birth weight, mode of delivery and obstetrical complications. Neonatal outcome, measured by neonatal intensive care unit admissions and by prevalence of respiratory distress syndrome, chronic lung disease, intra-ventricular hemorrhage, peri-ventricular leukomalacia and retinopathy, did not differ between cases and controls. Thus the major problem of aPL complicated pregnancy seems to be prematurity.

3. Short- and long-term development problems related to transplacental passage of maternal autoantibodies

Some maternal autoantibodies of IgG isotype cross the placenta and bind fetal antigens with consequent direct damage to the fetus or the newborn, for instance, in the children of women with myasthenia gravis exposed to anti-acetylcholine receptor antibodies or of women with thyrotoxicosis exposed to thyroid-stimulating antibodies, binding TSH receptor. In systemic autoimmune diseases, this pattern is typical of children of patients with anti-Ro/SS-A antibodies.

3.1. Anti-Ro/SS-A antibodies

A peculiar fetal/neonatal injury, called neonatal lupus syndrome (NLS), results from the transplacental passage of maternal IgG autoantibodies that react with intracellular soluble ribonucleoproteins SSA/Ro (52 or 60 kDa) and/or SSB/La (48 kDa) (Cimaz et al., 2003). Fetal/neonatal disease is independent from maternal disease: mothers can be affected by SLE, Sjogren Syndrome, or other autoimmune symptoms or can also be entirely asymptomatic (Buyon et al., 1998).

Permanent congenital heart block (CHB) and transient-cutaneous rash are the most common manifestations of NLS, initially named because of its resemblance to subacute cutaneous lupus. In both these conditions, the pathogenetic role of antibodies is shown by *in vivo* and *in vitro* experimental models (Buyon and Clancy, 2003).

CHB typically occurs "in utero" and can be detected during the second trimester. In some cases, CHB begins as first- or second-degree block and then progresses to third degree block (Sonesson et al., 2004). This finding has practical importance because it might indicate reversible situations where maternal treatment (with dexamethasone?) may be beneficial, avoiding progression to the fibrotic irreversible state of the complete CHB (Tseng and Buyon, 1997).

Although anti-Ro/SS-A and/or anti-La/SS-B antibodies were identified in more than 85% of the mothers of children with CHB, only about 2% of the first pregnancy of patients with anti-Ro/SS-A and/or anti-La/SS-B antibodies were found complicated by complete CHB (Brucato et al., 2001). This low frequency suggests that besides antibodies other factors are involved in the pathogenetic process.

Once established, complete CHB is irreversible and it may be linked to in utero increased morbidity and mortality (Buyon et al., 1998; Buyon et al., 2002). In women at risk, careful monitoring by serial fetal echocardiograms is now performed, starting at 18 weeks of gestation (Buyon and Clancy, 2003). The early diagnosis of the complete CHB usually can avoid the deterioration of the fetal cardiac function. Due to their important bradycardia, children born with complete CHB usually require an early implantation of the pacemaker.

Cutaneous manifestations of NLE appear as erythematosus, often annular, frequently photosensitive rash affecting eyes, face and scalp; the rash is rarely seen at birth, most often it occurs in the first 8 weeks after birth and lasts up to 22 weeks, resolving with the clearance of maternal antibodies (Neiman et al., 2000); in most cases it follows ultraviolet light exposure; it has been described in neonates from mother with antibodies against U1 RNP (Solomon et al., 1995).

Rarely, abnormalities of the liver or blood affect newborns exposed to maternal anti-SSA/Ro-SSB/La antibodies and are also grouped under the heading of NLS. Three types of hepatobiliary disease have been observed: liver failure at birth or in utero, transient conjugated hyperbilirubinemia or transient transaminase elevation during infancy (Lee et al., 2002). Hematologic abnormalities, consisting of thrombocytopenia, neutropenia or anemia, occur in about 27% of cases (Cimaz et al., 2003). It is uncommon for children with neonatal lupus to show the full expression of disease; rather they have only one or two organ systems involved.

To date, complete CHB is irreversible. In contrast, all the non-cardiac manifestations are transient, resolving by 6 months of life, coincident with the disappearance of maternal autoantibodies from the neonatal circulation.

The long-term prognosis of children who have NLE is still under investigation. Mortality in the first 5 years remains high. Some of these children may develop other autoimmune diseases later in childhood (Martin et al., 2002).

3.2. Anti-platelet antibodies

The passage of maternal platelet autoantibodies induces moderate or severe autoimmune thrombocytopenia in about 10% of newborns of mothers with immune thrombocytopenic purpura; although these infants are delivered with platelet counts below 50.000/mm^3 and counts often decrease during the first few days of life, intra-cranial hemorrhages occur in fewer than 1% of the children. The occurrence of intra-cranial hemorrhage is slightly higher than that observed in infants of healthy women (Payne et al., 1997).

3.3. Anti-phospholipid antibodies

Transplacental passage of aPL has been reported to cause, while rarely, thrombosis in neonates born to positive mothers with or without clinical features of anti-phospholipid syndrome. From 1987 to 2002, 13 neonatal thromboses related to aPL have been published; among them, arteries were involved 10 times (6 times in the cerebral territory), venous thrombosis 2 times and both arterial and venous thrombosis 1 time (Boffa et al., 2004). We described a fetal stroke associated with maternal aPL that was found, by ultrasound and CT scan, at 2 months of age, in a cerebral artery, likely due to an intra-uterine event (Lojacono et al., 1996). Obviously these, luckily rare, events, can have permanent consequence. The one we described developed West syndrome and left hemiparesis. To improve knowledge in this area, still rare and anecdotal, a European registry will collect clinical and biological data on this group of children (Boffa et al., 2004).

Certainly, thromboses reported in the offspring of mothers with aPL are extraordinarily rare compared to the number of pregnancies reported in this group of patients. Possible explanations are: children are protected from thrombosis because they do not have a concomitant risk factor. In fact, according to the two hit hypotheses, the presence of aPL is not enough to cause the thrombosis (Riboldi et al., 2004). Alternatively, placenta, might clear aPL because it carries a target antigen, diminishing the amount of antibodies reaching the fetus circulation (Avcin et al., 2002). Experimental work in progress will clarify these interesting aspects.

3.4. Maternal autoantibodies and brain development

The children of lupus mothers, according to the available follow-up studies, appear normal when compared with children born at same gestational age (Branch and Khamashta, 2003; Pollard et al., 1992). In the limited data available on long-term observation of these children, a high rate of learning disabilities occurs even if they have a normal intelligence (McAllister et al., 1997; Ross et al., 2003).

Dyslexia occurs in up to 45% of male children of SLE mothers, but much less frequently in female (Ross et al., 2003; Lahita, 1988). A suggested explanation of this finding is a higher immune response of the mother to a male fetus that may cause impairment in the brain development (Gualtieri and Hicks, 1985).

Interestingly, an increased frequency of anti-Ro/SS-A and anti-thyroid antibodies occur in mothers of children with development disorders, in particular dyslexia (Behan and Geschwind, 1985; Denenberg, 1991). The concentration of Ro antigen in the brain is particularly high (Wolin and Steitz, 1984).

In children born of patients with SLE, the influence of mothers' antibody profile was investigated only in two recent papers. According to one study, anti-Ro/SS-A, anti-La/SS-B antibodies during pregnancy significantly predicted learning disabilities in offspring (Ross et al., 2003). The second report underlined instead that the mothers of children with low score in specific learning tests were positive for aPL (Neri et al., 2004). This observation may also find support in the experimental models: *in vitro*, aPL were shown to bind brain endothelial cells (Meroni et al., 2003); *in vivo*, animals develop hyperactivity, anxiety and behavioral problems resembling human learning disabilities after a prolonged exposure to aPL (Ziporen et al., 1997).

4. Outcome of children exposed to immunosuppressive drugs in pregnancy

Some rheumatic diseases like SLE and SSc remain active or even flare during pregnancy and must be treated with drugs. Unfortunately, the number of controlled studies on pregnant women taking drugs is small and late effects in exposed offspring are largely unknown.

That it is possible to prescribe corticosteroids and some immunosuppressive drugs (azathioprine, cyclosporine-A) in pregnancy to control maternal autoimmune disease derives from observation of transplanted patients (Petri, 2003). Administration of such drugs can cause premature rupture of membranes, pre-term delivery, low birth weight and intrauterine growth restriction, but it is always difficult to separate the effect of drugs from the effect of maternal disease (Prevot et al., 2002).

In utero exposure to cyclosporine-A can induce autoimmunity in experimental animals, and seems to delay NK cell maturation in children of transplanted patients (Di Paolo et al., 2000). However, despite transient maturation defects shown in T, B and NK cells, follow-up study of 10 children from 0.5 to 9 years of age showed normal immune function (Pilarski et al., 1994). A recent study, focusing on children from mothers with connective tissue diseases, exposed and not exposed to immunosuppressive drugs during gestation, detected no difference in immunoglobulin level and lymphocyte subpopulations; these children also develop a satisfactory response to hepatitis B vaccinations (Cimaz et al., 2004).

Among corticosteroids, prednisone and prednisolone are suited for maternal treatment while dexamethasone and betamethasone are reserved for fetal treatment. Prednisone and prednisolone are inactivated by placenta hydroxylases; less than 10% of the mother's blood level reaches the fetus. In contrast, fluorinated corticosteroids (dexamethasone and betamethasone) are not inactivated and are helpful in fetal treatment, for example, when incomplete CHB is diagnosed (Buyon, 1999). A recent metaanalysis reports a significant increase of oral clefts after first trimester steroid exposure, even if the overall risk appears low (Park-Wyllie et al., 2000).

Prolonged fetal exposure to dexamethasone may impair cerebral development (Baud, 1999); multiple antenatal courses of dexamethasone but not betamethasone were associated with an increased risk of leukomalacia and neurodevelopmental abnormalities found at 2 years of age (Spinillo et al., 2004). On the other hand 11 children exposed to high antenatal dexamethasone doses because of CHB and studied at 1–11 years old were found completely normal at neuropsychological examination (Brucato et al., 2004). Although the real impact of in utero exposure to fluorinated corticosteroids remains to be clarified, according to the few available data, betamethasone seems safer for the children's long-term outcome and should be preferred in the treatment of these rare conditions (Jobe and Soll, 2004).

Antimalarial drugs are widely used in autoimmune rheumatic syndromes because of their beneficial effects on skin and joints. In addition, they can lower cholesterol and lipid levels and exert antiaggregant activity. Chloroquine crosses the placenta and accumulates in melanin-containing structures (Briggs et al., 2001). Abnormalities in the retina and in the inner ear have been reported in children born to women taking higher than recommended daily doses of drug throughout the pregnancy (Hart and Nauton, 1964; Panfique and Magnard, 1969).

Because of the long half-life of antimalarials (months), their discontinuation during pregnancy does not prevent fetal exposure, but may precipitate a maternal flare with harmful consequences for both mother and fetus. A recent case control study of 133 pregnancies in patients taking hydroxychloroquine shows no difference in pregnancy or neonatal outcome (Costedoat-Chalumeau et al., 2003), in agreement with other studies and with our collaborative experience (Borden and Parke, 2001; Tincani, 2005) (Table 1).

The safety of antimalarials is confirmed by ophthalmological examination of children that showed no particular problem during the first year of life (Motta et al., 2002). Also in our experience, 24 babies from mothers treated with hydroxychloroquine (13 also breast fed) and followed during the first year of life, showed normal motor quotient screening test and normal visual function (Motta et al., 2005).

5. Genetic background

In the families of patients affected by SLE, antiphospholipid syndrome, rheumatoid arthritis and other autoimmune disorders, it is not rare to find members affected by the same disease or other autoimmune syndrome (Ermann and Fathman, 2001). In monozygotic twins, autoimmune disease concordance rate is far from 100%, indicating that the disease penetrance is also linked to environmental factors. The lower concordance rate of siblings or dizygotic twins compared with monozygotic twins supports the concept of multiple gene involvement in autoimmune disease expression (Wandstrat and Wakeland, 2001).

Table 1

Pregnancy outcome of the patients with autoimmune diseases taking (study group) and not taking (control group) hydroxychloroquine

Pregnancy outcome	Study group 76 pregnancies	Control group 80 pregnancies	P
Spontaneous abortion, number (%)	3 (3.9)	3 (3.7)	NS
Fetal deaths, number (%)	2 (2.5)	0	NS
Live birth, number (%)	72 (94.7)	79 (98.7)	NS
Premature birth, number (%)	11 (14.4)	9 (11.2)	NS
Full-term birth, number (%)	60 (78.9)	68 (80.0)	NS
Gestational age, mean week (range)	38 (31–41)	37.5 (27–40)	$P<0.05$
Weight, mean in grams (range)	2990 (1420–3970)	2998 (990–4250)	NS

Table 2
Autoantibodies in children of anti-Ro/SS-A-positive patients

Autoantibody tests	29 cases, mean age 4 years (range 6 months to 13 years)	33 controls, mean age 7 years (1 month to 14 years)
ANA	4 (13.8%)	3 (9%)
Anti ds-DNA	0	0
Anti ss-DNA	0	0
Anti ENA	0	0
IgG anti cardiolipin	3 (10.3%)	0
IgM anti cardiolipin	0	0
IgG anti beta 2 glycoprotein I	8 (27.5%)	5 (15.1%)
IgM anti beta 2 glycoprotein I	0	0

In lupus-prone mice single alleles are linked to the capacity of animals to produce non-pathogenic anti-nuclear antibodies, while mice with two combined susceptibility alleles develop a systemic autoimmune disease, including a severe glomerulonephritis, fatal for 70% of the animal at 9 months (Morel, 2000). This model likely explains the observation that inheritance of autoimmune disease may vary from the acquisition of autoantibodies, to the more rare expression of a "complete" disease; in fact, relatives of SLE patients often present autoantibodies in the absence of clinical disease (Cimaz, 2004). Autoantibodies not related to the maternal disease are detectable in the sera children born of SLE patients (El-Roeiy et al., 1987), but the risk of developing SLE in these children seems to be small.

A recent study focused on the long-term prognosis of a group of 195 children (aged 4 months to 26 years) born of SLE patients, compared with 57 children from healthy mothers (Murashima et al., 2004). Two of 56 (4%) children undergoing clinical examination were diagnosed as having SLE. In addition, a significantly higher positive rate for anti-nuclear antibodies was found in these subjects (especially girls) compared with controls (27% vs. 7%). If anti-nuclear antibodies can be regarded as expression of the genetic background of these children, a close follow-up for the possible development of a connective tissue disease is strongly recommended. This suggestion is supported by the observation that the occurrence of SLE in children younger than 10 years or in males younger than 18 years may be related to maternal Ro/SS-A autoantibodies (Lehman et al., 1989).

The long-term outcome of babies with neonatal lupus is not well known. Despite early pacing, children with CHB have a high mortality during the first 12 months of life (Jaeggi et al., 2002). The risk of later development of a rheumatic disease in these babies is still uncertain: there have been few case reports of female children with neonatal lupus who developed an autoimmune disease, even after many years (Jackson and Gulliver, 1979; Hubscher et al., 1997). These cases may reflect the background of increased autoimmunity that exists in such families (Brucato et al., 1997). We have studied 29 children of mothers with anti-Ro/SS-A antibodies, mean age 4 years and 4 months, range 6 months to 13 years. As shown in Table 2, the autoantibodies occurrence in these children was not significantly increased when they were compared with a group of children from healthy mothers and comparable age. Further investigations are in progress.

Key points

- Maternal diseases and their flare-ups can influence the fetal/neonatal outcome.
- The presence of aPL, during pregnancy, is linked to an increased rate of repeated spontaneous abortions and fetal deaths.
- The major problem of aPL complicated pregnancy seems to be prematurity.
- The transplacental passage of aPL has been reported to cause, while rarely, thromboses in neonates.

- The presence of IgG anti-Ro/SS-A in the mother is known to be linked to "neonatal lupus syndrome" (NLS).
- Permanent congenital heart block and transient cutaneous rash disease are the most common manifestations of NLS.
- The presence of anti-Ro/SSA/La antibodies and aPL during pregnancy may be linked to the development of learning disabilities in offspring.
- The passage of maternal platelet autoantibodies can induce moderate or severe thrombocytopenia in about 10% of newborns even if intracranial hemorrhages have been shown in less than 1% of the children.
- Corticosteroids (prednisone and prednisolone) and some immunosuppressive drugs (mainly azatihoprine, cyclosporine-A) used in pregnancy to control maternal disease can cause pregnancy complications but do not seem to cause malformations or newborn immune system alteration.
- Betamethasone should be preferred to dexamethasone in the treatment of CHB because of the possible effect of dexamethasone on the cerebral development of the children.
- Hydroxychloroquine in pregnancy do not seem linked to the occurrence of neonatal malformation.
- In the families of patients affected by autoimmune disorders, members with a more or less expressed autoimmune syndrome are frequently found, to support the strong genetic component of these diseases.

References

Avcin, T., Cimaz, R., Meroni, P.L. 2002. Recent advances in antiphospholipid antibodies and antiphospholipid syndromes in pediatric populations. Lupus 11, 4–10.

Baud, O. 1999. Antenatal glucocorticoid treatment and cystic periventricular leukomalacia in very premature infants. New Engl. J. Med. 341, 1190–1196.

Behan, P., Geschwind, N. 1985. Dyslexia, congenital anomalies and immune disorders. The role of the fetal environment. Ann. NY Acad. Sci. 457, 13–18.

Boffa, M.C., Aurousseau, M.H., Lachassinne, E., Dauphin, H., Fain, O., Le Tomelin, P., Uzan, M., Piette, J.C., Derenne, S., Boinot, C., Avcin, T., Motta, M., Faden, D., Tincani, A. 2004. European register of babies born to mothers with antiphospholipid syndrome. Lupus 13, 713–717.

Borden, M.B., Parke, A. 2001. Antimalarial drugs in systemic lupus erythematosus: use in pregnancy. Drug Saf. 24, 1055–1063.

Branch, D.W. 2004. Pregnancy in patients with rheumatic diseases: obstetric management and monitoring. Lupus 13, 69–698.

Branch, D.W., Khamashta, M.A. 2003. Obstetric diagnosis, management, and controversies. Obstet. and Gynecol. 101, 1333–1344.

Branch, D.W., Silver, R.M., Blackwell, J.L., Reading, J.C., Scott, J.R. 1992. Outcome of treated pregnancies in women with antiphospholipid syndrome: an update of Utah experience. Obstet. Gynecol. 80, 614–620.

Briggs, G.G., Freeman, R.K., Yaffe, S.J. 2001. Drugs in Pregnancy and Lactation. 6th ed., Lippincott Williams & Wilkins, Baltimore.

Brown, A.N., Bolster, M.B. 2003. Scleroderma renal crisis in pregnancy associated with massive proteinuria. Clin. Exp. Rheumatol. 21, 114–116.

Brucato, A., Franceschini, F., Buyon, J.P. 1997. Neonatal lupus: long-term outcomes of mothers and children and recurrence rate. Clin. Exp. Rheumatol. 15 (5), 467–473.

Brucato, A., Frassi, M., Franceschini, F., Cimaz, R., Faden, D., Pisoni, M.P., Muscara, M., Vignati, G., Stramba-Badiale, M., Catelli, L., Lojacono, A., Cavazzana, I., Ghirardello, A., Vescovi, F., Gambari, P.F., Doria, A., Meroni, P.L., Tincani, A. 2001. Congenital heart block risk to newborns of mothers with anti-Ro/SSA/SSA antibodies detected by counterimmunoelectrophoresis. A prospective study of 100 women. Arthritis Rheum. 44, 1832–1835.

Brucato, A., Li Destri, M., Villa, P.M., Astori, M.G., Tincani, A., Chimini, L., Cimaz, R., Vaccai, R., Motta, M., Neri, F., Martinelli, S. 2004. Normal neuropsycological development of children with congenital complete heart block exposed or not exposed in utero to dexamethasone. Lupus 9 (13), 762.

Buyon, J.P. 1999. Neonatal lupus syndromes. In: R. Lahita (Ed.), Systemic Lupus Erythematosus, 3rd ed., Academic Press, San Diego CA, pp. 337–359.

Buyon, J.P., Clancy, R.M. 2003. Neonatal lupus: review of proposed pathogenesis and clinical data from the US-based research registry for neonatal lupus. Autoimmunity 36, 41–50.

Buyon, J.P., Hiebert, R., Copel, J. 1998. Autoimmune associated congenital heart block mortality, morbidity, and recurrence rates obtained from a national neonatal lupus registry. J. Am. Coll. Cardiol. 31, 1658–1666.

Buyon, J.P., Nugent, D., Mellins, E., Sandborg, C. 2002. Maternal immunologic disease and neonatal disorders. Neo. Rev. 3, 3.

Chin, A.J., Kaseba, C.M., Weaver, J.B.K. 1998. Scleroderma in pregnancy. J. Obstet. Gynecol. 18, 238–242.

Cimaz, R. 2004. Any increased risk of autoimmune disease?. Lupus 13, 736–739.

Cimaz, R., Meregalli, E., Biggioggero, M., Borghi, O., Tincani, A., Motta, M., Airo, P., Meroni, P.L. 2004. Alterations in the immune system of children from mothers treated with immunosuppressive agents during pregnancy. Toxicol. Lett. 149 (1–3), 155–162. Apr, 1.

Cimaz, R., Spence, D.L., Hornberger, L., Silverman, E.D. 2003. Incidence and spectrum of neonatal lupus erythematous: a prospective study of infant born to mothers with anti-Ro/SSA antibodies. J. Pediatr. 142, 678–683.

Clowse, M.E.B., Magder, L., Petri, M. 2003. Impact of the intensity and timing of lupus activity on pregnancy outcomes. Arthritis Rheum. 48, S435.

Costedoat-Chalumeau, N., Amoura, Z., Duhaut, P., Huong, D.L.T., Sebbough, D., Wechsler, B., Vauthier, D., Denjoy, I., Lupoglazoff, J.M., Piette, J.C. 2003. Safety of hydroxychloroquine in pregnant patients with connective tissue diseases. A study of one hundred thirty-three cases compared with a control group. Arthritis Rheum. 48, 3207–3211.

Denenberg, V.H. 1991. Effects of the autoimmune uterine/maternal environment upon cortical ectopia, behavior and autoimmunity. Brain Res. 563, 114–122.

Di Paolo, S., Schena, A., Morrone, L.F., Manfredi, G., Stallone, G., Derosa, C., Procino, A., Schena, F.P. 2000. Immunologic evaluation during the first year of life of infants born to cyclosporine treated female kidney transplant recipients: analysis of lymphocyte subpopulations and immunoglobulin serum levels. Transplantation 69, 2049–2054.

di Somone, N., Meroni, P.L., del Papa, N., Raschi, E., Calandro, D., De Carolis, C.S., Khamashta, M.A., Atsumi, T., Hughes, G.R., Balestrieri, G., Tincani, A., Casali, P., Caruso, A. 2000. Antiphospholipid antibodies affect trophoblast gonadotropin secretion and invasiveness by binding directly and through adhered β2-Glicoprotein I. Arthritis Rheum. 43, 140–150.

Doria, A., Vescovi, V., Laccarino, L., Faden, D., Ghirardello, A., Gorla, R., Zampieri, S., Taglietti, M., Casiglia, E., Gambari, P.F., Tincani, A. 2002. Pregnancy in SLE: it is possible to predict disease flare?. Arthritis Rheum. 812, S322.

El-Roeiy, A., Gleicher, N., Isenberg, D., Kennedy, R.C., Shoenfeld, Y. 1987. A common anti-DNA idiotype and other autoantibodies in sera of offspring of mothers with SLE. Clin. Exp. Immunol. 68, 528–534.

Ermann, J., Fathman, C.G. 2001. Autoimmune diseases: genes, bugs anf failed regulation. Nat. Immunol. 2, 759–761.

Gualtieri, T., Hicks, R.E. 1985. An immunoreactive theory of selective male affliction. Behav. Brain Sci. 8, 427–441.

Hart, C., Nauton, R. 1964. The ototoxicity of cloroquine phosphate. Arch. Otolaryngol. Heart Neck Surg. 80, 407–412.

Hubscher, O., Carrillo, D., Reichlin, M. 1997. Congenital heart block and subsequent connetive tissue disorder in adolescence. Lupus 6, 283–284.

Jackson, R., Gulliver, M. 1979. Neonatal lupus erythematosus progressing into systemic lupus erythematosus: a 15 years follow-up. Br. J. Dermatol. 101, 81–86.

Jaeggi, E.T., Hamilton, R.M., Silverman, E.D., Zamora, S.A., Homberger, L.K. 2002. Outcome of children with fetal, neonatal or childhood diagnosis of isolated congenital atrioventricular block. J. Am. Coll. Cardiol. 39, 130–137.

Jobe, A.H., Soll, R.F. 2004. Choice and dose of corticosteroid for antenatal treatments. Am. J. Obstet. Gynecol. 190, 878–881.

Kitridou, R.C. 1997. The mother in systemic lupus erythematosus. In: D.J. Wallace, B.H. Hahn (Eds.), Dubois' Lupus Erythematosus, 5th ed., Williams & Wilkins, Baltimore, pp. 967–1002.

Lahita, R.G. 1988. Systemic lupus erythematosus: learning disabilities in the male offspring of female patients and relationship to laterality. Psychoneuroendocrinology 13, 385–396.

Lee, kL.A., Sokol, R.J., Buyon, J.P. 2002. Hepatobiliary disease in neonatal lupus: prevalence and clinical characteristics in cases enrolled in a national registry. Pediatrics 109, 11.

Lehman, T.J.A., Reichlin, M., Santner, T.J. 1989. Maternal autoantibodies to Ro/SS-A are associated with both early onset of disease and male sex among children with systemic lupus erythematosus. Arthritis Rheum. 32, 1414–1420.

Lockshin, M., Sammaritano, L. 2003. Lupus pregnancy. Autoimmunity 36, 33–40.

Lockshin, M.D., Reinitz, E., Druzin, M.L., Murrman, M., Estes, D., et al. 1984. Lupus pregnancy: case-control prospective study demonstrating absence of lupus exacerbation during or after pregnancy. Am. J. Med. 77, 893–898.

Lojacono, A., Spatola, L., Faden, D., Bettini, P., Tanzi, P., Balestrieri, G., Tarantini, M., Pezzani, M., Escobar, R., Tincani, A. 1996. Fetal stroke associated with maternal antiphospholipid antibodies: a case report. Lupus 5 (5), 512.

Martin, V., Lee, L.A., Askanase, A.D., Katholi, M., Buyon, J.P. 2002. Long term follow-up of children with neonatal lupus and their unaffected siblings. Arthritis Rheum. 46, 2377–2383.

McAllister, D.L., Kaplan, B.J., Edworthy, S.M., Martin, L., Crawford, S.G., Ramsey Goldman, R., Manzi, R., Fries, S., Sibley, J. 1997. The influence of systemic lupus erythematosus of fetal development: cognitive, behavioral, and health trends. J. Int. Neuropsychol. Soc. 3, 370–376.

Meroni, P.L., Di Simone, N., Testoni, C., D'Asta, M., Acaia, B., Caruso, A. 2004. Antiphospholipid antibodies as cause of pregnancy loss. Lupus 13, 649–652.

Meroni, P.L., Riboldi, P. 2001. Pathogenic mechanisms mediating antiphospholipid syndrome. Curr. Opin. Rheumatol. 13, 377–382.

Meroni, P.L., Tincani, A., Sepp, N., Raschi, E., Testoni, C., Corsini, E., Cavazzana, I., Pellegrini, S., Salmaggi, A. 2003. Endothelium and brain. Lupus 12, 919–928.

Morel, L. 2000. Genetic reconstitution of systemic lupus erythematosus immunopathology with poly congenic murine strain. Proc. Natl. Acad. Sci. USA 97, 6670–6675.

Motta, M., Tincani, A., Faden, D., et al. 2002. Antimalarial agents in pregnancy. Lancet 359, 524–525.

Motta, M., Tincani, A., Faden, D., Zinzini, E., Lojacono, A., Marchesi, A., Frassi, M., Biasini, C., Zatti, S., Chirico, G. 2005. Follow-up of infants exposed to hydroxychloroquine given to mothers during pregnancy and lactation. J. Perinatol. 25 (2), 86–89.

Murashima, A., Fukazawa, T., Hirashima, M. 2004. Long term prognosis of children born to lupus patients. Ann. Rheum. Dis. 63, 50–53.

Neiman, A.R., Lee, L.A., Weston, W.L., Buyon, J.P. 2000. Isolated cutaneous manifestations of neonatal lupus: characteristics of mothers and children enrolled in a national registry. J. Pediatr. 137, 674–680.

Neri, F., Chimini, L., Bonomi, F., Filippini, E., Motta, M., Faden, D., Lojacono, A., Biasini Rebaioli, C., Frassi, M., Danieli, E., Tincani, A. 2004. Neuropsychological development of children born to patients with systemic lupus erythematosus. Lupus 13, 805–811.

Oshiro, B.T., Silver, R.M., Scott, J.R., Yu, H., Branch, D.W., et al. 1996. Antiphospholipid antibodies and fetal death. Obstet. Gynecol. 87, 489–493.

Panfique, L., Magnard, P. 1969. Retinal degeneration in 2 children following preventive antimalarial treatment of mother during pregnancy. Bull. Soc. Ophthalmol. Fr. 69, 466–467.

Park-Wyllie, L., Mazzotta, P., Pastuszak, A. 2000. Birth defects after maternal exposure to corticosteroids: prospective cohort study and meta-analysis of epidemiological studies. Teratology. 62, 385–392.

Payne, S.D., Resnik, R., Moore, T.R., Hedriana, H.L., Kelly, T.F. 1997. Maternal characteristics and risk of severe neonatal thrombocytopenia and intracranial hemorrhage in pregnancies complicated by autoimmune thrombocytopenia. Am. J. Obstet. Gynecol. 177, 149–155.

Petri, M. 2003. Immunosuppressive drug use in pregnancy. Autoimmunity 36, 51–56.

Petri, M. 2004. Prospective study of systemic lupus erythematosus pregnancies. Lupus 13, 688–689.

Petri, M., Howard, D., Repke, J. 1991. Frequency of lupus flare in pregnancy: the Hopkins Lupus Pregnancy Centre experience. Arthritis Rheum. 34, 1538–1545.

Pilarski, L.M., Yacyshyn, B.R., Lazarovits, A.I. 1994. Analysis of peripheral blood lymphocyte populations and immune function from children exposed to CsA or to azathioprine in utero. Transplantation 57, 133–144.

Pollard, J.K., Scott, J.R., Branch, D.W. 1992. Outcome of children born to women treated during pregnancy for the antiphospholipid pregnancy. Obstet. Gynecol. 80, 365–368.

Prevot, A., Martini, S., Guignard, J.P. 2002. In utero exposure to immunosuppressive drugs. Biol. Neonate. 81, 73–81.

Rand, J.H., Wu, X.X., Guller, S. 1994. Reduction of annexin V (placental anticoagulant protein I) on placental villi of women with antiphospholipid antibodies and recurrent spontaneous abortion. Am. J. Obstet. Gynecol. 171, 1566–1572.

Riboldi, P.S., Gerosa, M., Tincani, A., et al. 2004. Non organ specific autoimmunity involvement in cardiovascular disease. In: A. Doria, P. Pauletto (Eds.), The Heart in Systemic Autoimmune Diseases. Elsevier, Amsterdam, pp. 41–51.

Ross, G., Sammaritano, L., Nass, R., Lockshin, M. 2003. Effects of mothers' autoimmune disease during pregnancy on learning disabilities and hand preference in their children. Arch. Pediatr. Adolesc. Med. 157 (4), 397–402.

Ruiz Irastorza, G., Lima, F., Alves, J., Khamashta, M.A., Simpson, J., Hughes, G.R. 1996. Increased rate of lupus flare during pregnancy and puerperium: a prospective study of 78 pregnancies. Br. J. Rheumatol. 35, 133–138.

Salafia, C.M., Parke, A.L. 1997. Placental pathology in systemic lupus erythematosus. Rheum. Dis. Clin. North Am. 23, 85–97.

Solomon, B.A., Laude, T.A., Shalita, A.R. 1995. Neonatal lupus erythematosus: discordant disease expression of U1RNP-positive antibodies in fraternal twins—is this a subset of neonatal lupus erythematosus or a new distinct syndrome? J. Am. Acad. Dermatol. 32, 858–862.

Sonesson, S.E., Salomonsson, S., Jacobsson, L.A., Bremme, K., Herlenius, M. 2004. Signs of first-degree heart block occur in one-third of fetuses of pregnant women with anti–SSA/Ro 52-kd antibodies. Arthritis Rheum. 50, 1253–1261.

Spinillo, A., Viazzo, F., Colleoni, R., Chiara, A., Cerbo, R.M., Fazzi, E. 2004. Two-years infant neurodevelopmental outcome after single or multiple antenatal courses of corticosteroids to prevent complications of prematurity. Am. J. Obstet. Gynecol. 191, 217–224.

Steen, V.D. 1997. Scleroderma and pregnancy. Rheum. Dis. Clin. North Am. 23 (1), 133–147.

Steen, V.D., Brodeur, M., Conte, C. 1996. Prospective pregnancy study in women with systemic sclerosis. Arthritis Rheum. 39, 5151.

Steen, V.D., Conte, C., Day, N. 1989. Pregnancy in women with systemic sclerosis. Arthritis Rheum. 32, 151–157.

Tandon, A., Ibanez, D., Gladman, D.D., Urowitz, M.B. 2004. The effect of pregnancy on lupus nephritis. Arthritis Rheum. 12, 3941–3946.

Thureen, P.J., Anderson, M.S., Hay, W.W. 2001. The small-for-gestational-age infant. Neo. Rev. 2, e139–e149.

Tincani, A., Biasini, R.C., Frassi, M., Taglietti, M., Gorla, R., Cavazzana, I., Faden, D., Taddei, F., Lojacono, A., Motta, M., Trepidi, L., Meroni, P., Cimaz, R., Ghirardello, A., Doria, A., Pisoni, M.P., Muscarà, M., Brucato, A. 2005. Pregnancy and autoimmunity: maternal treatment and maternal disease influence on pregnancy outcome. Autoimmunity Rev. 4, 423–428.

Tincani, A., Branch, W., Levy, R.A., Piette, J.C., Carp, H., Rai, R.S., Khamashta, M., Shoenfeld, Y. 2003. Treatment of pregnant patients with antiphospholipid syndrome. Lupus 12 (7), 524–529.

Tincani, A., Faden, D., Tarantini, M., Lojacono, A., Tanzi, P., Gastaldi, A., Di Mario, C., Spatola, L., Cattaneo, R., Balestrieri, G., et al. 1992. Systemic lupus erythematosus and pregnancy: a prospective study. Clin. Exp. Rheumatol. 10 (5), 439–446.

Tincani, A., Lojacono, A., Taglietti, M., Motta, M., Biasini, C., Decca, L., Zatti, S., Frassi, M., Barbetti, L., Gorla, R., Danieli, E., Balestrieri, G., Chirico, G., Faden, D. 2002. Pregnancy and neonatal outcome in primary antiphospholipid syndrome. Lupus 11, 649.

Traub, Y.M., Shapiro, A.P., Rodnan, G.P. 1984. Hypertension and renal failure (scleroderma renal crisis) in progressive systemic sclerosis: report of a 25-year experience with 68 cases. Medicine 62, 335–352.

Tseng, C.E., Buyon, J.P. 1997. Neonatal lupus syndromes. In pregnancy and rheumatic disease. Rheum. Dis. Clin. North Am. 23, 31–54.

Wandstrat, A., Wakeland, E. 2001. The genetics of complex autoimmune diseases: non-MHC susceptibility genes. Nat. Immunol. 2, 802–808.

Wolin, S.L., Steitz, A. 1984. The Ro small cytoplasmic ribonucleoproteins: identification of the antigenic protein and its binding site on the Ro RNAs. Proc. Natl. Acad. Sci. USA 81, 1996–2000.

Ziporen, L., Shoenfeld, Y., Levy, Y., Korezyn, A.D. 1997. Neurological dysfunctions and hyperactive behavior associated with antiphospholipid antibodies. J. Clin. Invest. 100, 613–619.

Handbook of Systemic Autoimmune Diseases, Volume 4
Reproductive and Hormonal Aspects of Systemic Autoimmune Diseases
Michael Lockshin and D. Ware Branch, editors

CHAPTER 11

Contraception in Women with Autoimmune Diseases

Lisa R. Sammaritano*

Department of Medicine, Weill Medical College of Cornell University, Hospital for Special Surgery, New York, NY, USA

1. Introduction

A decision regarding method of contraception is a personal one for any woman, guided by perceived effectiveness, risk of side effects, stage in reproductive life, and personal beliefs. For a woman with autoimmune disease, underlying medical illness provides yet another variable involved in this decision. Up-to-date knowledge of the relative risks and benefits of various forms of contraception and their potential interaction with autoimmune disorders is critical for both the patient and her physician. In general, contraceptive methods are reversible or irreversible; the focus here will be on reversible methods of contraception, which may be hormonal or non-hormonal. Barrier methods, unlike others, provide some protection against sexually transmitted diseases.

1.1. Non-reversible contraception

Permanent sterilization (vasectomy or tubal ligation) is a common method of contraception used by couples nearing the end of their reproductive years. Vasectomy is used by 14% and tubal ligation by 19% of couples seeking contraception (Steinkampf et al., 1998). While surgical sterilization may be reversible in some cases, it is not considered a viable option for those seeking reversible contraception.

1.2. Reversible contraception

1.2.1. Non-hormonal methods

Reversible contraceptive methods fall into several broad categories: periodic abstinence, mechanical barrier methods, spermicides, intrauterine devices (IUDs), and hormonal contraception. Effectiveness of contraception is described in two ways: "method effectiveness" refers to risk of conception occurring with correct use of the contraceptive; "use effectiveness" refers to conception occurring with correct and incorrect use, i.e., "real life" likelihood of unintended pregnancy for most women. Method and use effectiveness are closest for those methods not directly related to coitus, e.g., oral contraceptive (OC) pills or intrauterine devices (Steinkampf et al., 1998; Chez and Strathman, 1999). Relative effectiveness rates for commonly used forms of contraception are listed in Table 1 (Hatcher et al., 1998). The highest continuation rates at the end of the first year of use are found with intrauterine devices, OCs, and depo-medroxyprogesterone acetate (DMPA) (Depo-provera); lower rates are seen with periodic abstinence, male condom, female condom, diaphragm, and spermicides (Pinter, 2002).

Periodic abstinence is the abstinence from intercourse during the days of the menstrual cycle when

*Corresponding author.
Department of Medicine, Weill Medical College of Cornell University, Hospital for Special Surgery, 535 East 70th Street, New York, NY 10021, USA.
Tel.: +1-212-606-1978; Fax: +1-212-774-2258.
E-mail address: sammaritan@hss.edu (L.R. Sammaritano).

DOI: 10.1016/S1571-5078(05)04011-0

Table 1
Methods of contraception with use and method effectiveness

Method	Useeffectiveness (%)	Method effectiveness (%)
No method	85	85
Sterilization		
Male	0.15	0.1
Female	0.5	0.5
Natural methods		
Withdrawal	19	4
Natural family planning	25	1–9
Barrier methods		
Male condom	14	3
Female condom	21	5
Diaphragm	20	6
Cervical cap	20–40	9–26
Spermicide	26	6
Intrauterine devices		
Copper T	0.8	0.6
Progesterone T	2	1.5
Hormonal		
Combined OC		
Estrogen/progestin	5	0.1
Progestin-only pill	5	0.5
DMPA injection	0.3	0.3

Note: DMPA, depo-medroxyprgesterone acetate; OC, oral contraceptive.
Source: Adapted from Hatcher et al. (1998).

an ovum can be fertilized, and can be determined by calendar rhythm, basal body temperature, cervical mucus, or symptothermal methods. The latter incorporates multiple indices to determine the fertile period. Use of techniques relying on physiologic change during the menstrual cycle is termed "natural family planning." Unintended pregnancy rates range from 1% to 25% (depending on the precise method) in the first year (Steinkampf et al., 1998; Chez and Strathman, 1999).

Barrier contraception methods include condoms, diaphragms, and cervical caps. The male condom is easily available and protects against a variety of sexually transmitted diseases including HIV. Use effectiveness is about 14% (i.e. 14% chance of unintended pregnancy in the first year of use). The relatively new female condom is composed of an inner and outer ring surrounding an inverted polyurethane condom, designed to protect against both pregnancy and sexually transmitted diseases. The diaphragm, a soft rubber cup surrounding a wound metal spring, is inserted vaginally and used with spermicide; unlike the condom, it must be prescribed and fitted by a health care professional. The cervical cap, similar to the diaphragm, is less commonly used due to difficulty with insertion and extraction but may remain in place for a greater number of hours. Spermicides are often used in combination with other methods, but may be used alone. The most common spermicidal agent is nonoxynol-9, which inactivates sperm by detergent activity and mechanically prevents sperm from entering cervical mucus.

The IUD is available in an unmedicated or a medicated form. The more commonly available medicated IUDs contain either copper or progesterone (levonorgestrel). Copper-containing IUDs, which are replaced every 10 years, significantly increase menstrual bleeding and dysmenorrhea. Progesterone-containing IUDs are associated with a 75% decrease in menstrual bleeding and dysmenorrhea, but must be replaced every 5 years. IUDs appear to prevent pregnancy by inducing an inflammatory endometrial response that is unfavorable to implantation. Complications of use (in addition to excessive bleeding and dysmenorrhea) include pelvic inflammatory disease (PID) and expulsion of the device. Contraindications to IUD use include current or previous pelvic infection, undiagnosed bleeding, uterine or cervical malignancy, history of ectopic pregnancy, and increased susceptibility to infection (including patients with malignancy, diabetes, valvular heart disease, AIDS or long-term corticosteroid therapy) (Steinkampf et al., 1998). In general, the IUD is not recommended for use in nulligravid women due to the risk of PID with tubal scarring and resulting infertility.

1.2.2. Hormonal methods

Hormonal contraception has evolved in a number of ways since the first birth control pill was approved for use in the United States by the FDA in 1960 (The Practice Committee of the American Society for Reproductive Medicine, 2004). The first oral contraceptive (OC) pill contained 150 mcg of the synthetic estrogen mestranol, 3–5 times the estrogen content of modern OCs. In addition to containing lower amounts of estrogen, current OCs may vary in progesterone components, and in dosage throughout the menstrual cycle. Use of extended hormonal contraception to prevent or delay menses is also on the horizon: in one recent study, an extended 49-day cycle of an OC containing 30 mcg ethinyl estradiol and 300 mcg norgestrel resulted in fewer days of bleeding with no increase in spotting and no significant differences in side effects (Miller and Notter, 2001).

Most OCs are combination products containing both an estrogen and a progestin. The synthetic estrogen is either ethinyl estradiol or mestranol (20–50 mcg); the progestin is one of multiple 17-α ethinyl analogs of 19-nortestosterone. Removal of the carbon at the C-19 position of ethisterone (an orally active testosterone derivative) confers progestational activity with some residual androgenic activity. The 19-nortestosterones include norethindrone, norethylnodrel, norethindrone acetate, ethynodiol diacetate, levonorgestrel, and norethindrone enanthate. Newer progestins include norgestimate, desogestrel, and gestodene. The specific progestin used in an OC may make a difference in potential side effects, since biologic effects vary, as shown in Table 2 (Schinder et al., 2003). In general, progestins are grouped according to a specific "generation"; most current OCs contain second- or third-generation progestins. Third-generation agents were developed to decrease androgenic effects such as acne, hirsuitism, nausea, and lipid changes while increasing progestational effects. Among available progestins, norgestimate has the greatest progestational effect and levonorgestrel the most androgenic activity. The recently developed drospirenone is an analog of the aldosterone-antagonist spironolactone and exhibits both progestational and anti-androgenic activity.

Initial combination OCs were monophasic, that is, the same dose of both hormones was taken daily for 21 days, followed by a medication-free period of 7 days to allow withdrawal bleeding. Multiphasic formulations allow either two (biphasic) or three (triphasic) different amounts of the estrogen and progestin over the course of the menstrual cycle in an attempt to reduce total amount of hormone while retaining efficacy and cycle control. The high effectiveness of combination OCs (use and method effectiveness are 5% and 0.1%, respectively) results from their multiple effects on the reproductive system. Ovulation is blocked due to inhibition of the mid-cycle surge of gonadotropins, and changes in cervical mucus retard sperm penetration. Uterine and tubal motility is altered, and inhibition of endometrial gland function impairs blastocyst survival (Steinkampf et al., 1998; Chez and Strathman, 1999).

Oral progestin-only contraceptives contain either norethindrone or norgestrel, and are used much less frequently due to irregular vaginal bleeding; however, they represent a viable option for those

Table 2
Biologic activities of common progestins

Progestin name	Progestogenic activity	Androgenic activity	Anti-androgenic activity	Anti-mineralocorticoid activity
Progesterone	(+)	(−)	(+/−)	(+)
Medroxy-progesterone acetate	(+)	(+/−)	(−)	(−)
Norethindrone[a]	(+)	(+)	(−)	(−)
Norethinodrel[a]	(+/−)	(+/−)	(−)	(−)
Levonorgestrel[a]	(+)	(+)	(−)	(−)
Norgestimate[b]	(+)	(+)	(+)	(−)
Desogestrel[b]	(+)	(+)	(−)	(−)
Gestoden[b]	(+)	(+)	(−)	(+)
Drospirenone[c]	(+)	(−)	(+)	(+)

Source: Adapted from Schinder et al. (2003).
[a] Second-generation progestin.
[b] Third-generation progestin.
[c] Spironolactone derivative.

patients in whom estrogen is contraindicated. Progestin-only preparations do not consistently inhibit ovulation (although other mechanisms of action are intact), and method and use effectiveness are slightly less than that with combination pills. Ingestion of the pills at the same time each day ensures stable serum levels and maximizes effectiveness (Chez and Strathman, 1999). The progesterone-only contraceptive DMPA, given as an intramuscular injection every 12 weeks, is a convenient estrogen-free alternative which requires little patient effort and has superior efficacy to the oral progestin-only preparations (Bigrigg et al., 2000).

Newer formulations of combination hormonal contraceptives include transdermal and intravaginal preparations. The recently approved transdermal combined estrogen–progestin patch delivers 20 mcg ethinyl estradiol and 150 mcg norelgestromin (an active metabolite of norgestimate) daily; the patch is changed weekly for 3 weeks followed by a no-patch week. Side effect profile and efficacy appear to be similar to OCs. The contraceptive vaginal ring (estrogen–progestin) releases 15 mcg ethinyl estradiol and 120 mcg etonogestrel (an active metabolite of desogestrel) daily and is used for 3 weeks continuously, followed by removal for 1 week. A 3-year implantable progestin contraceptive soon to be marketed in the U.S. consists of two rods containing levonorgestrel. The previous implantable contraceptive device, Norplant, was withdrawn from the market in 2002 due to complications associated with removal. Finally, although not recommended as a standard method of contraception, emergency OC regimens are effective if used within 72 h of unprotected intercourse. Two regimens are available, a combined estrogen–progestin medication and a progestin-only treatment; both require two doses 12 h apart. Efficacy ranges from 57% to 85% (The Practice Committee of the American Society for Reproductive Medicine, 2004).

1.2.3. Benefits of hormonal contraceptives

Unlike most medications, OCs are not intended to prevent or treat a disease, which makes scrutiny of side effects critical. Non-contraceptive benefits of OCs are occasionally the principle reason for use. The major non-contraceptive benefits include regulation of menstrual dysfunction, decrease in irregular bleeding from polycystic ovary syndrome, and decrease in blood loss from idiopathic menorrhagia. Primary dysmenorrheal pain, premenstrual symptoms, and peri-ovulatory discomfort are also diminished. Endometriosis may be treated with progestin alone or with a combination of estrogen and progestin. Regular use of OCs can prevent development of functional ovarian cysts and improve acne or hirsuitism caused by androgen excess. Although the mechanism is not clear, there is a decrease in the incidence of PID in OC users, possibly related to changes in cervical mucus. (Steinkampf et al., 1998).

An incidental benefit of OC use is a decreased risk of certain cancers. Endometrial cancer is less common in OC users, with risk reduction of >50% after 4 years. Benefit increases with longer duration of use, and persists after discontinuation (Schlesselman and Collins, 1999; Weiderpass et al., 1999). DMPA also protects against endometrial cancer, reducing risk by up to 80% at 8 years after discontinuation of medication (The WHO Collaborative Study of Neoplasia and Steroid Contraceptives, 1991). Ovarian cancer risk is similarly decreased. Incidence of ovarian cancer after 4 years is 41% lower in OC users than in non-users, and risk decreases further with additional years (The Cancer and Steroid Hormone Study of the Centers for Disease Control and the National Institute of Child Health and Human Development, 1987; Schildkraut et al., 2002). There is also preliminary evidence that OCs may protect against colorectal cancer (Fernandez et al., 2001). Combination OCs improve bone density in postmenopausal users, however, DMPA is associated with reversible bone loss in women of reproductive age due to lowered ovarian estrogen secretion (Berenson et al., 2001; Cundy et al., 1994). An uncertain suggested benefit of OCs is a protective effect on risk of developing rheumatoid arthritis (RA), discussed below.

1.2.4. Adverse effects of hormonal contraceptives

Mild side effects of combination OCs may be troublesome enough to prompt discontinuation, and include nausea, edema, chloasma (malar facial pigmentation), breast tenderness, and lactation. Estrogens affect tryptophan metabolism and decrease serotonin levels, possibly contributing to depression and mood changes. Abnormal uterine bleeding midcycle due to inadequate estrogen stimulation of the endometrium often resolves with substituting a pill that has greater estrogen content. Progestin-only medications are likely to cause irregular (or "breakthrough") menstrual bleeding and weight gain, leading to a high rate of discontinuation. Additional progestin-related symptoms include acne and amenorrhea (Steinkampf et al., 1998; Chez and Strathman, 1999). There is great interest in minimizing OC side effects while maintaining contraceptive benefit: one recently introduced OC promoted as enhancing "well-being" contains 30 mcg ethinyl estradiol with 3 mg drospirenone, a new progestin with both anti-mineralocorticoid and anti-androgenic effects. In addition to providing effective contraception, it is reported to show positive effects on mood, facial acne, and premenstrual syndrome symptoms (Mansour, 2002).

Other medical effects of OCs are varied. Impaired glucose tolerance may be seen with both combination and progestin-only oral preparations. Incidence of hypertension is increased, related primarily to type of progestin and patient age. DMPA, however, does not impair glucose tolerance or increase blood pressure. Development of benign hepatic adenomas, gallstones, and cholecystitis are rare with lower dose preparations. Net effect on the lipid profile results from opposing actions of the estrogen and progestin. In low-dose combination OCs, the resulting changes are not clinically significant for the majority of patients. Estrogen increases HDL and decreases LDL; progestins exert an opposite effect: the result is little clinical change. The more androgenic the progestin, the greater the negative effect; thus, the third-generation (less androgenic) progestin pills are least harmful with regard to lipid changes. DMPA has little effect on cholesterol levels (Steinkampf et al., 1998).

Serious complications of OCs are unusual, and may be limited with careful history and examination to exclude patients at high risk for side effects. Serious complications are primarily vascular, including venous thromboembolism, ischemic and hemorrhagic stroke, and myocardial infarction. There is also a slight increase in risk of breast and cervical cancers.

Although of concern, the increased relative risk for breast cancer with current OC use is quite small, RR 1.24 (95% CI, 1.15–1.33); risk declines and disappears within 10 years after discontinuation (Collaborative Group on Hormonal Factors in Breast Cancer, 1996). Breast cancers in OC users are in general less advanced than those in never-users, and there is no evidence for an increase in lifetime risk. Risk may be greater in OC users ages 25–34 years (RR 1.7, 95% CI, 2.3) (Rosenberg et al., 1996). Long-term OC use is also associated with an increased risk of cervical cancer, primarily in patients with human papilloma virus (HPV), the main causative agent in cervical neoplasia. Risk of cervical cancer in patients with HPV is increased with OC use for greater than 5 years (5–9 years of use, RR 2.82, 95% CI, 1.46–5.42; $\geqslant$10 years of use, RR 4.03, 95% CI, 2.09–8.02) (Moreno et al., 2002).

1.2.5. Effects of hormonal contraceptives on hemostasis

The effects of OCs on coagulation and fibrinolytic systems are numerous and complex. OC users have increased levels of prothrombin fragment 1 + 2 and thrombin–antithrombin complexes; plasma levels of all coagulation factors (except factor V) increase, while antithrombin III levels decrease. Plasma demonstrates APC resistance, an effect that is incompletely explained by the observed decrease in protein S. Finally, changes in the fibrinolytic system also occur. While estrogens induce activation of fibrinolysis through increased levels of tissue plasminogen activator (tPA) and decreased levels of plasminogen activator inhibitor (PAI), clot lysis time does not change due to increased thrombin activatable fibrinolysis inhibitor (TAFI) activity induced by increased thrombin levels. The ultimate result is an overall downregulation of fibrinolysis (Martinelli, 2001).

1.2.6. Hormonal contraceptives and venous thrombosis

The annual incidence of venous thromboembolism (VTE) in healthy women of reproductive age is 1 in

10,000; this is increased in women on current OC preparations by a factor of 3–5 (Martinelli, 2001). While the likelihood of VTE remains low given its rarity in the young female population, the large number of women worldwide who use OCs (over 100 million) makes the absolute number of events significant. The initial observed relative risk of VTE with early OCs was 10 times greater than normal; decreasing estrogen content from 150 to 50 mcg lowered risk to about 4 times that of non-users (Gerstman et al., 1991). Overall reported risk of VTE in studies of OC users compared with non-users ranges from three- to ninefold higher, depending on type of study, patient population, and particular progestin used (Martinelli, 2001). Recent studies make it clear that despite patient selection bias and other variables in early studies, third-generation OCs confer a greater risk of VTE than do second-generation formulations. A recent meta-analysis (Kemmeren et al., 2001) estimated an overall adjusted odds ratio of 1.7 (95% CI, 1.4–2.0) for development of VTE for third-vs. second-generation OC users. The progestin-induced mechanism is acquired APC resistance, which is more pronounced with the third-generation drugs (Rosing et al., 2001). Risk is also influenced by duration of use: risk is highest in the first year, decreases by more than 50% in later years, and disappears upon discontinuation of the drug (Martinelli et al., 2003; Lidegaard et al., 2002).

While thrombosis has been reported in numerous venous distributions, cerebral-vein thrombosis appears to be particularly increased with OC use. Martinelli et al. (1998) found an odds ratio of 22.1 (95% CI, 5.9–84.2) for cerebral-vein thrombosis in users of OCs; the same case–control study demonstrated an overall odds ratio of 4.4 (95% CI, 1.1–17.8) for deep-vein thrombosis. Non-oral hormonal preparations may have similar thrombotic risks: a recent report describes mesenteric vein thrombosis in an otherwise healthy woman using an intravaginal contraceptive (Voora and Vijayan, 2003).

Venous thrombosis risk is increased in the presence of certain risk factors: genetic or acquired thrombophilia, smoking (>10 cigarettes per day), age over 35 years, and obesity. A positive family history of thrombosis may also be a risk factor and often prompts a prothrombotic work-up, including factor V Leiden and prothrombin mutations, discussed in detail below (Martinelli, 2001). Obesity ($BMI \geqslant 25\,kg/m^2$), which increases risk of VTE by a factor of two in the non-OC individual, dramatically increases VTE risk in OC users by a factor of 10 (Abdollahi et al., 2003).

1.2.7. Hormonal contraceptives and arterial thrombosis

Risk of ischemic stroke is increased among all users of OCs by about twofold with current low-dose estrogen formulations (Kemmeren et al., 2002), but varies with presence or absence of concomitant risk factors. A case–control study of 203 young women with ischemic stroke (ages 19–49 years) calculated a relative risk of stroke in women using any type of OC as 2.3 (95%CI, 1.6 to 3.3). Unlike the risk of VTE, stroke risk in women using third-generation OCs was no different from those using second-generation drugs. A separate case-control study further suggested that users of third-generation OCs actually have a lower rate of stroke than do second-generation OC users: relative risk was 2.37 for second-generation and 1.32 for third-generation OCs (Lidegaard and Kreiner, 2002). This study also demonstrated a decrease in RR with decreasing estrogen content within the currently available formulations (50 mcg RR 2.65; 20 mcg RR 1.59). In contrast, Pettiti et al. (1996) did not find an increased risk of stroke in users of low dose OCs in a case–control study evaluating 295 women with stroke ages 15–44 years: after adjustment for other risk factors, RR was 1.18 (95% CI, 0.54–2.59). Risk of ischemic stroke appears increased with age older than 35, cigarette use, hypertension, and migraine. Risk of hemorrhagic stroke is also increased in OC users over the age of 35 (RR 2.2, 95% CI, 1.5–3.3) (Martinelli et al., 2003). In general, otherwise healthy normotensive and non-smoking women younger than 35 years using current low-dose estrogen combination pills probably have no increased risk of hemorrhagic or ischemic stroke (Pettiti et al., 1996).

Myocardial infarction, or MI (extremely rare among women of reproductive age) is increased among all users of OCs by twofold, even after controlling for usual cardiovascular risk factors

(Tanis et al., 2001). Risk for MI is greater in the presence of older age, smoking, hypertension, diabetes mellitus, hyperlipidemia, and obesity. In patients on OCs, risk of MI in a smoker over age 35 is 40 per 100,000; in contrast, for non-smokers over age 35, risk is 3 per 100,000, and risk for non-smokers under age 35 is 3 per million (World Health Organization Collaborative Study of Cardiovascular Disease and Steroid Hormone Contraception, 1997). Lewis et al. (1997) calculated an odds ratio of 2.35 (95% CI, 1.42–3.89) for second-generation and 0.82 (95% CI, 0.29–2.31) for third-generation OCs, again suggesting that third-generation drugs may be less likely to contribute to arterial thrombosis. Risk of peripheral arterial disease is also increased in OC users: the RATIO study demonstrated an adjusted odds ratio of 3.8 (95% CI, 2.4–5.8) for OC users vs. non-users (Van den Bosch et al., 2003).

At this time, absolute contraindications to use of combination OCs include history of thrombosis, cerebrovascular or coronary artery disease, uncontrolled hypertension, diabetes with vascular complications, age greater than 35 with cigarette smoking, estrogen-dependent neoplasia, breast cancer, pregnancy, active liver disease or liver tumor, and migraines with focal neurologic symptoms. Relative contraindications include prothrombotic risk factors, hyperlipidemia, prolactinoma, migraines, and prolonged immobilization (Steinkampf et al., 1998; Chez and Strathman, 1999).

1.3. Risks and benefits of contraceptive methods in autoimmune disease

Several specific issues are relevant when considering risks and benefits of contraception in patients with common autoimmune diseases. Presence of the acquired prothrombotic risk factor antiphospholipid antibody (aPL) is important in consideration of which hormonal methods may be used. A widely held perception that the immunostimulatory effects of estrogen promote flare of systemic lupus erythematosus (SLE) has limited use of OCs in these patients; however, recent well-designed studies demonstrate that clinical risks of OCs are not increased in stable lupus patients. A beneficial effect of OCs on disease activity has been suggested but not confirmed for patients with RA. Hormonal contraceptives interact with many other medications, an important consideration in patients with chronic disease. Finally, certain non-hormonal contraceptive methods may be physically difficult to use for some autoimmune disease patients.

1.3.1. Antiphospholipid antibody

aPL, widely recognized as a significant risk factor for thrombosis and fetal loss, represents an important acquired prothrombotic condition. While aPL are present in about 4% of the general population, titers are generally low with a low risk of complications. Within the SLE population, however, about 35% of patients have aPL. Patients with the primary antiphospholipid syndrome (PAPS) have the antibody and related complications without other underlying connective tissue disease. Although a relatively greater risk of thrombosis is seen in patients with high titers and the IgG isotype of anticardiolipin antibody (aCL), or the relatively more specific lupus anticoagulant (LA) or anti-$\beta 2$ Glycoprotein I (aβ2GPI) antibodies, the ability to predict risk of thrombosis for a given asymptomatic antibody-positive individual remains low (Asherson et al., 1999). Current theories suggest that thrombosis in these individuals is more likely to develop with a "second hit," that is, the presence of two or more risk factors which may be genetic or acquired. Well-recognized genetic factors include factor V Leiden, the prothrombin G20210A mutation, hyperhomocystinemia due to MTHFR mutations, and deficiencies of functional activity of proteins C, S, and antithrombin III. Lifestyle factors include cigarette smoking and combination OC use. Medical factors may include severe illness, surgery, other prolonged immobilization, malignancy, or pregnancy.

While aPL are rare in the general population, certain prothrombotic genotypes are surprisingly common. Prevalences of specific inherited thrombophilias vary. Deficiencies of protein C, protein S, and antithrombin III are relatively uncommon, affecting about 1% of the general population, and about 5% of patients with VTE. Factor V Leiden, a genetic variant which reduces susceptibility of factor V to inactivation by activated protein C, is more common: heterozygous factor V Leiden affects 2–15% of the Caucasian population, and accounts for up to 20% of first-time VTE (five- to sevenfold increased risk). The prothrombin G20210A mutation, which causes a 30% increase in plasma prothrombin levels, affects 2–4% of the Caucasian population and confers a two-to fourfold risk of VTE (Martinelli, 2001).

The combination of aPL with other prothrombotic conditions has been documented to increase risk of thrombosis. Forastiero et al. (2001) studied 105 unselected patients with aPL antibody for presence of common prothrombotic gene mutations. aPL-positive patients with the clinical syndrome of APS (i.e. thrombosis or fetal loss) were more likely to be positive for heritable risk factors (factor V Leiden, prothrombin G20210A, MTHFR, and the 4G/4G genotype of the PAI promoter) than were asymptomatic aPL subjects, and combinations of heritable thrombophilic genotypes were also more frequent in APS patients. In a series of 65 children with idiopathic ischemic stroke, Kenet et al. (2000) found an increased prevalence of thrombophilia markers, specifically factor V Leiden and aPL; six of the stroke patients, but none of the controls, had a combination of two or more thrombophilia markers. When thrombotic risk was analyzed in a cohort study of SLE patients, factor V Leiden and the prothrombin G20210A mutation were found to contribute to risk of VTE (but not arterial thrombosis) in SLE patients, and to potentiate the risk when combined with LA or aCL's. (Brouwer et al., 2004).

Use of OCs also exerts a marked additive effect on the risk of thrombosis in patients with hereditable risk factors, many of whom may not be aware of their genetic predisposition to thrombosis (Bloemenkamp et al., 2000; Pabinger et al., 1994). For women with antithrombin III deficiency, annual risk of VTE with OC is 27%; for carriers of protein C deficiency, it is 12%. Risk of thrombosis in heterozygous carriers of factor V Leiden using OCs is increased 20–30 times over non-carrier non-OC users; homozygous carriers' risk is 50–100 times greater (Martinelli, 2001). Heterozygous carriers of the prothrombin G20210A gene mutation on OCs have a 16-fold increase in VTE compared with non-carrier non-users (Martinelli et al., 1999), and risk for cerebral-vein thrombosis in carriers taking OCs has a staggering odds ratio of 149.3 (95% CI, 31.0–711.0). Vaya et al. (2003) have documented an increased risk of upper extremity venous thrombosis with OC use in patients who are carriers of the prothrombin G20210A gene mutation. Other genetic factors, not clinically tested or yet identified, may be important as well. For example, Bloemenkamp et al. (2002) reported a greater increase in plasma factor VII levels in OC users with the Q allele of the R/Q353 polymorphism in the factor VII gene, which may translate into increased likelihood of clot.

1.3.2. Hormonal contraceptives and aPLs

No well-designed studies have specifically studied the increase in thrombosis risk in aPL-positive patients on OCs, and the presumption of significantly higher thrombotic risk in patients with both aPL and OC makes a randomized trial unlikely. Multiple case reports, however, describe aPL-positive patients with thrombosis triggered by OCs (Asherson et al., 1988, 1993; Millan-Mon et al., 1993; Bacci et al., 1990; Girolami et al., 1996). Asherson et al. (1988) described seven women with aPL who had been on OCs before developing venous or arterial thrombosis. Julkunen's (1991) study of 31 SLE patients on OCs reported two episodes of DVT, both in patients with aPL. More recently, Girolami et al. (1996) reported three women who presented with VTE after starting OCs and were subsequently diagnosed with aPL.

Unlike factor V Leiden and the prothrombin G20210A mutations, aPL is associated with increased risk of arterial as well as venous thrombosis; use of OCs in aPL-positive patients will almost certainly increase risk of arterial events. Other factors which also increase risk of arterial complications, such as complicated migraines, atherosclerosis, or hyperlipidemia, may all be present or even increased in SLE patients with aPL, and may further increase risk of stroke or MI.

The aPL case reports as well as the more general demonstration of elevated thrombotic risk with multiple prothrombotic "hits" has generated significant concern regarding prescribing OCs to women with aPL, especially those with high titer antibody. In the recently completed SELENA (Safety of Estrogen in Lupus Erythematosus—National Assessment) study, designed to assess risk of flare in stable SLE patients on OCs, the study design specifically excluded patients with moderate to high titer IgG, IgM, or IgA aCLs or positive lupus anticoagulant, even those without a history of thrombosis. Although some patients in both OC and placebo groups presumably had low titer aCL (no numbers are reported), there was no increase in thrombotic complications in the OC patients: one OC-treated patient had a deep venous thrombosis, and two patients receiving placebo developed clots, an ocular thrombosis and a superficial thrombophlebitis (Petri et al., 2004). In a group of SLE patients studied by Sanchez-Guerrero et al. (2004), treatment with either combined or progestin-only OCs resulted in the same rate of thrombosis, two patients out of 54 in each group.

Although uncommon, non-thrombotic manifestations of aPL may also be affected by OCs. Chorea is associated with aPL and SLE, and risk may be increased further by addition of OCs (Asherson et al., 1986; Islander and Kahn, 1989). Although it has been recently suggested that OCs may induce development of aPLs in healthy women, specifically aβ2GPI IgG (Vad et al., 2003), this remains to be confirmed.

1.3.3. Systemic lupus erythematosus

Observations suggesting that estrogen therapy influences SLE disease activity include disease demographics (a 9:1 ratio of females to men during the reproductive years), alterations in estrogen metabolism in lupus patients, exacerbation of murine lupus with estrogen administration or androgen withdrawal, and scattered case reports of lupus flare following administration of OCs. Although the effects of sex hormones on the immune system are varied and complex, in general, estrogen appears to have an overall immunostimulatory effect that includes depression of cell-mediated immunity, natural killer function and immune surveillance (Ansar Ahmed et al., 1985; Grossman, 1988). Furthermore, effects of estrogen on the SLE immune system may differ from that of the normal immune system (Cutolo et al., 2001): for example, estradiol stimulates expression of CD40L in SLE T cells, but not control T cells (Rider et al., 2001). In addition to an increased immune system response to estrogen, SLE patients have a relatively greater estrogenic effect due to alterations in sex steroid levels and metabolism (Lahita et al., 1979; Inman et al., 1982): Lahita et al. (1979) demonstrated increased 16-hydroxylation of estrone in both males and females with lupus, which yields higher levels of 16 alpha-metabolites with more potent estrogenic activity.

Several murine lupus models also support an immunostimulatory effect of estrogen, although clearly these models are not necessarily analogous to human SLE (Steinberg et al., 1979). Castrated NZB/NZW F1 mice of both sexes show improved survival and lowered DNA antibody levels with androgen therapy, with the opposite effect observed with estrogen treatment. Treatment of the mice with 19-nortestosterone (nandrolone) had a similar beneficial effect (Roubinian et al., 1978; Verheul et al., 1981). This research has sparked attempts to treat lupus with both anti-estrogenic compounds, including tamoxifen (Sturgess et al., 1984), and androgenic compounds, including dehydroepiandrosterone (DHEA) (Petri et al., 2002; Chang et al., 2002). Recent studies of the latter suggest some clinical benefit.

It has been suggested that estrogen contributes to onset of SLE. Data are conflicting as to whether OCs induce antinuclear antibodies (Tarzy et al., 1972; Kay et al., 1971; Dubois et al., 1968; Bole et al., 1969). Scattered case reports describe onset of SLE after use of OCs, most often in patients with a predisposing condition such as arthritis or a biologic false-positive test for syphilis (Todd et al., 1985; Garovich et al., 1980; Travers and Hughes, 1978; Julkunen et al., 1991; Elias, 1973). Sanchez-Guerrero et al. (1997) demonstrated a slightly increased risk of developing SLE associated with past use of OC in the prospective Nurses' Health Study (RR 1.9; 95% CI, 1.1–3.3), although there was no relationship between duration of OC use or time since first use and the risk of developing SLE. A later population-based case control study of 240 SLE patients did not identify an association with OC use (Cooper et al., 2002), however, nor did a similar case–control study in a Swedish population (Bengtsson et al., 2002).

The bias against use of OCs in lupus is reflected in a 1993 cross-sectional study of contraceptive practices in Finland, where use of contraception was lower in SLE than in healthy women (59 vs. 77%, $p<0.001$), and barrier methods were more commonly used ($p<0.001$) (Julkunen et al., 1993). Several case reports have suggested flare with OC use (Table 3) (Pimstone, 1966; Hadida and Sayag, 1968; Chapel and Burns, 1971; Laugier et al., 1971; Miller, 1987). Conflicting results between early retrospective reports and later studies of OC effect on disease activity, however, are almost certainly due to variability in patient selection and method of evaluating flare (Table 4). For example, an early retrospective study by Jungers et al. (1982) that suggested increased risk of flare with OCs included only SLE patients with renal disease, some of whom had active disease at the time medication

Table 3
Case reports of flare in SLE with OC use

Case report	Oral contraceptive dose	Flare
Pimstone (1966)	50 mcg ethinylestradiol	Arthritis, fever, rash in 1 week
Hadida and Sayag (1968)	Norethindrone 5 mg (Note: progestin-only)	DLE→subacute LE 15 days
Chapel and Burns (1971)	Mestranol 100 mcg Mestranol 80 mcg	Arthritis (10 days) Rash (3 months)
Laugier et al. (1971)	Ethinyl estradiol	—
Miller (1987)	Ethinyl estradiol 30 mcg	Pulmonary hypertension (7 months)

Note: DLE, discoid lupus erythematosus; LE, lupus erythematosus.

Table 4
Studies on use of OCs in patients with SLE

Author	Type of study	No. SLE patients	OC	Outcome
Jungers et al. (1982)	Retrospective	20 with GN	30–50 mcg EE	43% flare (19% renal)
		11 with GN	Progesterone-only	No flares
Mintz et al. (1984)	Prospective	10	Norethisterone IM q 3 months	Same as controls
		15	Levonorgestrel 30 mcg/day	Same as controls
Julkunen (1991)	Retrospective interview	31	30–50 mcg EE	13% flare: Same as controls
Buyon et al. (1995)	Retrospective questionnaire	55	Not specified	13% self-reported flare rate
Petri et al. (2004)	Prospective (double-blind randomized placebo-controlled)	91	Triphasic 35 mcg EE	7.7% flare N.S.
		92	Placebo	7.6% flare
Sanchez-Guerrero et al. (2004)	Prospective (single-blind randomized)	54	30 mcg EE/levonorgestrel 150 mcg/day	0.92[a] N.S.
		54	Levonorgestrel 0.3 mg/day	0.90[a] N.S.
		54	Copper IUD	0.87[a]

Note: GN, glomerulonephritis; EE, ethinyl estradiol; N.S., not significant.
[a] Net probability of flare at 12 months.

was started; 12 patients had started on OCs prior to the diagnosis of SLE. Patients in Julkunen's later study (1991) that did not demonstrate OC-induced flare ranged from asymptomatic to those with active renal disease, but disease flare was evaluated on a clinical basis, with medical records examined where possible, and serologies other than aPL were not identified. Importantly, however, recognizing that some side effects of OCs could be confused with SLE activity, Julkunen specifically did not include mild arthralgia, LFT abnormalities, headache or migraine as SLE activity.

Newly released results of two well-designed randomized clinical trials suggest that OCs do not significantly increase the risk of lupus flare in a well-defined population of stable lupus patients (Petri et al., 2004; Sanchez-Guerrero et al., 2004). The SELENA trial was an equivalence trial specifically designed to test the hypothesis that OC use does not increase the risk of severe flare in SLE (Petri et al., 2004). The study randomized 183 lupus patients with inactive or stable-active disease to either OC (triphasic 35 mcg ethinyl estradiol/0.5–1 mg norethindrone for 12, 28 day cycles) or placebo. Patients with a history of thrombosis, moderate to high titer aCL, or LA were excluded. The 1-year severe flare rate was 0.084 for OC users and 0.087 for placebo. There was one severe renal flare in the OC arm and four in the placebo arm. Numbers of mild-to-moderate flares were equivalent in both groups, as were the numbers of patients experiencing three or more mild/moderate flares. Furthermore, there was no difference in the overall combined flare rate between the two groups.

Sanchez-Guerrero et al. (2004) compared several methods of contraception in SLE patients. They found disease activity to be similar among 162 lupus patients randomized to one of the three methods of contraception in a single-blind 12-month trial: combined OC, or COC (30 mcg ethinyl estradiol/levonorgestrel 150 mcg/day), progestin-only OC, or POC, (levoneorgestrel 0.3 mg/day) or a copper IUD. No difference was seen in global disease activity or flare rate, including rate of severe flare. POC users had a higher rate of discontinuation. Two thrombotic events were seen in each hormonal group, and two episodes of septic meningitis occurred in the IUD group.

1.3.4. Rheumatoid arthritis

In sharp contrast to SLE, it has been suggested that RA might benefit from treatment with OCs, based on improvement of RA symptoms in many patients during pregnancy (Ostensen and Husby, 1983), increase in risk of developing RA flare after pregnancy (Moskowitz et al., 1990), and demonstration of low androgen levels in RA patients. The latter has been suggested to be a possible factor in degree of disease activity, due to potential decrease in androgenic immunosuppression (James, 2003; Cutolo, 2002). Most research has actually centered on the question of whether OCs reduce risk of developing RA. Despite numerous studies, this question remains unresolved, likely because of differences in patient populations, source of controls, methodology, and OC content (Spector et al., 1990; Hannaford et al., 1990; Pladevall-Vila et al., 1996; Doran et al., 2004). An early report from the Royal College of General Practitioner's Oral Contraception Study (Anonymous, 1978) found the rate of RA development to be halved in current OC users, as compared to non-users and ex-users. Further studies demonstrated a protective effect, including an effect for previous OC users (Doran et al., 2004; Alleback et al., 1984; Hazes et al., 1991; Brennan et al., 1997). Hazes et al. (1991) demonstrated a relative risk of development of RA in current users to be 0.58 and 0.39 in ever-users, independent of dose, duration of use, or presence of HLA DR4. Other studies have suggested a duration-dependent effect (Spector and Hochberg, 1990), and some researchers contend that a possible reason for conflicting data is that the effect is most prominent for patients with severe or seropositive RA, rather than for RA in general (Van Zeben et al., 1990; Jorgensen et al., 1996; Van den Brouke et al., 1982). In contrast, a number of retrospective and prospective studies have found no reduction in risk, either in current or in ex-users (Linos et al., 1983; Del Junco et al., 1985; Vessey et al., 1987). Analysis from the Nurses' Health Study in 1990 did not show a protective effect of past use of OCs, although authors could not rule out a modest protective effect of current OC use (Hernandez-Avila et al., 1990). The question remains open, although the importance is obviously greatest for defining mechanisms of disease rather than intervention.

What about use of OCs to ameliorate disease course in RA? Several epidemiologic studies suggest a reduction in development of severe disease (Spector et al., 1990; Jorgensen et al., 1996), but therapeutic use of OCs in RA have not been well studied. This may be in part because hormone studies in patients show normal estrogen levels with low androgen levels. Low levels of both gonadal and adrenal androgens (testosterone and DHEA) have been demonstrated in serum and synovial fluid of both male and female RA patients (Masi et al., 1995; Cutolo et al., 1986, 2002) with a reduced androgen/estrogen ratio that suggests a reduction in net immunosuppressive effect. Men with RA have lower levels of bioavailable testosterone, and up to one-third are hypogonadal (Tengstrand et al., 2002). As a result, hormonal therapy attempts have focused on androgenic rather than estrogenic supplementation. Genetic factors may predispose to RA through sex hormone effects: for example, linkage to the locus for the estrogen synthase that catalyzes conversion of C19 androgens to C18 estrogens has been demonstrated in certain RA patients. Theoretically, enhanced activity of this enzyme could represent one genetic factor that would lead to reduced androgen levels and increased susceptibility to development of disease (John et al., 1999). Human macrophages have both cytoplasmic and nuclear receptors for androgens and estrogens, and can metabolize gonadal and adrenal androgens precursors to active metabolites (Cutolo et al., 1992). Interestingly, intra-articular testosterone has shown significant inhibitory effects on synovial hyperplasia and cartilage erosion in animal models of RA (Sterward and Bayley, 1992). Despite normal serum levels of estrogen in RA, recent work also suggests increased estrogen metabolites within the joint itself may activate synovial cell inflammation (Cutolo et al., 2003). Clinical attempts at using androgen therapy to treat RA has had mixed results. Early testosterone therapy showed improvement in disease activity, but complications of masculinization and menstrual disturbances (Margolis and Caplan, 1951). Treatment with the anabolic androgenic steroid nandrolone (19-nortestosterone) was not helpful in reducing disease activity (Bird et al., 1987). A more recent double-blind placebo-controlled study of testosterone in postmenopausal RA patients suggested a response in pain score, ESR and disability; 21% of patients showed improvement that was not statistically significant (Booij et al., 1996). Effects of androgen therapy in male patients are unresolved (Cutolo et al., 1991; Hall et al., 1996). Postmenopausal use of estrogen therapy has been evaluated in RA patients with no significant effect on disease activity, but improvement in bone mineral density (Van der Brink et al., 1993; Hall et al., 1994).

Thus, although treatment with OCs is unlikely to produce a beneficial effect on course of disease activity in RA, certainly no evidence suggests that use might exacerbate disease, and OCs seem an attractive contraception alternative for RA patients. Although purely theoretical, a case could be made for use of OCs containing relatively more androgenic progestin components. Effects of progestin-only OCs on RA have not been specifically evaluated. Although use of barrier methods should be safe in patients with RA, insertion of a cervical cap or diaphragm may be difficult for patients with severe arthritis affecting the hands or hip joints.

1.3.5. Other connective tissue diseases

OC therapy in patients with other autoimmune diseases has been paid scant attention. Estrogen therapy, however, has been evaluated in several cases of severe Raynaud's phenomenon associated with systemic sclerosis: intravenous administration of estrogen improved endothelial function in 10 female patients with systemic sclerosis and Raynaud's phenomenon with a significant increase in endothelium-dependent dilatation (Lekakis et al., 1998), and reversed cold-induced myocardial ischemia on nuclear imaging in a patient with Raynaud's due to systemic sclerosis (Lekakis et al., 1996). Use of oral estrogen in the form of OCs has not been demonstrated to affect patient-reported frequency, severity, or duration of Raynaud's attacks, although some patients report improvement in symptoms during pregnancy (Bartelink et al., 1992).

There is no specific data on effects of estrogen in patients with vasculitis, but one should obviously avoid OCs in patients with atherosclerosis or vasculitis who have increased risk for ischemia or

Table 5
Significant medication interactions with OCs

Medication	Effect with concomitant OC
Anticonvulsants	
Carbamazepine, barbiturates	↓ OC efficacy due to ↑ hepatic metabolism
Phenytoin	↑ Phenytoin concentration due to ↑ metabolism
Antibiotics	
Penicillins, cepalosporins, macrolides, metronidazole, sulfa, tetracyclines	↓ OC efficacy due to ↑ intestinal transport and ↓ enterohepatic reabsorption
Rifampin	↓ OC efficacy due to ↑ hepatic metabolism
Griseofulvin	↓ OC efficacy due to ↑ hepatic metabolism
Corticosteroids	↑ Steroid concentration due to ↓ metabolism
Cyclosporin	↑ Cyclosporine concentration due to ↓ metabolism
Warfarin	↑ or ↓ warfarin effect due to alteration in metabolism
Thyroid hormone	↓ Levels of free thyroxine due to ↑ levels of thyroxine-binding globulin

Source: Adapted from Fotherby (1990).

stroke. Takayasu's, in particular, affects women during the reproductive years when use of OCs might be desired. Although there are no reports of benefit or adverse effects of OCs in myositis, there is interesting animal data showing that estrogen may influence the degree of disruption in skeletal muscle after ischemia-reperfusion induced damage, suggesting some theoretical potential for estrogen to positively influence rate of skeletal muscle recovery (Tiidus, 2001).

There are general points relevant to most patients with autoimmune disease considering various modes of contraception. Potential interactions with medications are well recognized, and may interfere with efficacy of OCs; since many CTD patients are on multiple medications, it is imperative to check for pharmacologic interactions before prescribing OCs (Table 5). Medications commonly used in patients with connective tissue disorders that have potential interactions with OCs include anti-convulsants, corticosteroids, warfarin, and cyclosporine (Fotherby, 1990). While use of IUDs is discouraged in women who have not completed childbearing, IUD use is also generally contraindicated in women on immunosuppressive medications. Finally, prolonged immobilization is not uncommon in patients with rheumatologic illness, whether due to flare of disease, surgery, or other hospitalization; OCs should be discontinued during these periods if possible, and prophylactic heparin therapy added to reduce risk of VTE. This is obviously of critical importance in patients with prothrombotic conditions.

Key points

Although many questions remain unanswered, some important points regarding specific contraceptive methods in patients with autoimmune diseases are summarized below.

- Barrier methods of contraception are low-risk alternatives that reduce risk of sexually transmitted disease, but have lower use effectiveness than other methods.
  - The diaphragm and cervical cap may be difficult to insert properly for patients with hand or hip arthritis.
- IUDs are a very effective method of contraception, but are discouraged in nulligravid women due to increased risk of tubal infection and scarring.
  - Menstrual blood flow is increased with copper IUDs, which may be an issue for patients on anticoagulation therapy.
  - IUDs are generally contraindicated in patients who are on chronic corticosteroid or immunosuppressives, ruling them out as alternatives for many autoimmune disease patients.

- Combined OCs are the most effective form of reversible birth control.
  - Recent studies demonstrate no increase in risk of flare in lupus patients with inactive or stable disease who do not have moderate or high titer aPL or other standard contraindications.
  - OCs are contraindicated in all patients with moderate to high titer aPL, although use in patients on concurrent warfarin is an open question. Decisions regarding patients with borderline or low titer aPL are less clear, although screening for other prothrombotic risk factors seems a logical way to rule out other contraindications.
  - Interactions of OCs with other medications must be carefully researched, as this may reduce efficacy of either drug, or increase drug toxicity.
  - OCs should be held, and/or prophylactic anticoagulation given, to patients at prolonged bed rest especially if they are aPL-positive.
- Progestin-only contraception is a good alternative for patients with contraindications to estrogen-containing preparations.
  - The oral progestin pill is less effective than depot-medroxyprogesterone, and represents more of a challenge for patient compliance since it must be taken at the same time each day to be effective.
  - DMPA is associated with good compliance and does not represent a prothrombotic risk, although it can cause osteoporosis, an important issue for patients already on corticosteroid.
  - DMPA is an effective way to decrease menstrual blood flow and prevent anemia in patients on warfarin, while providing effective contraception.

References

Abdollahi, M., Cushman, M., Rosendaal, F.R. 2003. Obesity: risk of venous thrombosis and the interaction of coagulation factor levels and oral contraceptives. Thromb. Haemost. 89, 493.

Alleback, P., Ahlbom, A., Ljungstrom, K., Allander, E. 1984. Do oral contraceptives reduce the incidence of rheumatoid arthritis? A pilot study using the Stockholm County medical information system. Scand. J. Rheumatol. 13, 140.

Anonymous, 1978. Reduction in incidence of rheumatoid arthritis associated with oral contraceptives. Royal College of General Practitioners' Oral Contraception Study. Lancet i (8064), 569.

Ansar Ahmed, S., Penhale, W.J., Talal, N. 1985. Sex hormones, immune responses, and autoimmune diseases. Mechanisms of sex hormone action. Am. J. Pathol. 121, 531.

Asherson, R.A., Buchanan, N., Baguley, E., Hughes, G.R.V. 1993. Post-partum bilateral renal vein thrombosis in the primary antiphospholipid syndrome. J. Rheumatol. 20, 874.

Asherson, R.A., Cervera, R., Lie, J.T. 1999. The antiphospholipid syndromes. In: R.G. Lahita (Ed.), Systemic Lupus Erythematosus. Academic Press, San Diego, CA, p. 829.

Asherson, R.A., Harris, E.N., Hughes, G.R.V., Farquaharson, R.G. 1988. Complications of oral contraceptives and aPL: reply to the letter by Bruneau et al. Arthritis Rheum. 31, 575.

Asherson, R.A., Harris, N.E., Gharavi, A.E., Hughes, G.R.V. 1986. Systemic lupus erythematosus, antiphospholipid antibodies, chorea and oral contraceptives. Arthritis Rheum. 29, 1535.

Bacci, S., Urquiola, G., del Medico, P., et al. 1990. Budd-Chiari syndrome, pulmonary thromboembolism, and deep venous thrombosis associated with the "lupus anticoagulant" and recent use of oral contraceptives. Gen 44, 237.

Bartelink, M.L., Wollerheim, H., van de Lisdonk, E., Thien, T. 1992. Raynaud's phenomenon: subjective influence of female sex hormones. Int. Angiol. 11, 309.

Bengtsson, A.A., Rylander, L., Hagmar, L., Nived, O., Sturfelt, G. 2002. Risk factors for developing systemic lupus erythematosus: a case-control study in southern Sweden. Rheumatology 41, 563.

Berenson, A.B., Radecki, C.M., Grady, J.J., Rickert, V.I., Thomas, A. 2001. A prospective controlled study of the effects of hormonal contraception on bone mineral density. Obstet. Gynecol. 98, 576.

Bigrigg, A., Evans, M., Gbolade, B., et al. 2000. Depo provera. Position paper on clinical use, effectiveness and side effects. Br. J. Fam. Plann. 26, 52.

Bird, H.A., Burkinshaw, L., Pearson, D., et al. 1987. A controlled trial of nandrolone decanoate in the treatment of rheumatoid arthritis in postmenopausal women. Ann. Rheum. Dis. 46, 237.

Bloemenkamp, K.W., deMaat, M.P., Dersjant-Roorda, M.C., Helmerhorst, F.M., Kluft, C. 2002. Genetic polymorphisms modify the response of factor VII to oral contraceptive use: an example of gene-environment interaction. Vasc. Pharmacol. 39, 131.

Bloemenkamp, K.W.M., Rosendaal, F.R., Helmerhorst, F., Vandenbrouke, J.P. 2000. Higher risk of venous thrombosis during early use of oral contraceptives in women with inherited clotting defects. Arch. Int. Med. 160, 49.

Bole, G.G., Jr., Friedlaender, M.H., Smith, C.K. 1969. Rheumatic symptoms and serological abnormalities induced by oral contraceptives. Lancet 1 (7590), 323.

Booij, A., Biewenga-Booij, C.M., Huber-Brunning, O., et al. 1996. Androgens as adjuvant treatment in postmenopausal patients with rheumatoid arthritis. Ann. Rheum. Dis. 55, 811.

Brennan, P., Bankhead, C., Silman, A., Symmons, D. 1997. Oral contraceptives and rheumatoid arthritis: results from a primary care-based incident case-control study. Sem. Arthritis Rheum. 26, 817.

Brouwer, J.L., Bijl, M., Veeger, N.J., Kluin-Nelemans, H.C., van der Meer, J. 2004. The contribution of inherited and acquired thrombophilic defects, alone or combined with antiphospholipid antibodies, to venous and arterial thromboembolism in patients with systemic lupus erythematosus. Blood 104, 143.

Buyon, J.P., Kalunian, K.C., Skovron, M.L., et al. 1995. Can women with systemic lupus erythematosus safely use exogenous estrogens?. J. Clin. Rheumatol. 1, 205.

Chang, D.M., Lan, J.L., Lin, H.Y., Luo, S.F. 2002. Dehydroepiandrosterone treatment of women with mild-to - moderate systemic lupus erythematosus: a multi-center randomized, double-blind, placebo-controlled trial. Arthritis Rheum. 46, 2924.

Chapel, T.A., Burns, R.E. 1971. Oral contraceptives and exacerbation of lupus erythematosus. Am. J. Obstet. Gynecol. 110, 366.

Chez, R.A., Strathman, I. 1999. Contraception and sterilization. In: J.R. Scott, P.J. DiSaia, C.B. Hammond, W.N. Spellacy (Eds.), Danforth's Obstetrics and Gynecology. Lippincott, Williams & Wilkins, Philadelphia, PA, p. 553.

Collaborative Group on Hormonal Factors in Breast Cancer, 1996. Breast cancer and hormonal contraceptives: collaborative reanalysis of individual data on 53,297 women with breast cancer and 100,239 women without breast cancer from 54 epidemiological studies. Lancet 347 (9017), 1713.

Cooper, G.S., Dooley, M.A., Treadwell, E.L., St. Clair, E.W., Gilkeson, G.S. 2002. Hormonal and reproductive risk factors for development of systemic lupus erythematosus: results of a population based, case–control study. Arthritis Rheum. 46, 1830.

Cundy, T., Cornish, J., Evans, M.C., Roberts, H., Reid, I.R. 1994. Recovery of bone density in women who stop using medroxyprogesterone acetate. BMJ 308, 247.

Cutolo, M. 2002. Sex hormone adjuvanting therapy in rheumatoid arthritis. Lupus 11, 670.

Cutolo, M., Accardo, S., Villaggio, B., et al. 1992. Evidence for androgen receptors in the synovial tissue of rheumatoid arthritis patients and healthy controls. Arthritis Rheum. 35, 1007.

Cutolo, M., Balleiri, E., Giusti, M., et al. 1991. Androgen replacement therapy in male patients with rheumatoid arthritis. Arthritis Rheum. 34, 1.

Cutolo, M., Balleiri, E., Giusti, M., Monachesi, M., Accardo, S. 1986. Sex hormone status in women suffering from rheumatoid arthritis. J. Rheumatol. 15, 561.

Cutolo, M., Capellino, S., Montagna, P., et al. 2003. New roles for estrogens in rheumatoid arthritis. Clin. Exp. Rheumatol. 21, 687.

Cutolo, M., Carruba, G., Villaggio, B., et al. 2001. The phorbol diester 12-0-tetradecanoylphorbol 13-acetate (TPA) upregulates the espression of receptors in human THP-1 leukemia cells. J. Cell Biochem. 83, 390.

Cutolo, M., Seriolo, B., Villaggio, B., et al. 2002. Androgens and estrogens modulate the immune and inflammatory responses in rheumatoid arthritis. Ann. NY Acad. Sci. 966, 131.

Del Junco, D.J., Annegers, J.F., Luthra, H.S., Coulam, C.B., Kuralnd, L.T. 1985. Do oral contraceptives prevent rheumatoid arthritis?. JAMA 254, 1938.

Doran, M.F., Crowson, C.S., O'Fallon, W.M., Gabriel, S.E. 2004. The effect of oral contraceptives and estrogen replacement therapy on the risk of rheumatoid arthritis: a population-based study. J. Rheumatol. 31, 207.

Dubois, E.L., Strain, L., Ehn, M., Bernstein, G., Friou, G.J. 1968. LE cells after oral contraceptives. Lancet 2 (7569), 679.

Elias, P.M. 1973. Erythema nodosum and serological lupus erythematosus. Simultaneous occurrence in a patient using oral contraceptives. Arch. Dermatol. 108, 716.

Fernandez, E., La Vecchia, C., Balducci, A., et al. 2001. Oral contraceptives and colorectal cancer risk: a meta-analysis. Br. J. Cancer. 84, 722.

Forastiero, R., Martinuzzo, M., Adamczuk, Y., et al. 2001. The combination of thrombophilic genotypes is associated with definite antiphospholipid syndrome. Haematologica 86, 735.

Fotherby, K. 1990. Interactions with oral contraceptives. Am. J. Obstet. Gynecol. 163, 2153.

Garovich, M., Agudelo, C., Pisko, E. 1980. Oral contraceptives and systemic lupus. Arthritis Rheum. 23, 1396.

Gerstman, B.B., Piper, T.M., Tomita, D.K., et al. 1991. Oral contraceptive estrogen dose and the risk of venous thromboembolic disease. Am. J. Epidemiol. 133, 32.

Girolami, A., Zanon, E., Zanardi, S., Saracino, M.A., Simioni, P. 1996. Thromboembolic disease developing during oral contraceptive therapy in young females with antiphospholipid antibodies. Blood Coag. Fibrino. 7, 497.

Grossman, C.J. 1988. The importance of hormones in the regulation of the immune system. Immunol. Allergy Pract. 10, 104.

Hadida, M., Sayag, J. 1968. Lupus erythemateus subanu apparu après une cure du Norfutin chez une malade atteinte de lupus erythematreux chronique. Soc. Franc. Derm. Syph. Bull. 74, 616.

Hall, G.M., Daniels, M., Huskisson, E.C., et al. 1994. A randomized controlled trial of the effect of hormone replacement therapy on disease activity in postmenopausal. RA. Ann. Rheum. Dis. 53, 112.

Hall, G.M., Larbre, J.P., Spector, T.D., et al. 1996. A randomized trial of testosterone therapy in males with rheumatoid arthritis. Br. J. Med. 35, 568.

Hannaford, P.C., Kay, C.R., Hirsch, S. 1990. Oral contraceptives and rheumatoid arthritis: new data from the Royal

College of General Practitioners' oral contraceptive study. Ann. Rheum. Disease 49, 744.

Hatcher, R.A., Trussel, J., Stewart, et al. 1998. Contraceptive Technology. 17th Revised ed., Irvington Publishers, New York.

Hazes, J.M., Dijkmans, B.C., Vanddenbroucke, J.P., de Vries, R.R., Cats, A. 1991. Reduction of the risk of rheumatoid arthritis among women who take oral contraceptives. Arthritis Rheum. 34, 498.

Hernandez-Avila, M., Liang, M.H., Willett, W.C., et al. 1990. Exogenous sex hormones and the risk of rheumatoid arthritis. Arthritis Rheum. 33, 947.

Inman, R.D., Jovanovic, L., Markenson, J., et al. 1982. Systemic lupus erythematosus in men: genetic and endocrine features. Arch. Int. Med. 142, 1813.

Islander, M.K., Khan, M. 1989. Chorea as the initial presentation of oral contraceptive related systemic lupus erythematosus. J. Rheumatol. 16, 850.

James, W.H. 2003. Oral contraceptives, rheumatoid arthritis, and androgens. Ann. Rheum. Dis. 62, 279.

John, S., Myerscough, A., Eyre, S., et al. 1999. Linkage of a marker in intron D of the estrogen synthase locus to rheumatoid arthritis. Arthritis Rheum. 42, 1617.

Jorgensen, C., Picot, M.C., Bologna, C., Sany, J. 1996. Oral contraception, parity, breast feeding, and severity of rheumatoid arthritis. Ann. Rheum. Diseases 55, 94.

Julkunen, H., Kaaja, R., Joouhikainen, T., et al. 1991. Malignant hypertension and antiphospholipid antibodies as presenting features of SLE in a young women using oral contraceptives. Br. J. Rheumatol. 30, 471.

Julkunen, H.A. 1991. Oral contraceptives in systemic lupus erythematosus: side effects and influence on the activity of SLE. Scand. J. Rheumatol. 20, 427.

Julkunen, H.A., Kaaja, R., Friman, C. 1993. Contraceptive practice in women with systemic lupus erythematosus. Br. J. Rheumatol. 32, 227.

Jungers, P., Dougados, M., Pelissier, C., et al. 1982. Influence of oral contraceptive therapy on the activity of systemic lupus erythematosus. Arthritis Rheum. 25, 618.

Kay, D.R., Bole, G.G., Ledger, W.J. 1971. Antinuclear antibodies, rheumatoid factor and C-reactive protein in serum of normal women using oral contraceptives. Arthritis Rheum. 14, 239.

Kemmeren, J.M., Algra, A., Grobbee, D.E. 2001. Third-generation oral contraceptives and risk of venous thrombosis: meta-analysis. BMJ 323, 131.

Kemmeren, J.M., Tanis, B.C., van den Bosch, M.A., et al. 2002. Risk of arterial thrombosis in relation to oral contraceptives (RATIO) study: oral contraceptives and the risk of ischemic stroke. Stroke 33, 1202.

Kenet, G., Sadetzki, S., Murad, H., et al. 2000. Factor V Leiden and antiphospholipid antibodies are significant risk factors for ischemic stroke in children. Stroke 31, 1283.

Lahita, R.G., Bradlow, H.L., Kunkel, H.G., Fishman, J. 1979. Alterations of estrogen metabolism in systemic lupus erythematosus. Arthritis Rheum. 22, 1195.

Laugier, P., Orusco, P., Chatelanat, F., et al. 1971. Lupus erythemateux dissemine induit par estrogenes. Bull. Soc. Fr. Dermatol. Syphiligr. 78, 623.

Lekakis, J., Mavrikakis, M., Emmanuel, M., et al. 1996. Acute estrogen administration can reverse cold-induced coronary Raynaud's phenomenon in systemic sclerosis. Clin. Exp. Rheumatol. 14, 421.

Lekakis, J., Mavrikakis, M., Papamichael, C., et al. 1998. Short-term estrogen administration improves abnormal endothelial function in women with systemic sclerosis and Raynaud's phenomenon. Am. Heart J. 136, 905.

Lewis, M.A., Heinnemann, L.A.J., Spitzer, W.O., MacRae, K.D., Bruppacher, R. 1997. The use of oral contraceptives and the occurrence of acute myocardial infarction in young women. Results from the Transnational Study on Oral Contraceptives and the Health of Young Women. Contraception 56, 129.

Lidegaard, O., Edstrom, B., Kreiner, S. 2002. Oral contraceptives and venous thromboembolism: a five-year national case-control study. Contraception 65, 187.

Lidegaard, O., Kreiner, S. 2002. Contraceptives and cerebral thrombosis: a five-year national case–control study. Contraception 65, 197.

Linos, A., Worthington, J.W., O'Fallon, W.M., Kurland, L.T. 1983. Case-control study of rheumatoid arthritis and prior use of oral contraceptives. Lancet 1 (8337), 1299.

Mansour, D. 2002. Experience with Yasmin: the acceptability of a novel oral contraceptive and its effect on well-being. Eur. J. Contracep. Reprod. Health Care 7, 35.

Margolis, H.M., Caplan, P.S. 1951. The effect of some steroids (testosterone prionate, desoxycorticosterone acetate and ascorbic acid, and 21-acetoxy-5-pregnenolone artisone acetate) in rheumatoid arthritis. Ann. Int. Med. 34, 61.

Martinelli, I. 2001. Risk factors in venous thromboembolism. Thromb. Haemost. 86, 395.

Martinelli, I., Battaglioli, T., Mannucci, P.M. 2003. Pharmacologic aspects of the use of oral contraceptives and the risk of thrombosis. Pharmacogen 13, 589.

Martinelli, I., Sacchi, E., Landi, G., et al. 1998. High risk of cerebral vein thrombosis in carriers of a prothrombin gene mutation and in users of oral contraceptives. New Engl. J. Med. 338, 1793.

Martinelli, I., Taioli, E., Bucciarelli, P., Akhavan, S.S., Mannucci, P.M. 1999. Interaction between the G20210A mutation of prothrombin gene and oral contraceptive use in deep vein thrombosis. Arterioscler. Thromb. Vasc. Biol. 19, 700.

Masi, A.T., Feigenbaum, S.L., Chatterton, R.T., et al. 1995. Integrated hormonal-immunological-vascular systems interactions in the rheumatic diseases. Clin. Exp. Rheumatol. 13, 203.

Millan-Mon, A., Porto, J.L., Novo, C., Garcia-Martin, C., Guitan, D. 1993. Hepatic infarction in a pregnant patient with 'primary' antiphospholipid syndrome. Lupus 2, 275.

Miller, L., Notter, K.M. 2001. Menstrual reduction with extended use of oral combination contraceptive pills: randomized controlled trial. Obstet. Gynecol. 98, 771.

Miller, M.H. 1987. Pulmonary hypertension, systemic lupus erythematosus, and the contraceptive pill: another report. Ann. Rheum. Dis. 46, 159.

Mintz, G., Gutierrez, G., Deleze, M., Rodriguez, E. 1984. Contraception with progestagens in systemic lupus erythematosus. Contraception 30, 29.

Moreno, V., Bosch, F.X., Munoz, N., et al. 2002. Effect of oral contraceptives on risk of cervical cancer in women with human papilloma virus infection: the IARC multicentric case-control study. Lancet 359 (9312), 1085.

Moskowitz, M.A., Jick, S.S., Burnside, S., et al. 1990. The relationship of oral contraceptive use to rheumatoid arthritis. Epidemiology 1, 153.

Ostensen, M., Husby, G. 1983. A prospective study of the effect of pregnancy on rheumatoid arthritis and ankylosing spondylitis. Arthritis Rheum. 26, 1155.

Pabinger, I., Schneider, B., and the GTH study group, 1994. Thrombotic risk of women with hereditary antithrombin III, protein C- and protein S-deficiency taking oral contraceptive medication. Thromb Haemost. 71, 548.

Petri, M., Buyon, J.P., Kim, M., et al. 2004. Combined oral contraceptives (OC) are not associated with an increased rate of flare in SLE patients in SELENA. Arthritis Rheum. 50, S239.

Petri, M.A., Lahita, R.G., Van Vollenhoven, et al. 2002. Effects of prasterone on corticosteroid requirements of women with systemic lupus erythematosus: a double-blind, randomized, placebo-controlled trial. Arthritis Rheum. 46, 1820.

Pettiti, D.B., Sidney, S., Bernstein, A., et al. 1996. Stroke in users of low dose contraceptives. New Engl. J. Med. 335, 8.

Pimstone, B. 1966. Systemic lupus erythematosus. S Afr. J. Obstet. Gynaecol. 40, 62.

Pinter, B. 2002. Continuation and compliance of contraceptive use. Eur. J. Contracep. Reprod. Health Care 7, 178.

Pladevall-Vila, M., Delclos, G.L., Varas, C., et al. 1996. Controversy of oral contraceptives and risk of rheumatoid arthritis: met-analysis of conflicting studies and review of conflicting meta-analysis with special emphasis on analysis of heterogeneity. Am. J. Epidemiol. 144, 1.

Rider, V., Jones, S., Evans, M., et al. 2001. Estrogen increases CD40 ligand expression in T cells from women with systemic lupus erythematosus. J. Rheumatol. 28, 2644.

Rosenberg, L., Palmer, J.R., Rao, R.S., et al. 1996. Case–control study of oral contraceptive use and risk of breast cancer. Am. J. Epidemiol. 143, 25.

Rosing, J., Curvers, J., Tans, G. 2001. Oral contraceptives, thrombosis, and hemostasis. Eur. J. Obstet. Gynecol. Reprod. Biol. 95, 193.

Roubinian, J.R., Talal, N., Greenspan, J.S., Goodman, J.R., Siiteri, P.K. 1978. Effect of castration and sex hormone treatment on survival, anti-nucleic acid antibodies, and glomerulonephritis in NZB/NZW F1 mice. J. Exp. Med. 147, 1568.

Sanchez-Guerrero, J., Karlson, E.W., Liang, M.H., et al. 1997. Past use of oral contraceptives and the risk of developing systemic lupus erythematosus. Arthritis Rheum. 40, 804.

Sanchez-Guerrero, J., Mestanza, M., Jiminez, M.L., et al. 2004. Safety of use and effect on disease activity of three contraceptive methods in women with systemic lupus erythematosus: a one year follow-up clinical trial. Arthritis Rheum. 50, S689.

Schildkraut, J.M., Calingaert, B., Marchbanks, P.A., Moorman, P.G., Rodriguez, G.C. 2002. Impact of progestin and estrogen potency in oral contraceptives on ovarian cancer risk. J. Natl. Cancer Inst. 94, 32.

Schinder, A.E., Campagnoli, C., Druckmann, R., et al. 2003. Classification and pharmacology of progestins. Maturitas. 4651, S7.

Schlesselman, J.J., Collins, J.A. 1999. The influence of steroids on gynecologic cancers. In: I.S. Fraser, R.P.S. Jansen, R.A. Lobo, M.I. Whitehead (Eds.), Estrogens and Progestins in Clinical Practice. Churchill Livingstone, London, p. 831.

Spector, T.D., Hochberg, M.C. 1990. The protective effect of the oral contraceptive pill on rheumatoid arthritis: an overview of the analytic studies using meta-analysis. J. Clin. Epidemol. 43, 1221.

Spector, T.D., Roman, E., Silman, A.J. 1990. The pill, parity, and rheumatoid arthritis. Arthritis Rheum. 33, 782.

Steinberg, A.D., Melez, K.A., Raveche, E.S. 1979. Approach to the study of the role of sex hormones in autoimmunity. Arthritis Rheum. 22, 1170.

Steinkampf, M.P., Carr, B.R., Blackwell, R.E., 1998. Contraception. In: Carr, B.C., Blackwell, R.E. (Eds.), Textbook of Reproductive Medicine. 2nd ed., Appleton and Lange, Stamford, p. 707.

Sterward, A., Bayley, D.L. 1992. Effects of androgen in animal models of rheumatoid arthritis. Agents Actions 35, 268.

Sturgess, A.D., Evans, D.T., Mackay, I.R., Riglar, A. 1984. Effects of the oestrogen antagonist tamoxifen on disease indices in systemic lupus erythematosus. J. Clin. Lab. Immunol. 13, 11.

Tanis, B.C., van den Bosch, M.A., Kemmeren, J.M., et al. 2001. Oral contraceptives and the risk of myocardial infarction. New Engl. J. Med. 345, 1787.

Tarzy, B.J., Garcia, C.R., Wallach, E.E., et al. 1972. Rheumatic disease, abnormal serology and oral contraceptives. Lancet 2 (7776), 501.

Tengstrand, B., Carlstrom, K., Hafstron, I. 2002. Bioavailable testosterone in men with rheumatoid arthritis—high frequency of hypogonadism. Rheumatology 41, 285.

The Cancer and Steroid Hormone Study of the Centers for Disease Control and the National Institute of Child Health and Human Development, 1987. The reduction in risk of ovarian cancer associated with oral contraceptive use. New Engl. J. Med. 316, 650.

The Practice Committee of the American Society for Reproductive Medicine, 2004. Hormonal contraception: recent advances and controversies. Fertil. Steril. 82, 520.

The WHO Collaborative Study of Neoplasia and Steroid Contraceptives, 1991. Depot-medroxyprogesterone acetate (DMPA) and risk of endometrial cancer. Int. J. Cancer 49, 186.

Tiidus, P.M. 2001. Oestrogen and sex influence on muscle damage and inflammation: evidence from animal models. Curr. Opin. Clin. Nutr. Metabol. Care 4, 509.

Todd, G.R., McAteer, E.J., Jack, C.M., et al. 1985. Pulmonary hypertension, systemic lupus erythematosus, and the contraceptive pill. Ann. Rheum. Dis. 44, 266.

Travers, R.L., Hughes, G.R.V. 1978. Oral contraceptive therapy and systemic lupus erythematosus. J. Rheumatol. 5, 448.

Vad, S., Lakos, G., Kiss, E., et al. 2003. Antiphospholipid antibodies in young women with and without oral contraceptive use. Blood Coag. Fibrinol. 14, 57.

Van den Bosch, M.A., Kemmeren, J.M., Tanis, B.C., et al. 2003. The RATIO study: oral contraceptives and the risk of peripheral arterial disease in young women. J. Thromb. Haemost. 1, 439.

Van der Brink, H.R., van Everdingen, A.A., van Wijk, M.J.G., et al. 1993. Adjuvant estrogen therapy does not influence disease activity in postmenopausal female patients with RA. Ann. Rheum. Dis. 52, 862.

Van den Brouke, J.P., Valkenburg, H.A., Boersma, J.W., et al. 1982. Oral contraceptives and rheumatoid arthritis: further evidence for a preventive effect. Lancet ii (8303), 839.

Van Zeben, D., Hazes, J.M., Vandenbroucke, J.P., Dijkmans, B.A., Cats, A. 1990. Diminished incidence of severe rheumatoid arthritis associated with oral contraceptive use. Arthritis Rheum. 33, 1462.

Vaya, A., Mira, Y., Mateo, J., et al. 2003. Prothrombin G20210A mutation and oral contraceptive use increase upper-extremity deep vein thrombotic risk. Thromb. Haemo. 89, 452.

Verheul, H.A., Stimson, W.H., den Hollander, F.C., Schuurs, A.H. 1981. The effects of nandrolone, testosterone and their decanoate esters on murine lupus. Clin. Exp. Immunol. 44, 11.

Vessey, M.P., Villard-Mackintosh, L., Yeates, D. 1987. Oral contraceptives, cigarette smoking, and other factor factors in relation to arthritis. Contraception 35, 457.

Voora, D., Vijayan, A. 2003. Mesenteric vein thrombosis associated with intravaginal contraceptives: a case report and review of the literature. J. Thomb. Thrombolysis 15, 105.

Weiderpass, E., Adami, H.O., Baron, J.A., et al. 1999. Use of oral contraceptives and endometrial cancer risk (Sweden). Cancer Cause Control 10, 277.

World Health Organization Collaborative Study of Cardiovascular Disease and Steroid Hormone Contraception, 1997. Acute myocardial infarction and combined oral contraceptives: results of an international, multicentre, case–control study. Lancet 349 (9060), 1202.

Handbook of Systemic Autoimmune Diseases, Volume 4
Reproductive and Hormonal Aspects of Systemic Autoimmune Diseases
Michael Lockshin and D. Ware Branch, editors

CHAPTER 12

Gynecologic Problems in Women with Autoimmune Diseases

Kjersti M. Aagaard-Tillery[a,*], Calla M. Holmgren[a], James R. Scott[b]

[a]*Division of Maternal-Fetal Medicine, Department of Obstetrics and Gynecology, University of Utah Health Sciences Center, Salt Lake City, UT, USA*

[b]*Division of General Obstetrics and Gynecology, Department of Obstetrics and Gynecology, University of Utah Health Sciences Center, Salt Lake City, UT, USA*

1. Introduction

As the recognition of autoimmune disorders among women expands, primary care physicians, rheumatologists, dermatologists, and obstetrician-gynecologists are called upon to evaluate, diagnose, and treat an array of common gynecologic conditions. While these conditions are not limited to this population of women, real or perceived prevalence and incidence are increased, as well as severity. In this chapter, wewill approach the issues of management of vulvar, vaginal, and cervical conditions and sexuality and sexual dysfunction.

2. Vulvar disorders

2.1. Contact dermatitis

The most common benign lesion of the external genitalia is contact dermatitis. Most cases are due to local irritants, such as "feminine hygiene" products, bath soaps, powders, and synthetic clothing. Obviously, the treatment involves identifying and eliminating the offending agent(s). The local application of fluorinated hydrocorticosteroidism, used sparingly, will provide symptomatic relief.

2.2. Lichen sclerosis

Lichen sclerosis, an inflammatory disease of unknown etiology and poorly characterized pathogenesis, is a rather common vulvar disorder and can affect all age groups from 6 months to late adulthood. In women, vulvar and perineal involvement are most common with symptoms including pruritis, burning pain, dyspareunia, dysuria, vaginal discharge, anal or genital bleeding. An eruption of lichen sclerosis begins as white papules that coalesce into plaques. Advanced cases may present with labial stenosis and fusion (Chernosky et al., 1957). Histological examination finds a compact hyperkeratosis, usually overlying a thin epidermis, underlying collagenization, and an inflammatory infiltrate.

While the pathogenesis of lichen sclerosis is not fully understood, there appears to exist an infectious and an inflammatory component. Atypical mycobacterium and certain viral conditions have been implicated in the pathogenesis (Jorgensen and Svensson, 1993). Torok et al. (1975) evaluated biopsy specimens and noted tubular particles in endothelial cells and fibrocytes that resemble paramyxovirus-like inclusion bodies. It was thought

*Corresponding author.
Division of Maternal-Fetal Medicine, Department of Obstetrics and Gynecology, 30 North 1900 East, Rm 2B200 SOM, University of Utah Health Sciences Center, Salt Lake City, UT 84132, USA.
Tel.: 801-581-7260.
E-mail address: kjersti.aagaard@hsc.utah.edu (K.M. Aagaard-Tillery).

DOI: 10.1016/S1571-5078(05)04012-2

that these were not of viral origin, but perhaps represented aberrant cytoplasmic tubules, instituting the idea that an autoimmune response was responsible. Recent investigation has shown that there may be an immune-based association linking lichen sclerosis and scleroderma. Thus, others have demonstrated that a subpopulation of dermal fibroblasts will proliferate following incubation with serum from patients with scleroderma. These findings suggest that those factors yielding inflammation and fibrosis in lichen sclerosis and scleroderma present in serum, bear bioidentical function (Stoughton and Wells, 1950; Frances et al., 1983).

The mainstay of therapy for lichen sclerosis is steroid-based. Topical clobetasol propionate is applied at a strength of 0.025% once a day for 5 days of each week until resolution of symptoms, typically for 3 months. By contrast, topical estrogen and testosterone have been used with mixed results. Thus, patients treated with estrogen note variable degrees of symptomatic relief. With topically applied testosterone, the patients demonstrated clinical improvement, but at the expense of side affects like clitoralmegaly, acne, hirsutism, and menstrual irregularities.

The differential diagnosis of white lesions of the vulva includes several less common problems. Hyperplastic dystrophy is characterized by a particularly thick keratin layer overlying a thinning or thickened epithelial layer and with an underlying chronic inflammatory infiltrate. It is also treated with topical steroids. Extramammary Paget disease, appearing as white, hyperkeratotic lesions on a reddened epidermal background, requires excisional treatment and has a tendency to recur locally. Finally, intraepithelial neoplasia usually presents as pruitic scaly white (or red) vulvar lesions. It is imperative that all vulvar lesions are biopsied to establish the diagnosis, and rule out neoplasia.

2.3. Lichen planus

Another inflammatory condition that affects skin and mucous membranes is lichen planus. Isolat ed vulvar involvement is considered uncommon, occurring in only 5% of women presenting with lichen planus. However, if lichen planus is present in other parts of the body, vulvar disease can be found in up to 50% of patients (Jensen et al., 2004). When lichen planus involves the skin of the vulvar area, it commonly appears as an eruption of shiny, flat, polygonal, violaceous papules with white striae; when it occurs on mucosal surfaces, it typically will result in white reticulate lesions. The etiology of lichen planus is unknown, but it has been proposed that an autoimmune mechanism involving activated T-cells directed against basal keratinocytes is responsible (Scully et al., 1998). A form of the disorder can be drug-induced. Medications for hypertension, including β-blockers, α-methyldopa, and ACE inhibitors have been implicated, as well as several drugs used to treat autoimmune disease like NSAIDS, gold, and quinidine.

Patients presenting with lichen planus will often complain of vulvar soreness and vaginal discharge. Significant pruritis and burning are also often present. It is unusual, but some patients are completely asymptomatic. On physical examination, one of three types of lichen planus may affect the vulva: papulosquamous, hypertrophic, and erosive. Treatment of lesions is with topical steroid cream, as per aforementioned dosing regimens. Oral steroids may be employed in refractory cases, or among patients with severe symptoms.

2.4. Autoimmune disorders that may affect the vulva

A number of autoimmune disorders have been associated with vulvar disease. Psoriasis is a common, generalized skin disease of unknown etiology that involves the vulva in approximately 20% of patients. The disease is chronic, relapsing with an unpredictable course. Typically, manifesting as red papules that enlarge and become well circumscribed, a gentle scraping of observed affected tissue will confirm the diagnosis. Treatment involves topical hydrocortisone cream and occasionally oral retinoids. Reiter's syndrome, in classic form, typically consists of a triad of arthritis, urethritis, and conjunctivitis, and is uncommon in females. However, a case of atypical Reiter's syndrome is reported in the literature consisting of the above findings in conjunction with severe ulcerative vulvitis (Lotery et al., 2003). Widespread pustules, erosions, and erythema affected the groin, labia majora, labia minora, and perineum. *Lupus* has also been associated with idiopathic genital ulcers, as has *Behcet's* disease, a multisystem vascular disease consisting of a triad of genital and oral ulcers with an associated uveitis. Lastly, although uncommon, vulvar and perineal manifestations of *Crohn's* disease may occur and, in rare instances, precede the gastrointestinal symptoms.

Autoimmune bullous dermatoses are composed of a variety of blistering diseases, some of which involve the vulva. They can be extremely incapacitating and occasionally fatal. Most are extremely rare and mentioned here as a matter of completeness. Examples include pemphigus vulgaris, paraneoplastic pemphigus, bullous pemphigoid, cicatricial pemphigoid, dermatitis herpetiformis, and linear IgA dermatosis (Marren et al., 1993).

Pemphigus vulgaris is a rare disorder that is more common in women of Jewish or Mediterranean descent. Clinical features associated with condition are flaccid blisters or crushed erosions located in intertriginous areas and mucosa. The lesions are typically painful and carry a risk of infection in untreated cases, resulting (albeit infrequent) in sepsis and mortality. Diagnosis is made under direct light visualization, displaying suprabasilar blister with acantholysis. The primary modes of treatment focus on immunosuppression with corticosteroids or azathioprine, methotrexate, cyclophosphomide. In extreme conditions, plasmapheresis may be indicated (Marren et al., 1993).

Paraneoplastic pemphigus is extremely rare, with age of onset approximating 60 years. As its nomenclature would suggest, paraneoplastic pemphigus must be considered to be associated with a lymphoid malignancy unless proven otherwise. The disease is characterized by extensive painful mucocutaneous erosions resembling pemphigus vulgaris, but with the presence of a neoplasm. Treatment necessitates diagnosis and therapy for the underlying neoplasm (Marren et al., 1993).

Bullous pemphigoid is equally prevalent among men and women, again with onset in the mid to late 6th decade. It is typified by tense bullae, with the concomitant presence of clear fluid or erosions. Sentinel lesions frequently manifest as erythematous urticarial pruritic plaques localized in the groin, and rarely involve the underlying mucosa. Diagnosis may be made with light displaying subepidermal blister with mixed superficial inflammation. As with the majority of cutaneous dermatopathologies, treatment involves the use of corticosteroids alone or with azathioprine, mycophenolate mofetil or a tetracycline. The anticipated natural course is usually self-limiting, but may last from months to years (Marren et al., 1993).

Cicatricial pemphigoid is similarly rare, again occurring in women during the 4th and 5th decades of life. In this disorder, the blistering of the skin characterized by severe, erosive lesions of the skin as well as the underlying mucosal membranes. The blisters are subepidermal and surrounded by an inflammatory cell infiltrate of mononuclear cells, histiocytes, and plasma cells. Diagnosis is established with direct immunofluorescence, with linear deposition of C3 and IgG along the basement membrane. Topical and oral steroids are the mainstays of therapy.

Dermatitis herpetiformis is a chronic skin disease characterized by papulovesicular lesions, urticarial wheals, and intense pruritis. It is too rare, with an incidence of 10–39 cases per 1,00,000. Typical initial stage of onset occurs in the 3rd decade of life. On examination, findings are notable for a symmetric distribution along extensor surfaces including elbows, knees, buttocks, shoulders, and the sacral area. The mucous membranes are rarely affected. Direct immunofluorescence will confirm the diagnosis upon lesion biopsy, and treatment is with dapsone or sulfapyridine. Of note, a gluten-free diet has also been found to improve skin lesions (Bickle et al., 2002).

The final observed autoimmune bullous disease that may affect the vulva is a condition known as *linear* IgA *disease*. It is characterized histopathologically by deposition of IgA along the basement membrane. The lesions are pruritic; annual papules, vesicles, and bullae are found in groups.

As with other immune-mediated dermatoses, it too occurs most frequently on extensor surfaces. While the majority of cases present in the 3rd decade of life, it is of note that there does exist a similar chronic bullous disease of childhood. Treatment is typically rapid with dapsone or sulfaprindine; patients may also require low-dose prednisone to suppress blister formation (Marren et al., 1993).

2.5. Vulvar disorders resulting from systemic therapy or systemic illness

As reviewed above, autoimmune conditions may result in organ-specific damage to the vulva; in addition, vulvar dystrophies and dermatoses may result as secondary manifestations. Most commonly, systemic immunosuppression resulting from the treatment of autoimmune disorders or the presence of an underlying vasculitis can predispose patients to vulvar disease. In fact, any chronic medical condition or use of immunosuppressant medication increases the likelihood of secondary infection, with implications for the female genitalia and specifically, the vulva. A particularly common vulvar disorder influenced by systemic therapy is infection due to *Candida albicans*; this is discussed under the vaginitis section of this chapter.

Vulvar dysplasia is seen more frequently in these patients with impaired cell-mediated immunity, i.e., HIV-positive or transplant recipients on immunosuppressive therapy (Conley et al., 2002). In recent years, premalignant changes of the vulva are seen with increasing frequency in young patients, possibly a result of increased human papillomavirus (HPV) infections in this group. This observation is supported by the findings of Crum et al., demonstrating that HPV DNA is involved in the development in a group of vulvar carcinomas that occur in younger patients (Crum, 1992). HPV is discussed more extensively in latter sections of this chapter.

Patients with *premalignant or malignant atypias of the vulva* will present most often with irritation or itching, occasionally, a mass or lesion. The vulva typically appears whitish due to a thickened keratin layer; a mass that may or may not be present. Alternatively, vulvar regions may occasionally appear red or atypically pigmented. Given the marked clinical variability, biopsy should be performed with a Keyes dermal punch when such a condition is suspected. Treatment and therapy is ultimately dependent upon biopsy results. If vulvar dysplasia is encountered, therapy is focused on eradicating the area of premalignant neoplasia, usually with surgery. If vulvar condylomata without dysplasia are noted indicative of low-risk strains of HPV, management is variable and controversial. Suffice it to say, while in the general population vulvar condylomas may be considered for conservative management with observation, treating only large and symptomatic lesions, certain experts in the field would suggest more aggressive ablative therapy among immunosuppressed patients. Treatment with CO_2 laser vaporization, fulgration or trichloroacetic acid is typically indicated and after treating the lesions, monitoring of the area with tri or biannually is recommended (Ferenczy et al., 2003).

Several vulvar problems characterized by erosions or ulcers are also infectious in nature. Diseases like *syphilis, chancroid, herpes*, and *hidrandenitis suppurativa* are associated with an infectious etiology that may be exacerbated with the use of immunosuppressive therapy. Appropriate cultures and supportive tests are indicated to make a specific diagnosis and treatment should be tailored to that diagnosis.

3. Vaginitis

Vaginitis is one of the most common infections in women, is a frequent reason for physician–patient visits and can be a recurrent problem in all age groups. Furthermore, evidence suggests that vaginitis is an even greater problem for patients that suffer from chronic illness and immunosuppression. It is important that vaginitis should be evaluated, diagnosed, and treated in a systematic and suitable way in this patient population.

The vagina is a complex environment of microflora, hormones, and specific pH levels. Numerous organisms are present in the vagina, mostly yeast, Gram-positive and Gram-negative aerobic organisms, as well as anaerobic bacteria. These organisms, particularly *Lactobacillus acidophilus*, exist together to establish an equilibrium with a vaginal pH level between 3.8 and 4.2. Lactobacilli are extremely important to suppress the growth of the other components of the vaginal flora and to produce hydrogen peroxide, which is toxic to anaerobes. Pathological situations in which the vaginal pH rises may result in suppression of the growth of lactobacilli and overgrowth of potentially pathogenic bacteria or yeast. This leads to vaginitis (Priestley et al., 1997).

An alteration in the vaginal ecosystem described above can result from numerous factors. Antibiotics, hormones, contraceptives, douches, vaginal medication, sexual intercourse, concomitant sexually transmitted diseases, and stress can all contribute to a change in vaginal pH and the growth of pathogenic organisms. Immunocompromised states such as diabetes mellitus, HIV and presumably, autoimmune disease, placed women at increased risk for this disorder (Hillier, 1998).

Vaginitis can present in several ways, forms, the most common being *Candidal vaginitis*, bacterial vaginosis and *Trichomonas vaginalis* (Table 1). Vaginitis can also be caused by atrophy, resulting in vaginal dryness or burning, but this is usually secondary to hormone deficiency and will not be discussed at length here.

Candidal vaginitis is an extremely common vaginal infection, and frequently presents with a component of vulvar involvement (Haefner, 1999). By age 25, half of all college age women will have experienced at least one clinically diagnosed episode of vulvovaginal candidiasis (Foxman et al., 2000). Approximately 30% of healthy women have Candida as a part of their normal vaginal ecosystem (Giraldo et al., 2000). Although there are several types of Candida, the most common offending organism is *Candida albicans*. Patients with an overgrowth of Candida will present complaining of pruritis, increased vaginal discharge, and burning affecting both the vulva and vagina (Table 1). On physical examination, there will usually be a non-malodorous, thick, white discharge. The vagina may be edematous and erythematous, and vulvar signs are similar and may include excoriations secondary to scratching. Diagnosis is achieved by pelvic examination, pH determination and a wet-mount preparation with potassium

Table 1
Vaginitis: etiology, findings on physical examination, diagnosis, and treatment

Vaginosis	Organism	Physical examination findings	Diagnosis	Treatment
Yeast infection	*Candida (albicans, glabrata, topicalis)*	Non-malodorous thick white discharge	Wet preparation and KOH preparation with presence of pseudohyphae or budding pH <4.5	Antifungal agents Oral Topical See text
Bacterial vaginosis	Polymicrobial	Malodorous "fishy" vaginal discharge	Amsel's criteria: thin gray vaginal discharge	Metronidazole or clindamycin Oral Topical
		Discharge may be thin, homogeneous	Positive "whiff" test clue cells pH >4.5	See text
Trichomonas	*Trichomonas*	Copious yellow-gray or green discharge	Fresh wet-mount with presence of mobile flagellated organisms	Single oral 2 gm dose of metronidazole or 500 mg BID for 7 days
		Foul odor Vulvovaginal irritation Dysuria "Strawberry cervix"	PH >4.5–4.7	Treat sexual partners

hydroxide (KOH). The vaginal pH level may not be altered with Candida, but the microscopic evaluation of the KOH wet-mount should show hyphae or budding yeast cells. Some yeast infections will not show these findings on wet-mount, but *in these instances*, clinical correlation is important. *Confirmation of Candidal vaginitis* using culture is not recommended (Haefner, 1999). Uncomplicated candidal infections can be treated with one of many different antifungal therapies, as summarized in Table 2. Most Candida will be sensitive to topical clotrimazole or miconazole.

Recurrent vaginal candidiasis, several or more episodes of infection per year, may be more common in women with systemic autoimmune conditions such as systemic lupus erythematosus (SLE). Authorities currently believe that recurrent infections are likely the result of host factors, though infection with resistant fungal organisms other than *C. albicans* is a possibility (Sobel and Chaim, 1997). The use of chronic steroids has been implicated as a potential likely etiologic factor, as have repeated courses of antibiotics. Mycologic culture may play a role in the diagnosis and management of recurrent candidal infection. Treatment may require decreasing glucocorticoid dose, when possible. An initial regimen of oral therapy is recommended and continued for approximately 14 days so as to ensure clinical remission and a negative fungal culture. Immediately after achievement of these treatment goals, a maintenance regimen is indicated. Several possible regimens to consider include ketoconazole, 100 mg daily for 6 months, itraconazole, 50–100 mg daily for 6 months, and fluconazole, 100 mg weekly once for 6 months. One topical regimen that is useful is clotrimazole, 500 mg vaginal suppositories, administered weekly once.

A second common cause of vaginitis is *bacterial vaginosis*. This condition is caused by an overgrowth of several bacterial species. It is very common, found in 10–25% of patients in general clinics and up to 64% of those in STD clinics (Eschenbach et al., 1988). Patients with bacterial vaginosis may be asymptomatic, but frequently patients will present with a malodorous vaginal discharge that is typically thin and dull gray in color (Table 1). Vulvar pruritis may be present. Diagnosis is made with the aid of a good physical examination. A "whiff" test is performed by treating a drop of the discharge with KOH to produce a fishy amine odor when bacterial vaginosis is present. A wet-mount can be done to detect the presence of clue cells (vaginal leukocytes with adherent bacteria) and to ascertain the makeup of the vaginal flora. The pH of the vagina is typically elevated. Cultures are not necessary. Treatment of bacterial vaginosis involves the use of antibiotics,

Table 2
Treatment of yeast vaginitis: medications, dosage regimens, and duration of therapy

Antifungal medications	Dosage	Duration
Over the counter		
Clotrimazole	1 applicator qhs (1% cream)	7 days
	1 tablet vaginally qhs (100 mg)	7 days
Miconazole	1 applicator qhs (2% cream)	7 days
	1 suppository vaginally qhs (100 mg sup)	7 days
Prescription		
Fluconazole	1 tablet orally (150 mg)	One time
Butoconazole	1 applicator qhs (2% cream)	3 days
Clotrimazole	1 applicator qhs (100 mg tablet)	7 days
	1 tablet vaginally (500 mg tablet)	One time
	1 applicator qhs (1% cream)	7 days
Miconazole	1 suppository vaginally qhs (200 mg sup)	3 days
Tioconazole	1 applicator (6.5% ointment)	One time
Terconazole	1 applicator qhs (0.8% cream)	3 days
	1 suppository vaginally qhs (80 mg sup)	3 days

specifically those effective against anaerobes. Topical and oral regimens are available (Table 1). It is unclear as to whether or not there is a relationship between immunosuppression and bacterial vaginosis.

Lastly, vaginitis can be caused by an infection with *Trichomonas vaginalis*, a sexually transmitted protozoan. Trichomonas infection presents with a copious, yellow or green discharge and vulvar–vaginal irritation. A wet-mount with saline allows the identification of flagellated, mobile organisms confirming the diagnosis. Occasionally, the diagnosis can be made without wet-mount, if the organism is detected on the Papanicolaou (Pap) smear. Treatment is done with metronidazole, with the most widely used regimen being a single oral 2 gm dose. Again, there is little evidence to suggest that autoimmune disease is related to this infection, but to be thorough, it is mentioned here.

4. Cervical disorders

There are no specific autoimmune disorders that affect the cervix. However, the presence of systemic autoimmune disease and immunosuppression may create susceptibility to alterations of the cervix. Most of the cervical manifestations of autoimmune disease appear to be a result of increased infectious risk stemming from immunosuppression or the presence of an underlying chronic vasculitis. Infections that affect the cervix specifically are HPV, leading to cervical dysplasia. Other STDs, such as, Herpes simplex virus (HSV), Gonorrhea, and Chlamydia can also play an infectious role in the cervix of these patients.

4.1. Human papillomavirus and precancerous lesions of the cervix

Human papillomavirus is the most common sexually transmitted disease in the United States (Moscicki, 1998). It is a double-stranded DNA virus and a common pathogen of immunocompetent individuals. HPV is highly tropic for epithelial cells of the skin and mucous membranes; in fact, transmission likely occurs via skin to skin contact, perhaps facilitated by disruption in the skin (Bosch et al., 1995). Over 80 types of HPV have been identified (Ho et al., 1998). These have been associated with a range of disorders from asymptomatic infection to genital warts. Most concerning has been the identification of high-risk oncogenic types of HPV, particularly 16, 18, 31, and 33, which have demonstrated an association between HPV and premalignant and malignant disorders of the vulva and cervix (Nobbenhuis et al., 1999). The relationship between HPV types 16 and 18 to neoplasia appears to be a factor of the expression of E6 and E7 oncoproteins. E6 oncoprotein binds to P53 tumor suppressor protein, which is postulated to result in a loss of suppressor function. E7 oncoprotein links to the protein of the retinoblastoma (Rb) susceptibility gene. In addition to this evidence, epidemiologic studies have shown that HPV detection is associated with a 10-fold greater risk of cervical neoplasia when compared with controls, and over 75% of high-grade intraepithelial lesions are positive for high- or intermediate-risk HPV types (Saito et al., 1999).

An association between abnormal Pap smears, HPV, and autoimmune disease has been suggested in the literature after evaluation of abnormal cervical cytology in women with SLE. Dhar et al., 2001 studied the prevalence of abnormal Pap smears, in which women with SLE were compared to a large control population and founded that women with lupus have an increased prevalence of cervical dysplasia (Dhar et al., 2001). This was confirmed by another group of investigators who noted that patients with SLE not only had more abnormal Pap smears, they also had an increased proportion of high-risk HPV infections when compared with controls. In addition, this finding appeared to be independent of the use of immunosuppressant agents (Tam et al., 2004). Factors associated with abnormal Pap smears in patients with SLE were evaluated by Bernatsky et al. After utilizing a logistic regression model, this study suggested that a history of STDs and the use of oral contraceptives are associated with abnormal cervical cytology, but immunosuppressive exposure may confer further risk to those patients with SLE (Bernatsky et al., 2004).

Immunosuppression and increased risk of abnormal cervical cytology has also been evaluated by studies involving renal transplant patients and those patients with HIV (Clarke and Chetty, 2002; Sun et al., 1997; Birkeland et al., 2000). An abundant literature suggests that the presence of immunosuppression, whether iatrogenic or infectious (HIV), creates an increased risk for cervical dysplasia and carcinoma, likely secondary to the presence of HPV. A study by Birkeland et al. (1995) showed an increased ratio of expected (3.6) to observed (39) cases of cervical cancer in patients who were being treated with immunosuppressive agents after renal transplantation. Also noted was that the cumulative prevalence of malignancy increased with the duration of follow-up. The HIV Epidemiology Research Study group collected data on HPV infection from those women with and without HIV. Of patients that tested positive for HIV, 78% also tested positive for the presence of HPV. In contrast, HPV was found in only 27% of those that tested negative for HIV (Jamieson et al., 2002). The authors also found that one of the most important risk factors for HPV infection in an HIV-positive patient was the low CD4 count, establishing a relationship between infection and the degree of immunosuppression (Ahdieh et al., 2001).

4.1.1. Diagnosis and management

Cervical HPV infection and precancerous lesions are typically asymptomatic. Because of this, detection of cervical HPV infection often occurs through the process of cervical cytologic screening with a Pap smear. The widespread use of cervical cancer screening with the Pap smear has been associated with a 70% decrease in the incidence of and mortality from cervical cancer in the United States (WHO Databank). Most of the decrease is likely secondary to the early detection of cervical dysplasia.

As noted above, several types of HPV are associated with the development of cervical dysplasia and cervical squamous cell cancer. Given this relationship, the frequency of Pap smear screening in immunosuppressed patients, such as those with autoimmune disease, is an area of concern. The best studied immunocompromised group is the HIV population, and important clues as to optimal management of other immunocompromised patients can be derived from Pap studies in women with HIV. Importantly, it appears that the level of accuracy with the Pap smear in HIV-infected patients is comparable with that of uninfected, immunocompetent women, particularly if the ThinPrep® method is utilized. Currently, the USPHS/IDSA recommends that immunocompromised women, such as those with HIV, have a Pap smear every 6 months for the first year after diagnosis, followed by annual cytology if those screening tests are normal (WSPHS/IDSA guidelines). In the general population, 5–7% of patients will have an abnormal Pap smear. The majority of these abnormal tests will be secondary to "atypical squamous cells of undetermined significance" (ASCUS), the most common and perhaps least serious abnormality recognized by the current Bethesda Pap Smear scoring system. However, in immunocompromised individuals, such as those with HIV, the prevalence of ASCUS Pap smears is increased (25% in HIV-positive women compared with 9% in uninfected women) (Wright et al., 1994). Moreover, although an ASCUS Pap smear result is considered minimally abnormal in healthy women, 12% of the HIV patients with ASCUS were found to have a high-grade intraepithelial dysplasia upon colposcopic evaluation (Wright et al., 1994; Holcomb et al., 1999). Given this, it is reasonable to conclude that all patients infected with HIV, and by extension, immunocompromised women in general, with Pap smears showing minimally abnormal results should be referred immediately for more extensive evaluation of the cervix, including colposcopy and possibly biopsy. When the colposcopy is performed, the entire genital tract must be evaluated because dysplasia and cancer of the entire lower genital tract is significant in immunocompromised patients with HIV.

The natural course of cervical dysplasia is also likely different in the immunocompromised patient than in those with an intact immune response. In a healthy population, mild dysplasia of the cervix is likely to regress spontaneously in up to 60% of patients (Holowaty et al., 1999) and very unlikely to progress to cancer (<0.5% in 2 years) (Bos et al., 1997). Moderate dysplasia also has a considerable chance of regression, but a higher likelihood of progression to more serious forms of dysplasia and carcinoma. In contrast, HIV-infected women have a lower regression rate for low-grade intraepithelial cervical lesions than immunocompetent women (Fruchter et al., 1996).

Treatment for cervical dysplasia involves either excision or ablation of the abnormal cells. Excisional therapies include loop electrosurgical excisional procedure (LEEP) or conization with a scalpel. Ablation involves either cryotherapy or laser therapy. Currently, lesions that are determined to be high-grade or those that are low-grade and persistent usually mandate treatment with one of the above methods. Though these procedures are usually curative in healthy women, it appears that the likelihood of recurrence is increased in women with HIV and in immunocompromised women (Holcomb et al., 1999). Because of this, the importance of close surveillance cannot be overemphasized. Exact surveillance protocols differ, but it is reasonable to follow a patient with a prior treated lesion every 3 months with Pap smear screening. A suggested protocol is shown in Fig. 1.

4.2. Herpes simplex virus

Herpes simplex virus is another virus that can affect the cervix, and this is particularly true in the immunocompromised patient. HSV is a double-stranded DNA virus with two strains: HSV-1 and HSV-2. Both may be associated with genital tract disease and transmission is secondary to mucous membrane contact. Lesions can present as grouped vesicles on an erythematous base and resolve within 2 weeks without treatment in an immunocompetent host. Recurrent lesions are common, though they tend to have a shorter clinical course. With impaired immune function, these lesions may become chronic, painful ulcerations at risk for superimposed bacterial infection. Although the diagnosis is most frequently made by the typical presentation and recurrent lesions, culture of the

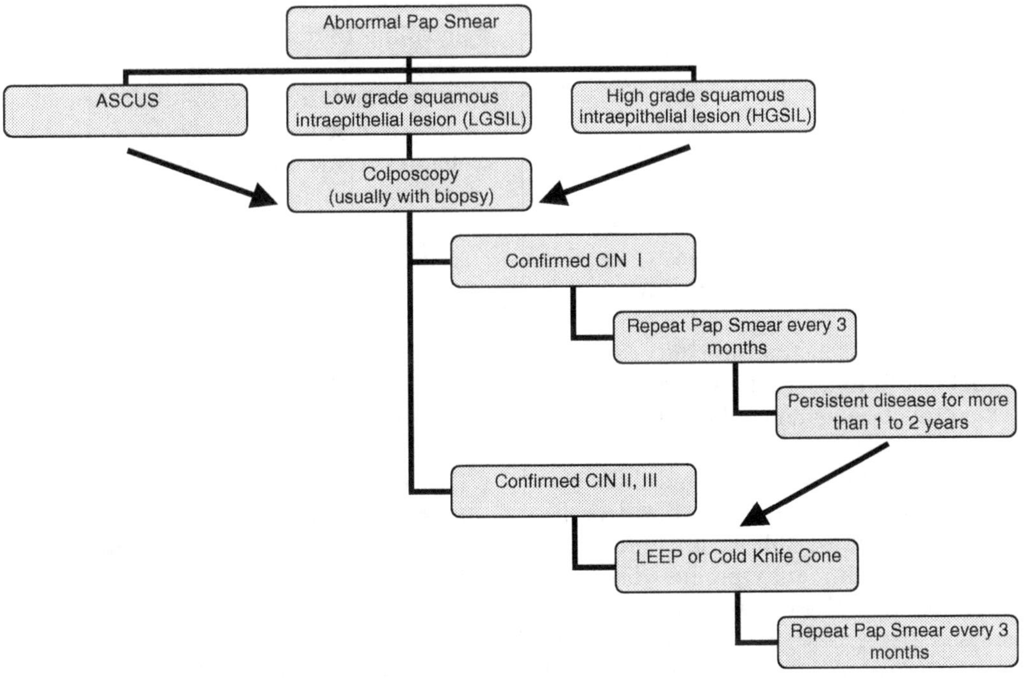

Figure 1. Proposed management algorithm for abnormal Pap smear (or equivalent cervical cytology).

lesion(s) or PCR-based assays may be used to definitively diagnose HSV infection. Although there is scant literature documenting HSV and autoimmune disorders, HIV-infected women tend to have more HSV infections. In addition, these infections tend to be of increased severity and prolonged healing time (Cejtin, 2003). Treatment for HSV in the immunocompromised population is the same as that for those that are immunocompetent. Acute and recurrent episodes of HSV may be treated with antiviral agents such as acyclovir, famciclovir, and valacyclovir. The same agents may be used for long-term suppressive therapy. HSV does not increase the risk of cervical cancer.

4.3. Other cervical infections

As with HPV and HSV, infections caused by *Neisseria gonorrhea* and Chlamydia are a potential problem in a patient who is immunosuppressed or chronically ill. Early reports of pelvic inflammatory disease in HIV-infected women suggested a possible earlier need for surgical intervention and increased mortality rate, but more recent literature does not support this, and the current recommendations for the treatment of upper genital tract infections for HIV patients are the same as for the general population. Again, it would seem reasonable to apply this rational to the immunocompromised patient with autoimmune disease.

5. Sexuality and sexual dysfunction

Sexuality is an essential tenet of humanity, integral to health, quality of life, and interactive behavior. Healthy sexual functioning and behavior improves self-image and increases the motivation for an individual to address health concerns, and thus promotes a healthier lifestyle. When one considers the obvious importance of overall health and well-being among those with autoimmune disorders alongside the fact that those with chronic illness are at increased risk for sexual dysfunction, the need for health care providers to be both well versed and competent in this arena is apparent.

In recent years, issues of sexual dysfunction have become prevalent topics among health practitioners and patients alike. A number of surveys, interviews, and questionnaires have attempted to better grasp the scope of the issue by establishing prevalence and incidence. Utilizing a variety of interactive and non-interactive techniques with random sampling methods, recent data suggests that 38–50% of women have concerns regarding sexual function (Geiss et al., 2003). In a Web-based survey of 3807 women, the reported incidence of a single sexual function complaint was 77%. Of note, although 40% of survey responders reported that they did not seek help from a physician for these complaints, 54% reported that they would like to do so. Among those participants that did seek help from their care provider, 52% felt that their physician did not want to hear about their sexual concern, and 60% felt that their physician did not appreciate the significance of the problem. While one might certainly question whether any health-related issue with a prevalence well-over 50% can truly be considered a "disorder," it is undoubtedly true that sexual concerns among patients are prevalent, and physicians are generally perceived by their patients as being ill-equipped or unwilling to discuss these concerns. However, the majority of patients consider sexual matters to be an appropriate topic for their primary care clinician to discuss. It is beyond the scope of this chapter to include a discussion of the normal sexual response in women and how hormones and neurotransmitters are involved. The interested reader has referred appropriate reviews.

5.1. Classification and diagnosis of female sexual dysfunction

The first issue in classifying sexual dysfunction is delineating what actually constitutes a sexual disorder. In essence, the debate among experts in the field of sexual dysfunction hinges on avoiding over diagnosis of sexual disorders in women whose sexual responses are satisfying to them but not to their partners. As noted in one recent review, the authors noted that "Although modifications were made to the DSM-IV system, ... from a clinical perspective, the current system still lacks both therapeutic and prognostic significance, and from a research perspective, it is atheoretical with regard to the determinants of female sexual function". With this concern in mind, the DSM-IV states that sexual dysfunctions are "disturbances in sexual desire and in the psychophysiologic changes that characterize the sexual response cycle and cause marked distress and interpersonal difficulty." While such a definition fails to provide objective and non-ambiguous criteria for the degree of impairment necessary to warrant a diagnosis, it nevertheless acknowledges the need for psychological stressors.

The DSM-IV delineates sexual disorders into four categories: disorders of desire, arousal, orgasm, and pain; these are summarized in Table 3. Of these classified disorders, the most common categories are the sexual desire and arousal disorders, followed by orgasmic disorders, and least often are women affected by the sexual pain disorders. Basson suggests further subtypes of sexual arousal disorder (Basson, 2001). Further subclassification into generalized sexual arousal disorder versus genital arousal disorder is based upon the delineation as to whether there is a reduction in sexual desire, or whether there is reduced vaginal blood flow. Moreover, in certain instances where the vasocongestive response is awry, a dysphoric or missed arousal may exist. These classifications are perhaps best utilized clinically, as they may herald discrete physiologic etiologies to the observed dysfunction.

5.1.1. Screening

While certainly some patients will self-initiate an evaluation of sexual dysfunction, the vast majority will not volunteer this information. It is therefore incumbent upon a treating physician to screen for sexual dysfunction. For most clinicians, a simple statement initiating such dialog will focus on legitimizing the need to discuss sexual function in a professional capacity. Clarifying confidentiality while expressing legitimate interest and concern will further facilitate open dialog. With respect to patients with chronic medical conditions, it is important to answer four essential questions. First, is the dysfunction lifelong or onset within the context of diagnosis or new symptom manifestation? Second, does the dysfunction correlate with recent addition of medications? Third, is the dysfunction situational or global? Fourth, what other seemingly unrelated symptoms are present? With respect to the latter, in patients with autoimmune disorders abrupt or recent onset sexual dysfunction may herald thyroid dysfunction or hyperprolactinemia or sicca. In addition to a thorough and directed medical and sexuality history, formal assessment tools such as the Female Sexual Function Index may be utilized to narrow and subclassify the sexual dysfunctions.

5.2. Sexual dysfunction among patients with autoimmune disorders

Numerous chronic medical conditions have long been associated with sexual dysfunction. However, it is often difficult to differentiate between predisposing, precipitating, and maintaining factors. Thus, the disorder may result from the pathophysiology of the disease itself, surgery, medications, normal age-related declines in sexual functioning, or alterations in perceived or real-body image. This is especially true in the autoimmune disorders, both as a result of the disorder as well as the treatments employed in their management. While there are actually limited data to support the true prevalence or treatment of sexual dysfunction among these patients, extrapolations from other populations provide potential insight.

In the context of chronic disease, studies suggest that changes in body image are accompanied by changes in the perception of self, which in turn reconstructs the social and sexual aspects of life. In such circumstances, a women's sexuality must be viewed and eventually reconstructed alongside her prior experiences, potential dysfunctions, increasing relationship demands, changing body image, and expectations. As others have noted after interviews and therapy sessions with women afflicted with multiple sclerosis (MS), "Sexuality has multiple meanings that are shaped and influenced by

Table 3
Classification of female sexual dysfunction

Disorder	DSM-IV definition	Possible etiologic factors
Sexual desire disorder Hypoactive sexual desire disorder	Persistently or recurrently deficient (or absent) sexual fantasies and desire for sexual activity. The disturbance causes marked distress or interpersonal difficulty	Interpersonal issues (partner sexual dysfunction) Depression Medications[a] Substance abuse Premature loss of testosterone/androgen Psychodynamic Fatigue Prior abuse history Absence of sexual stimuli Hypothyroidism/hyperthyroidism Hyperprolactinemia
Sexual arousal disorder	Persistent or recurrent inability to attain, or to maintain until completion of the sexual activity, an adequate lubrication-swelling response of sexual excitement. The disturbance causes marked distress or interpersonal difficulty	Lack of adequate stimulus Depression Medications[a] Premature loss of testosterone/androgen Prior abuse history Vascular disease Hypoestrogeneic Hypothyroidism/hyperthyroidism Hyperprolactinemia Conditions interfering with autonomic stimulation Diabetes mellitus Multiple sclerosis Pelvic surgery (radical or sacral) Spinal cord injury
Orgasmic disorder	Persistent or recurrent delay in, or absence of, orgasm following a normal excitement phase. The disturbance causes marked distress or interpersonal difficulty	Primary: lack of experience, psychosocial inhibitions Secondary: medications, neurologic disease, pelvic surgery
Pain Disorder Dyspareunia	Recurrent or persistent genital pain associated with sexual intercourse. The disturbance causes marked distress or interpersonal difficulty	Hypoestrogeneic Infection Vulvar vestibulitis Interstitial cystitis Vulvar dystrophies Anatomic changes s/p surgery or trauma Endometriosis
Vaginismus	Recurrent or persistent involuntary spasm of the musculature of the outer-third of the vagina that interferes with sexual intercourse.	Psychologic stress Fear of vaginal entry Secondary to vulvar vestibulitis syndrome

[a] Medications associated with sexual dysfunction are further delineated in Table 5.

life experiences. When MS intrudes in a woman's life, sexuality is reshaped against a foundation of previous sexual experiences and expectations. Constructions of sexuality encompassed physical sexual responses, perceptions of appearance and attractiveness to self and others, communication and relationships, self-image and self-esteem, and the sense of affirmation and acknowledgment that women experienced from other in their everyday lives".

5.2.1. Multiple sclerosis

As the best characterized autoimmune disorder with respect to both female and male sexuality, sexual dysfunction has been well documented in

MS patients. Prevalence may be as high as 73.1% among patients with relapsing–remitting MS, with roughly one-third manifesting as desire disorder, one-third as arousal disorder, and one-third as orgasmic disorder. There is further evidence that sexual dysfunction adversely affects established relationships and marriage in patients with MS: associated marital and relationship problems occurred in a large fraction of MS patients with sexual dysfunction (McCabe et al., 2003). Moreover, as MS frequently gives rise to alterations in cognition, speech, and role activities, affected individuals report additional adverse influences and stresses among their relationships and partnerships (Hakim et al., 2000; Gagliardi, 2003).

Changes in sexual function in MS patients are commonly associated with bladder and bowel dysfunction; however, in controlled studies no specific urodynamic pattern has been shown to be of predictive value (Litwiller et al., 1999; DasGupta and Fowler, 2002; Zivadinov et al., 2003). In a recent study, investigators employed MRI imaging to calculate lesion load and brain parenchymal fraction (Zivadinov et al., 2003). Subsequent analysis demonstrated a statistical association between symptoms of sexual dysfunction and age, cognitive function, disability, anxiety, depression, and parenchymal atrophy in the pons. These findings are consistent with the notion that CNS lesions of the pons may directly affect sexual function among MS patients. In support of this hypothesis, other authors have demonstrated that women with MS were more likely to experience difficulties in masturbating as well as a lack of sensation or numbness during sexual intercourse. These findings are further supported by recent findings demonstrating limited benefit among MS patients with sildenafil therapy. In this randomized, controlled trial, there was noted to be an improvement in vaginal lubrication when comparing sildenafil to placebo; however, no improvement in orgasm or desire was observed.

Taken together, the available evidence would suggest that sexual dysfunction in MS patients reflects the physiologic symptomology of MS, albeit the likely contributions of somatic, psychological, and social difficulties are difficult to gauge. It is reasonable to conclude that the predominant complaints of MS patients (reduced desire, decreased lubrication, reduced sensation, dyspareunia, and secondary orgasmic disorder) have their roots in both the neuropathology and psychology of the disorder. Thus, successful treatment ought to be multifaceted.

5.2.2. Systemic lupus erythematosus

There are a number of presumptive sexual issues unique to women with SLE. First, as a result of both dosage and duration of systemic steroid therapy, patients may develop a cushinoid habitus with associated androgen alterations; often accompanying are psychological manifestations of depression, mania, and rare psychosis. In addition, women utilizing steroid therapy may develop avascular necrosis. Resulting pain and limitations in range of motion might limit positioning during intercourse. Second, cutaneous manifestations of SLE may lead to significant body image alterations. Third, as with all vascular diseases, there exists the potential for sexual arousal disorders. With this in mind, one might anticipate a number of sexual disorders among SLE patients to arise.

Compared to age-matched controls, women with SLE have statistically significantly higher rates of abstention, low frequency of masturbation, less frequent sexual activity among those who were sexually active, diminished vaginal lubrication, poorer general sexual adjustment, and depression; although, orgasm was attained among a similar number of cases when compared to controls (Curry et al., 1994). The same authors found that among patients with greater SLE disease severity was associated with higher sexual impairment. Modifiers of this association included age, relationship "quality," body image perceptions, depression, and premorbid sexual adjustment (Curry et al., 1993, 1994). Others have similarly documented adverse emotional and "physical," i.e., affectionate and/or sexual behaviors intimacy among lupus patients, and found that women who sought support and intimacy from their partners during disease exacerbations were more likely to subjectively report relationship satisfaction as measured by an established quality of marriage index (Druley et al., 1997).

With respect to sexual dysfunction among SLE patients, pain, fatigue, and decreased activity and productivity contribute to alterations from the premorbid lifestyle. Since these symptoms are not amenable to management with pharmacologic means, investigators have assessed behavioral methods for their impact in affecting such parameters among lupus patients. In some of their work, others have shown in both prospective and randomized controlled trials that biofeedback-assisted/cognitive-behavioral treatments (Braden et al., 1993; Greco et al., 2004) and graded exercise therapy (Tench et al., 2003).

5.2.3. Systemic sclerosis

Known manifestations of the systemic connective tissue diseases include decreased tactile sensation secondary to cutaneous thickening and articular contractures, genital ulcerations or fissures (primarily in Behcet's syndrome), and esophageal reflux symptoms (Clements et al., 1990). In the largest case series examining gynecologic complications and obstetric outcomes among these patients, 150 patients were reviewed, and comparisons were drawn from their history prior to the onset and diagnosis of the systemic sclerosis condition and after. Of those queried, 37% of those sexually active reported vaginal dryness and dyspareunia. This complaint was almost exclusive to the subset with *cutaneous xerosis* (skin thickening with atrophy of the sebaceous and sweat glands). Other investigators compared symptoms related to sexual dysfunction among systemic sclerosis patients to those of lupus and rheumatoid arthritis patients, and controlled for age and duration of disease. Among these 83 patients, analysis of subjective indexes of sexual function as well as frequency of sexual intercourse and satisfaction revealed a significantly greater incidence of dyspareunia in systemic sclerosis patients. Disease-related symptoms shown to cause problems during coitus in this population over controls, included skin tightness (33% vs. 0%), reflux symptoms (38% vs. 6%), contractures (42% vs. 18%), and muscle weakness (28% vs. 6%). Articular pain and fatigue were equally prevalent among cases and controls. To overcome these problems, patients had altered their physical approach to sexual intercourse by change in position, lubrication, and light meals prior to intercourse. In addition, systemic sclerosis patients also reported breast manifestations (hypomastia, hardening of the nipple with hyperthesia), irritation of the urethra and incontinence, and anorectal bleeding as barriers to sexual function. There are no prospective studies to date on therapeutic interventions in this population.

5.2.4. Sjogren's syndrome

In Sjogren's syndrome, often a secondary disorder among SLE and other connective tissue disease patients, the salivary and lacrimal glands are progressively destroyed by lymphocytes and plasma cells. Thus, the disorder is characterized gynecologically by the absence of vaginal lubrication (Lehrer et al., 1994). Such symptoms may respond to vaginal moisturizer and lubricant therapy (Astroglide, Replens, Gyne-Moistrin, MoistAgain). Women with Sjogren's syndrome report sexual arousal and orgasmic dysfunction.

5.2.5. Rheumatoid arthritis and ankylosing spondylitis

A number of lines of evidence suggest that presence and subtype of sexual dysfunction among patients with rheumatoid arthritis may be highly variable. The range of affects involves interest disorders (fatigue), as well as dyspareunia and secondary orgasmic dysfunction.

In one of the more comprehensive studies to date, social function, relationships, and sexual activity was examined among a cohort of adults with juvenile idiopathic arthritis (Packham et al., 2002). In this study, 246 adult patients were interviewed to ascertain age of first sexual encounter and sexual problems; physical function was ascertained from a validated health assessment questionnaire, mood from an anxiety and depression scale, and social support network with a social support questionnaire. In some of their findings, while individuals were more likely than their siblings to be single and living outside a stable partnership or marriage, the level of satisfaction with an individual's social support was high. Even in the face of high levels of physical disability, the majority of patients were sexually active. As might be anticipated in this population, the majority of sexual problems were related to physical disability and pain, and physical disability correlated strongly with a delay in sexual activity. Thirty percent of those who were not sexually active felt that this was attributable to disease status. Physical disability accounted for 8.3% of these; 66.6% were related to body image, and 25% felt they were not generally regarded by others as sexual beings (Packham et al., 2002).

5.3. Treatment of uncomplicated sexual disorders

5.3.1. General principles

While the intensity and complexity of therapy necessary for the successful treatment of sexual dysfunction is beyond the scope of most primary care physicians, the initial recognition and management is not. Treatment of sexual dysfunction is ultimately based on the underlying factors, which lend themselves to being addressed. These include psychological, relationship, medication, and physiologic factors. As an initiation point, one might consider employment of the PLISSIT (permission, limited information, specific strategies, intensive therapy) model in defining appropriate levels of intervention. Additional resources that may be helpful are listed in Table 4.

Psychotherapeutic interventions have been the mainstay of sexual dysfunction therapy. Such "sex therapy" rests on the premise that a comprehensive evaluation of the woman and her partner be performed by a qualified therapist prior to initiating a treatment plan. Thereafter, a number of interventions are commonly employed. These may include education about female sexuality, communication training among partners, and non-demand genital and non-genital sensual stimulation, and encouragement of masturbation in an effort to develop a "pleasure-focused" approach to sex (Leiblum and Wiegel, 2002). In addition, some experts advocate utilization of erotica and sexual tools, such as vibrators, notably in instances of sexual arousal disorders. The FDA-approved mechanical devise Eros-Clitoral Therapy Device—a clitoral vacuum engorgement device—has been employed in both arousal and orgasmic disorders (Billups, 2002).

5.3.2. Sexual desire disorders

As reviewed earlier (Table 3), hypoactive sexual desire disorder is the most common form of female sexual dysfunction, and results from a combination of factors. As such, therapy must be multimodal. Medications may be reviewed and revised where appropriate and feasible (Table 5). Potential underlying co-morbidities should be sought and addressed. The possibility of alcohol abuse should be considered.

Hormonal therapy may be entertained, once contraindications (thrombophilia, history of hormone-responsive malignancy, hepatic disease, hyperlipidemia) have been excluded. With respect to the various forms of testosterone, commercially available forms include estrogen combinations (Estratest [esterified estrogen 1.25 mg/methyltestosterone 2.5 mg] and Estratest HS [esterified estrogen 0.625 mg/methyltestosterone 1.25 mg]). In addition, compounded topical testosterone has been utilized, typically in the form of a 1–2% gel

Table 4
Resources for sexual dysfunction

Professional resources	American Psychological Association website: www.apa.org American Association of Sex Educators, Counselors, and Therapists website: www.aasect.org National Vulvodynia Association website: www.nva.org
Patient resources	American College of Obstetricians and Gynecologists. ACOG patient pamphlets AP020 and AP072. website: www.acog.org Berman and Berman. For Women Only. New York: Henry Holt and Company; 2001

Table 5
Medications associated with sexual dysfunction and their alternatives

Disorder	Medication	Possible Alternative
Sexual desire disorder	Appetite suppressants (amphetamines) Antidepressants (SSRIs,tricyclics, clomipramine, imipramine, trazadone, St. John's Wort) Mood stabilizers (lithium) Antihypertensives (β-blockers,digoxin, Aldomet, reserpine, spironolactone, clonidine)	Antidepressants least likely to interfere with sexual desire response: Central noradrenergic acting agents (mirtazipine, buproprion, venlafaxine) Dopaminergic agents (buproprion, venlafaxine) 5-HT_{1A} agonists (buspirone)
	Gastrointestinal (H_2-antagonists/cimetidine, metoclopramide, niacin)	Antihypertensives least likely to interfere with sexual desire response:Antihypertensives least likely to interfere with sexual desire response: ACE inhibitors Calcium-channel blockers
	Neural/Pain (benzodiazepines, indomethicin,tricyclics, clomipramine, imipramine, trazadone)	
	Tamoxifen	
Sexual arousal disorder	Anticholinergics Antidepressants (SSRIs,tricyclics, clomipramine, imipramine, trazadone, MOIs, St. John's Wort) Mood stabilizers (lithium) Antihypertensives (β-blockers,digoxin, Aldomet, reserpine, spironolactone, clonidine)	Antidepressants least likely to interfere with sexual arousal response: Central noradrenergic acting agents (mirtazipine, buproprion, venlafaxine) Dopaminergic agents (buproprion, venlafaxine) 5-HT_{1A} agonists (buspirone)
	Steroids Tamoxifen	Antihypertensives least likely to interfere with sexual arousal response: ACE inhibitors Calcium-channel blockers
Orgasmic disorder	Amphetamines Antidepressants Mood stabilizers Antihypertensives Gastrointestinal Neural/Pain (trazadone, methadone)	Note as above

or ointment with one-fourth teaspoon may be applied genitally daily. Long-term use is discouraged secondary to the risk of clitoralmegaly and hyperstimulation. Prior to initiation of testosterone therapy, a specimen for cervical cytology, mammogram, a fasting lipid panel, baseline testosterone (total and unbound), and hepatic transaminases should be obtained. These should be repeated every 3–4 months for 1 year and yearly thereafter.

A transdermal patch of testosterone alone is currently undergoing Phase III trials for the treatment of androgen insufficiency in women, with anticipated release in 2005. Available data suggests treatment benefits for sexual dysfunction among women following oopherectomy. Women require an approximate 20-fold lower dosing requirement than men (150–300 μg/day as compared to 2.5–10 mg/day). This lower required delivery rate enables a tolerable twice-weekly administration in an alcohol-free matrix patch (Shifren, 2002). At a higher dosage (300 μg/day) the percentages of women with improved sexual fantasy, masturbation, and frequency was two- to three-fold higher than controls. Studies thus far show that adequate free concentrations of testosterone are attainable without significant adverse effects on acne or hirsutism, nor examined lipids, hepatic enzymes or carbohydrates. Whether such findings will hold true in a non-surgical population is unknown.

In postmenopausal women, several clinical trials have looked at improved sexual desire with estrogen replacement therapy in the absence of testosterone. This data are summarized in a recent systematic review (Modelska and Cummings, 2003). In sum, a single trial has provided Level I (randomized and placebo controlled) evidence regarding efficacy (Sherwin, 2000). These authors found that postmenopausal women had improved desire and arousal on therapy, when compared with prior; no effect on orgasm was observed. Estrogen replacement for sexual desire has not yet been specifically tested in a chronic disease population.

Non-hormonal pharmacologic therapy most often employs alterations in existing SSRI regimens (Table 5), or addition of bupropion in non-depressed women. There are a number of studies exploring the use of sildenafil and other agents in reversing SSRI-mediated sexual dysfunction. With respect to sildenafil, results in premenopausal women without underlying chronic disease appears promising (reviewed by Warnock and Morris, 2002), though sildenafil has been yet to be proven efficacious in MS or other autoimmune disorders. Other authors have investigated the affects of mirtazipine, yohimbine, or olanzipine with placebo as an antidote to SSRI-mediated desire and orgasmic disorder; none was shown to be effective (Michelson and Kociban, 2002).

5.3.3. *Sexual arousal disorders*

The complexity of women's sexual arousal disorders precludes a simplistic focus on medication to enhance genital response. Nevertheless, the number of elementary interventions may be of assistance among patients with primary or secondary sexual arousal disorder.

Since vaginal lubrication is perceived by many as testament to sexual arousal, utilization of vaginal moisturizers and lubricants is both a necessary and an appropriate initial intervention among affected individuals. Available products include Astroglide, Replens, Gyne-Moistrin, and MoistAgain. In addition, estrogen creams and suppositories have been used by some clinicians. Currently available vaginal cream regimens include conjugated equine estrogens (Premarin) and estradiol (Estrace). Use is employed daily for 2 weeks, then twice a week thereafter. Low-dose estrogen is available in a vaginal tablet containing 10 μg of estradiol (Vagifem); it is administered daily for 2 weeks and twice weekly thereafter. Finally, 6–9 mcg of estradiol is available as a silicon-based vaginal ring (Estring). Meant to be placed by either the patient or physician, it is proven efficacious for 3 month intervals and is not an impediment to intercourse. Clinicians should recognize that while local estrogen preparations create lower circulating estrogen levels than systemic therapy, they should not be used when estrogen is otherwise contraindicated. Many experts suggest intermittent progesterone withdrawal for the risk of endometrial hyperplasia and subsequent neoplasia. Thus, women using vaginal creams and suppository long term should receive a 5 mg of oral progesterone for 10 days of every 1–3 months.

5.3.4. *Orgasmic disorder*

Of the female sexual disorders, secondary orgasmic dysfunction is the most difficult to treat. As a general rule, non-pharmacologic modalities are more effective than pharmacologic therapies. In the instance of neuropathic secondary orgasmic dysfunction, few if any therapies have yet been proven successful. We recommend seeking the assistance of experts in sexual dysfunction for the treatment of orgasmic disorders.

5.3.5. Sexual pain disorders

The mainstay of therapy for dyspareunia is improved lubrication or abstinence in the instance of ulcerations or fissures. Vaginal lubricants have been previously discussed in this chapter.

Deep dyspareunia (pain associated with thrusting) is often related to pelvic disease. With acute onset of deep dyspareunia, timely gynecologic evaluation for the presence of an infectious process (PID or tuboovarian abcess) or other pelvic disorder is warranted.

Treatment of *vaginismus* consists of progressive focused pelvic relaxation with biofeedback, vaginal dilation, and extensive counseling (Ragucci and Culhane, 2003). Vaginismus is best treated by physicians and therapists with extensive experience, as inappropriate therapy can exacerbate pain.

5.3.6. Resources

While the intensity and complexity of therapy necessitated for the successful treatment of sexual dysfunction is undoubtedly beyond the scope of most primary care physicians, the initial recognition and management is not. Treatment of sexual dysfunction is ultimately based on the underlying factors that lend themselves to being addressed in any given population. Clearly, these include psychologic, relationship, medication, and physiologic factors. Additional resources that may be helpful are listed in Table 4.

References

Ahdieh, L., Klein, R.S., et al. 2001. Prevalence, incidence, and type-specific persistence of human papillomavirus in human immunodeficiency virus (HIV)-positive and HIV-negative women. J. Infect. Dis. 184 (6), 682–690.

Basson, R. 2001. Are the complexities of women's sexual function reflected in the new consensus definitions of dysfunction? J. Sex Marital Ther. 27 (2), 105–112.

Bernatsky, S., Ramsey-Goldman, R., et al. 2004. Factors associated with abnormal Pap results in systemic lupus erythematosus. Rheumatology (Oxford) 43 (11), 1386–1389.

Bickle, K., Roark, T.R., et al. 2002. Autoimmune bullous dermatoses: a review. Am. Fam. Physician 65 (9), 1861–1870.

Billups, K.L. 2002. Re: Long-term efficacy of sildenafil and tachyphylaxis effect. J. Urol. 168 (1), 204–205.

Birkeland, S.A., Lokkegaard, H., et al. 2000. Cancer risk in patients on dialysis and after renal transplantation. Lancet 355 (9218), 1886–1887.

Birkeland, S.A., Storm, H.H., et al. 1995. Cancer risk after renal transplantation in the Nordic countries, 1964–1986. Int. J. Cancer 60 (2), 183–189.

Bos, A.B., van Ballegooijen, M., et al. 1997. Non-progression of cervical intraepithelial neoplasia estimated from population-screening data. Br. J. Cancer 75 (1), 124–130.

Bosch, F.X., Manos, M.M., et al. 1995. Prevalence of human papillomavirus in cervical cancer: a worldwide perspective. International biological study on cervical cancer (IBSCC) Study Group. J. Natl. Cancer Inst. 87 (11), 796–802.

Braden, C.J., McGlone, K., et al. 1993. Specific psychosocial and behavioral outcomes from the systemic lupus erythematosus self-help course. Health Educ. Q. 20 (1), 29–41.

Cejtin, H.E. 2003. Gynecologic issues in the HIV-infected woman. Obstet. Gynecol. Clin. North Am. 30 (4), 711–729.

Chernosky, M.E., Derbes, V.J., et al. 1957. Lichen sclerosus et atrophicus in children. AMA Arch. Dermatol. 75 (5), 647–652.

Clarke, B., Chetty, R. 2002. Postmodern cancer: the role of human immunodeficiency virus in uterine cervical cancer. Mol. Pathol. 55 (1), 19–24.

Clements, P.J., Lachenbruch, P.A., et al. 1990. Skin score. A semiquantitative measure of cutaneous involvement that improves prediction of prognosis in systemic sclerosis. Arthritis Rheum. 33 (8), 1256–1263.

Conley, L.J., Ellerbrock, T.V., et al. 2002. HIV-1 infection and risk of vulvovaginal and perianal condylomata acuminata and intraepithelial neoplasia: a prospective cohort study. Lancet 359 (9301), 108–113.

Crum, C.P. 1992. Carcinoma of the vulva: epidemiology and pathogenesis. Obstet. Gynecol. 79 (3), 448–454.

Curry, S.L., Levine, S.B., et al. 1994. The impact of systemic lupus erythematosus on women's sexual functioning. J. Rheumatol. 21 (12), 2254–2260.

Curry, S.L., Levine, S.B., et al. 1993. Medical and psychosocial predictors of sexual outcome among women with systemic lupus erythematosus. Arthritis Care Res. 6 (1), 23–30.

DasGupta, R., Fowler, C.J. 2002. Sexual and urological dysfunction in multiple sclerosis: better understanding and improved therapies. Curr. Opin. Neurol. 15 (3), 271–278.

Dhar, J.P., Kmak, D., et al. 2001. Abnormal cervicovaginal cytology in women with lupus: a retrospective cohort study. Gynecol. Oncol. 82 (1), 4–6.

Druley, J.A., Stephens, M.A., et al. 1997. Emotional and physical intimacy in coping with lupus: women's dilemmas of disclosure and approach. Health Psychol. 16 (6), 506–514.

Eschenbach, D.A., Hillier, S., et al. 1988. Diagnosis and clinical manifestations of bacterial vaginosis. Am. J. Obstet. Gynecol. 158 (4), 819–828.

Ferenczy, A., Coutlee, F., et al. 2003. Human papillomavirus and HIV coinfection and the risk of neoplasias of the lower genital tract: a review of recent developments. Cmaj 169 (5), 431–434.

Foxman, B., Barlow, R., et al. 2000. Candida vaginitis: self-reported incidence and associated costs. Sex Transm. Dis. 27 (4), 230–235.

Frances, C., Wechsler, J., et al. 1983. Investigation of intercellular matrix macromolecules involved in lichen sclerosus. Acta Dermatol. Venereol. 63 (6), 483–490.

Fruchter, R.G., Maiman, M., et al. 1996. Multiple recurrences of cervical intraepithelial neoplasia in women with the human immunodeficiency virus. Obstet. Gynecol. 87 (3), 338–344.

Gagliardi, B.A. 2003. The experience of sexuality for individuals living with multiple sclerosis. J. Clin. Nurs. 12 (4), 571–578.

Geiss, I.M., Umek, W.H., et al. 2003. Prevalence of female sexual dysfunction in gynecologic and urogynecologic patients according to the international consensus classification. Urology 62 (3), 514–518.

Giraldo, P., von Nowaskonski, A., et al. 2000. Vaginal colonization by Candida in asymptomatic women with and without a history of recurrent vulvovaginal candidiasis. Obstet. Gynecol. 95 (3), 413–416.

Greco, C.M., Rudy, T.E., et al. 2004. Effects of disease activity, pain, and distress on activity limitations in patients with systemic lupus erythematosus. J. Rheumatol. 31 (2), 260–267.

Haefner, H.K. 1999. Current evaluation and management of vulvovaginitis. Clin. Obstet. Gynecol. 42 (2), 184–195.

Hakim, E.A., Bakheit, A.M., et al. 2000. The social impact of multiple sclerosis—a study of 305 patients and their relatives. Disabil. Rehabil. 22 (6), 288–293.

Hillier, S.L. 1998. The vaginal microbial ecosystem and resistance to HIV. AIDS Res. Hum. Retroviruses 14 (Suppl. 1), S17–S21.

Ho, G.Y., Bierman, R., et al. 1998. Natural history of cervicovaginal papillomavirus infection in young women. New Engl. J. Med. 338 (7), 423–428.

Holcomb, K., Abulafia, O., et al. 1999. The significance of ASCUS cytology in HIV-positive women. Gynecol. Oncol. 75 (1), 118–121.

Holcomb, K., Matthews, R.P., et al. 1999. The efficacy of cervical conization in the treatment of cervical intraepithelial neoplasia in HIV-positive women. Gynecol. Oncol. 74 (3), 428–431.

Holowaty, P., Miller, A.B., et al. 1999. Natural history of dysplasia of the uterine cervix. J. Natl. Cancer Inst. 91 (3), 252–258.

Jamieson, D.J., Duerr, A., et al. 2002. Characterization of genital human papillomavirus infection in women who have or who are at risk of having HIV infection. Am. J. Obstet. Gynecol. 186 (1), 21–27.

Jensen, J.T., Bird, M., et al. 2004. Patient satisfaction after the treatment of vulvovaginal erosive lichen planus with topical clobetasol and tacrolimus: a survey study. Am. J. Obstet. Gynecol. 190 (6), 1759–1763, discussion 1763–1765.

Jorgensen, E.T., Svensson, A. 1993. The treatment of phimosis in boys, with a potent topical steroid (clobetasol propionate 0.05%) cream. Acta Dermatol. Venereol. 73 (1), 55–56.

Lehrer, S., Bogursky, E., et al. 1994. Gynecologic manifestations of Sjogren's syndrome. Am. J. Obstet. Gynecol. 170 (3), 835–837.

Leiblum, S.R., Wiegel, M. 2002. Psychotherapeutic interventions for treating female sexual dysfunction. World J. Urol. 20 (2), 127–136.

Litwiller, S.E., Frohman, E.M., et al. 1999. Multiple sclerosis and the urologist. J. Urol. 161 (3), 743–757.

Lotery, H.E., Galask, R.P., et al. 2003. Ulcerative vulvitis in atypical Reiter's syndrome. J. Am. Acad. Dermatol. 48 (4), 613–616.

Marren, P., Wojnarowska, F., et al. 1993. Vulvar involvement in autoimmune bullous diseases. J. Reprod. Med. 38 (2), 101–107.

McCabe, M.P., McKern, S., et al. 2003. Changes over time in sexual and relationship functioning of people with multiple sclerosis. J. Sex Marital Ther. 29 (4), 305–321.

Michelson, D., Kociban, K., et al. 2002. Mirtazapine, yohimbine or olanzapine augmentation therapy for serotonin reuptake-associated female sexual dysfunction: a randomized, placebo controlled trial. J. Psychiatr. Res. 36 (3), 147–152.

Modelska, K., Cummings, S. 2003. Female sexual dysfunction in postmenopausal women: systematic review of placebo-controlled trials. Am. J. Obstet. Gynecol. 188 (1), 286–293.

Moscicki, A.B. 1998. Genital infections with human papillomavirus (HPV). Pediatr. Infect. Dis. J. 17 (7), 651–652.

Nobbenhuis, M.A., Walboomers, J.M., et al. 1999. Relation of human papillomavirus status to cervical lesions and consequences for cervical-cancer screening: a prospective study. Lancet 354 (9172), 20–25.

Packham, J.C., Hall, M.A., et al. 2002. Long-term follow-up of 246 adults with juvenile idiopathic arthritis: predictive factors for mood and pain. Rheumatology (Oxford) 41 (12), 1444–1449.

Priestley, C.J., Jones, B.M., et al. 1997. What is normal vaginal flora? Genitourin. Med. 73 (1), 23–28.

Ragucci, K.R., Culhane, N.S. 2003. Treatment of female sexual dysfunction. Ann. Pharmacother. 37 (4), 546–555, quiz 603–604.

Saito, J., Fukuda, T., et al. 1999. High-risk types of human papillomavirus associated with the progression of cervical dysplasia to carcinoma. J. Obstet. Gynaecol. Res. 25 (4), 281–286.

Scully, C., Beyli, M., et al. 1998. Update on oral lichen planus: etiopathogenesis and management. Crit. Rev. Oral Biol. Med. 9 (1), 86–122.

Sherwin, B.B. 2000. Oestrogen and cognitive function throughout the female lifespan. Novartis Found. Symp. 230, 188–196, discussion 196–201.

Shifren, J.L. 2002. Androgen deficiency in the oophorectomized woman. Fertil. Steril. 77 (Suppl. 4), S60–S62.

Sobel, J.D., Chaim, W. 1997. Treatment of Torulopsis glabrata vaginitis: retrospective review of boric acid therapy. Clin. Infect Dis. 24 (4), 649–652.

Stoughton, R., Wells, G. 1950. A histochemical study on polysaccharides in normal and diseased skin. J. Invest. Dermatol. 14 (1), 37–51, illust.

Sun, X.W., Kuhn, L., et al. 1997. Human papillomavirus infection in women infected with the human immunodeficiency virus. N. Engl. J. Med. 337 (19), 1343–1349.

Tam, L.S., Chan, A.Y., et al. 2004. Increased prevalence of squamous intraepithelial lesions in systemic lupus erythematosus: association with human papillomavirus infection. Arthritis Rheum. 50 (11), 3619–3625.

Tench, C.M., McCarthy, J., et al. 2003. Fatigue in systemic lupus erythematosus: a randomized controlled trial of exercise. Rheumatology (Oxford) 42 (9), 1050–1054.

Torok, E., Orley, J., et al. 1975. Lichen sclerosus et atrophicus in children. Clinical and pathological analysis of 33 cases. Mod. Probl. Paediatr. 17, 262–271.

Warnock, J.K., Morris, D.W. 2002. Adverse cutaneous reactions to antidepressants. Am. J. Clin. Dermatol. 3 (5), 329–339.

Wright, T.C., Jr., Koulos, J., et al. 1994. Cervical intraepithelial neoplasia in women infected with the human immunodeficiency virus: outcome after loop electrosurgical excision. Gynecol. Oncol. 55 (2), 253–258.

Zivadinov, R., Zorzon, M., et al. 2003. Sexual dysfunction in multiple sclerosis: a MRI, neurophysiological and urodynamic study. J. Neurol. Sci. 210 (1–2), 73–76.

Handbook of Systemic Autoimmune Diseases, Volume 4
Reproductive and Hormonal Aspects of Systemic Autoimmune Diseases
Michael Lockshin and D. Ware Branch, editors

CHAPTER 13

The Climacteric and Osteoporosis in Women with Autoimmune Diseases

Felicia Tenedios*

Hospital for Special Surgery, Weill Medical College of Cornell University, New York, NY, USA

1. Osteoporosis

Menopause, or the climacteric, represents a transition from the reproductive to the nonreproductive years, the end of fertility, resulting from the ovaries' decreased production of estrogen and progesterone. Menopause can occur naturally or as the result of medical or surgical intervention. Menopause can be physiologic, induced, or premature. Physiologic (natural) menopause refers to the end of menstruation, which has traditionally been confirmed after 12 consecutive months without a menstrual period. Induced menopause is the result of removal of both ovaries or as a result of medical treatment. Premature menopause refers to the gradual or abrupt cessation of menstruation before 40 years. The primary symptoms of menopause are hot flashes and vaginal atrophy. The estrogen deficiency associated with menopause can contribute to the development of osteoporosis, decreased high-density lipoprotein (HDL) levels, increased low-density lipoprotein (LDL) levels, increased triglyceride levels, and associated with an increased incidence of cardiovascular disease (CVD).

The onset of menopause has a pivotal role in the bone health of women. Peak bone mass in women is attained between the ages of 25 and 35 and is the result of many factors, including genetics, diet, smoking and alcohol use, calcium intake, and exercise. Bone mineral density (BMD) declines slowly after peak bone mass is attained, 0.3% a year before the onset of menopause. Women arrive at the time of menopause with close to the highest BMD of their lifetimes. Estrogens directly promote BMD as osteoblasts and osteoclasts have estrogen receptors. Estrogens reduce bone resorption by osteoclasts. Estrogens act on bone marrow stromal and mononuclear cells to decrease the amount of interleukins and tumor necrosis factor when an adequate amount of estrogen is present, and increase the amount of cytokines produced in the absence of estrogen (Steinweg, 2002).

The loss of estrogen during the menopausal period has a profound effect on bone density and is associated with increased bone resorption. Bone loss in postmenopausal women is the result of increases in the rate of bone remodeling and the imbalance between osteoclasts and osteoblasts. This pattern of accelerated bone loss in women primarily affects trabecular bone and results in irreversible bone loss. The bone loss occurs in two phases. The rapid phase produces a loss of about 3% per year in the spine and lasts about 5 years. A slower phase of bone loss begins at about age 55 (Steinweg, 2002).

During the early, rapid phase indices of bone resorption are twice those in the premenopausal phase. The bone loss is qualitative and quantitative and can lead to trabecular meshwork loss and

*Corresponding author.
Hospital for Special Surgery, Weill Medical College of Cornell University, 535 East 70th Street, New York, NY 10021, USA.
Tel.: +1-212-774-2935; fax: +1-212-606-1519.
E-mail address: tenediosf@hss.edu (F. Tenedios).

DOI: 10.1016/S1571-5078(05)04013-4

irreversibly weakened structural integrity. The loss of estrogen has a dramatic acceleration on bone loss, with as much as 20% of a woman's bone mass lost 5–7 years after menopause. This period of accelerated bone loss, in addition to the lower BMD in women compared to men, is believed to explain the higher incidence of osteoporosis and related fractures in women (Steinweg, 2002).

The impetus for prevention, diagnosis, and treatment of osteoporosis is its devastating complications. From a public health perspective, the problem is rapidly increasing in the face of an aging population. Approximately 1.5 million fractures annually are associated with this disease. Within a physician's practice, one in three women aged 50 or older has osteoporosis. Eventually, one out of two women over age 50 will have an osteoporosis-related fracture. Only one-third of patients with hip fractures ever regain their prefracture levels of function, with many patients unable to walk independently or perform activities of daily living. Approximately 20% of women who suffer hip fracture will die in the following year as an indirect consequence of the fracture. Direct financial costs for treatment of osteoporosis-related fractures are estimated at $10–14 billion annually (Steinweg, 2002). Unfortunately, only 1 in 10 patients of the 30 million Americans with osteoporosis is diagnosed and treated (Repa-Eschen, 2000).

Certain diseases and treatments concomitantly accelerate bone loss. Generalized osteoporosis is a well-known phenomenon in rheumatoid arthritis (RA), demonstrated by decreased BMD and the increased risk of fracture. Independent of glucocorticoids, RA causes regional and generalized bone loss, and RA patients are at higher risk for fracture (Cooper et al., 1995). There is focal bone loss affecting the immediate subchondral bone at the joint margins, the erosions, and the periarticular osteopenia adjacent to inflamed joints. It has been suggested that both local and systemic bone destruction are mediated by osteoclast activation because it has been shown that several cells at the bone–pannus interface in RA express receptor activator of nuclear factor kappa B ligand (RANKL), a factor stimulating osteoclast differentiation (d'Elia et al., 2003).

Rheumatoid arthritis patients on glucocorticoids generally have lower BMD than their nonuser counterparts. Bone loss resulting in fractures is the most incapacitating problem of long-term glucocorticoid therapy (Dequecker and Westhovens, 1995; Saag, 1997). It is suspected that long-term steroid therapy may cause or exacerbate osteoporosis and lead to excess fractures in up to 50% of patients, (Lukert and Raisz, 1990; Adami et al., 1991), although the true incidence is unknown. Cross-sectional studies in patients with RA, sarcoidosis, vasculitides, systemic lupus erythematosus (SLE), or asthma, and in patients undergoing organ transplant show lower bone mass in patients treated with glucocorticoids than those who did not receive this therapy.

Community surveys indicate that glucocorticoids are used by an estimated 0.2–0.5% of the general population. The cumulative prevalence of vertebral fracture with glucocorticoids has been derived from cross-sectional studies; rates as high as 28% have been reported. Estimates of vertebral fracture incidence with glucocorticoids, derived from the calcium-treated arms of recent randomized trials range from 13 to 22% in the first year of therapy. The incidence appears to be particularly low in premenopausal women and highest in postmenopausal women (Rheumatology, 2004; Sambrook, 2004).

RA patients constitute the largest group of glucocorticoid users overall. An increased rate of fractures has been observed in cross-sectional and longitudinal studies (Saag et al., 1994). A large observational study of RA patients by Michel et al. (1993) indicated that a woman taking an average dose of 8.6 mg of prednisone had a nearly 33% chance of a self-reported clinical fracture after 5 years of follow-up. Other observational studies suggest that over 40% of long-term users will ultimately have a fracture. Placebo arms of randomized controlled trials document about a 15% incidence of morphometrically defined vertebral fractures after 1 year in patients on median doses of less than 10 mg/day (Saag et al., 1998; Cohen et al., 1999).

Longitudinal studies show that the most rapid bone loss occurs in the first 6 months after initiation of glucocorticoid therapy (LoCascio et al., 1984), with subsequent loss being slower but continual.

During the first 6–12 months of glucocorticoid therapy, there is an initial rapid loss of 3–27% of BMD. Trabecular bone is preferentially affected, followed by losses in cortical bone. The literature is divided, however, on whether trabecular bone is lost most rapidly from the trochanter or the lumbar spine. Bone loss may be potentially reversible by lowering or cessation of the glucocorticoid. After approximately 2 years of glucocorticoid therapy, there is a slow rate of bone loss in many patients. However, BMD continues to be lost at a rate higher than with normal aging (Saag, 2003).

There is also a relationship between rate of bone loss and the dose of glucocorticoid used for treatment. Corticosteroid doses as low as 7.5 mg/day have been associated with bone loss. It is unclear whether cumulative steroid dose correlates to more bone loss, with Reid et al. (1992) suggesting this relationship at doses of more than 12.5 mg/day. There is much debate on whether peak or cumulative dose is most strongly associated with bone loss (Trence, 2003). Alternate-day therapy has no benefit on bone preservation over daily therapy (Gluck et al., 1981). The cumulative glucocorticoid dose seems more important than peak dose based on a number of studies (Hall et al., 1993). In contrast to these data, a secondary analysis of the large United Kingdom General Practice Research Database (GPRD) found that adverse effects of glucocorticoids on bone occurred rapidly and were most strongly related to daily rather than cumulative dose. In this study, an association was identified between clinical fractures and glucocorticoid dose up to 20 mg/day that increased in a more exponential fashion thereafter. However, most of the glucocorticoid users in GPRD did not have inflammatory diseases requiring chronic doses of glucocorticoids, as evidenced by median glucocorticoid duration of approximately 30 days. Therefore, it seems the presence of fractures with even low-dose oral therapy further argues against a 'safe' glucocorticoid dose from the standpoint of bone (van Staa et al., 2000).

The most comprehensive study of osteoporosis in SLE was published by Ramsey-Goldman et al. (1999), who found that 86 (12%) of 702 women with SLE had suffered at least one self-reported fracture since the onset of SLE. The standardized morbidity ratio for fracture was 4.7 (3.8–5.8). Associations with time from lupus diagnosis to fracture are very reminiscent of the risk factors for CVD: older age at diagnosis, longer disease duration, longer duration of steroid use, postmenopausal status, and, in this case, less use of oral contraceptives. Furthermore, Ramsey-Goldman and Manzi (2001) showed an association between decreased BMD and both an increased carotid plaque index and the presence of coronary artery calcification in a pilot study of 65 patients with SLE. This supports the concept that inflammatory and immune-mediated mechanisms involved in SLE may also contribute to the development of atheroma and osteoporosis (Gordon, 2002).

Kipen et al. (1997) studied 97 female SLE patients with mean age of 44.2 years and found that there was low bone mass (>1 SD below adult mean) in the spine and femoral neck in over 40% of the patients. There was an osteoporotic level BMD (>2.5 SD below the young adult mean) in the spine of 13% of the patients and in the femoral neck of 6% of the patients. There was a much clearer inverse relation between steroid use ever and the spine BMD result than the femoral neck BMD (Gordon, 2002).

The etiology of glucocorticoid-induced osteoporosis (GIOP) is multifactorial and occurs concomitantly with normal age and menopause-associated bone loss. There are two major pathways by which glucocorticoids lead to abnormalities in bone metabolism: (1) a reduction in bone formation and (2) an increase in bone resorption (Adachi et al., 1993). Although the pathogenesis of GIOP is somewhat unsettled, direct inhibition on osteoblast activity by glucocorticoids is the most favored mechanism. Histologically, this is indicated by reduced trabecular wall thickness. Glucocorticoids cause a decrease in the absolute number of osteoblasts and their premature death by apoptosis. Glucocorticoids modulate osteoblasts' response to skeletal growth factors such as IGF-1, IGF-2, IGF-binding proteins, and cytokines TGF-beta and PDGF-beta. Osteoblast inhibition is evident by decreases in serum osteocalcin levels. Osteoblast dysfunction results in incomplete repair of the bone remodeling lacunae (Manolagas and Weinstein, 1999).

Enhanced osteoclast-mediated bone resorption is the other mechanistic pathway to GIOP. Limited data show that glucocorticoids significantly inhibit calcium absorption through the gastrointestinal tract, increased renal calcium loss, or diminished sex hormone production, all of which could lead to increased bone resorption. Effects on calcium may be mediated partially by direct effects on glucocorticoids on vitamin D receptors. Another even more compelling mechanism of bone resorption is the suppression of osteoprotegerin (OPG) by glucocorticoids and the concurrent stimulation OPG ligand production by osteoblastic lineage cells (Sasaki et al., 2001).

The osteoporosis of glucocorticoid therapy is attributable to several metabolic changes. Gonadal hormone function is altered through inhibition of pituitary gonadotrophin secretion and therefore the inhibition of estrogen and testosterone production. Lukert and Raisz (1994), found that suppression of adrenal androstenedione further contributes to decreased circulating gonadal hormone levels. Mineral metabolism is affected through a classic model of decreased intestinal calcium absorption, with increased compensatory secretion of parathyroid hormone (PTH). Glucocorticoids can exert a direct effect on bone, with inhibition of osteoclast cell numbers, lifespan, and function (Jee et al., 1977; Dempster et al., 1983). Overall, the primary effect is the inhibition of bone formation.

The risk factors for osteoporosis with glucocorticoid therapy are not the same as those typically associated with osteoporosis. Men and women of all ethnic backgrounds and ages are at risk for glucocorticoid osteoporosis. Lane and Lukert (1998) showed that fracture risk remains highest in postmenopausal women, presumably owing to lower bone mass at initiation of therapy. A cross-sectional study of postmenopausal women found that the risk factors for steroid-induced osteoporosis included duration of steroid use but also age and body mass index (Thompson et al., 1997).

Fracture risk with glucocorticoids is determined by several factors including (Fig. 1): Age: this is a risk factor for vertebral fracture, independent of BMD.

BMD: both the initial value before glucocorticoid therapy and the amount of subsequent glucocorticoid-induced loss are important. Bone loss of 10% from a baseline T score of 0 (as in a premenopausal woman) has a weaker influence on fracture risk than a similar bone loss from a baseline T score of −2 (as for example in a postmenopausal woman). The greatest risk of vertebral fracture is in older postmenopausal women.

Glucocorticoid dose: bone loss is dependent both on cumulative and mean daily dose.

Duration of exposure: a short course of glucocorticoids will cause bone loss that is largely reversible on ceasing glucocorticoids, but long-term therapy causes a sustained reduction in BMD due to decreased bone formation increasing the likelihood that a fracture will occur eventually.

The underlying diseases for which glucocorticoids are prescribed, which may be independently associated with increased fracture risk (Rheumatology, 2004).

There needs to be high suspicion for potential bone loss among all patients initiating or chronically using glucocorticoids. The most accurate way to determine osteoporosis status is to assess bone mass, typically through the use of dual-energy X-ray absorptiometry (DEXA). Despite the precision of this approach and the vast benefits of DEXA, the use of different DEXA devices and disparities between the sites of measurements limit this technique (Hansen et al., 1999).

DEXA measures a combination of trabecular and cortical bone, and trabecular bone is lost more rapidly than cortical bone in glucocorticoid-induced bone loss. In comparison to quantitative computerized tomography (QCT), which measures trabecular bone more directly, DEXA is less expensive, easily accessible, and is associated with less radiation exposure (Lukert and Raisz, 1994). If only one site can be measured, then the preferred site in women younger than age 60 should be the lumbar spine. In older patients the femoral neck should be measured to minimize the potential effect of osteophyte formation at vertebral bodies affecting density readings. DEXA of the spine in the lateral position may be a more sensitive indicator of glucocorticoid-induced bone loss than the anteroposterior position (Reid et al., 1992). Ideally, DEXA should be performed before the initiation of glucocorticoid therapy and although the optimal

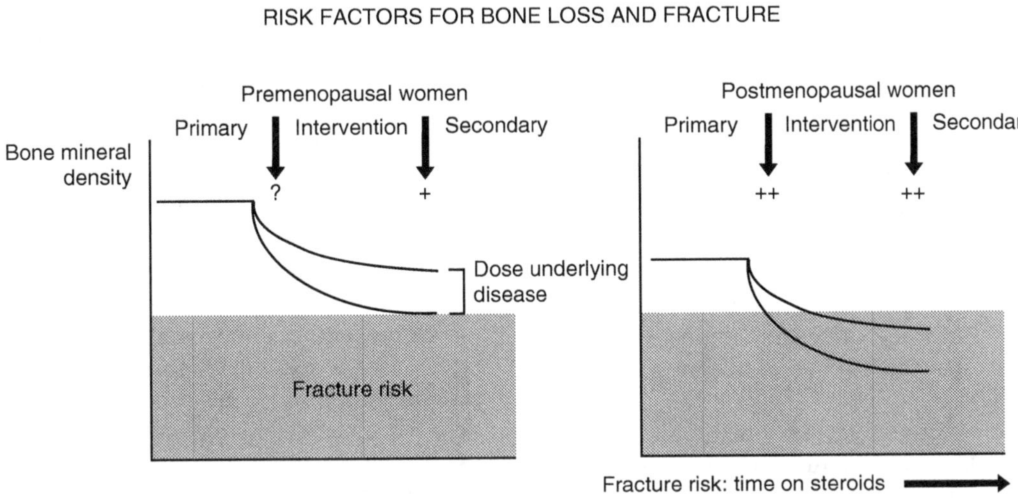

Figure 1. Risk factors for bone loss and fracture. (Adapted from Rheumatology, 2004, Fig. 199.6.)

interval for follow-up DEXA remains unclear, the American College of Rheumatology recommends repeating them at yearly intervals (ACR, 2001).

Recommendations for bone mass measurement of patients on glucocorticoids have been proposed by different medical societies and ad hoc panels and are reimbursed under the US Bone Mass Measurement Act. Most guidelines suggest a BMD test if the patient will receive treatment with greater than physiologic glucocorticoid usage (>7.5 mg of prednisone or its equivalent per day) and treatment for at least 1–6 months. The lumbar spine and trochanter demonstrate rapid bone loss with glucocorticoids and respond reliably to effective GIOP interventions and thus are sensitive imaging sites. Poor precision and localized effects of arthritis may limit the use of peripheral BMD measurements in the wrist, fingers, and heels. QCT can also be used but may overestimate the effects of glucocorticoid on bone because glucocorticoids increase bone marrow fat (Saag, 2003).

Although a decline in BMD correlates strongly with fracture risk and BMD is the best measurable predictor currently known, the rate of bone turnover, bone quality, and other factors play important independent roles in fracture risk (Peel et al., 1995). A high value of a bone resorption marker such as urinary *N*-telopeptides or deoxypyridinoline cross-links may identify patients with particularly rapid bone turnover or substantiate a lack of response to antiresorptive agents. An elevated 24-h urinary calcium-to-creatinine ratio is also indicative of rapid bone turnover, such as seen among patients newly using glucocorticoid.

Among patients who are assumed to have osteoporosis on the basis of chronic glucocorticoid use, postmenopausal status, and inflammatory condition, selective screening for other causes of bone loss need to be considered. Hyperparathyroidism, hyperthyroidism, osteomalacia due to poor dietary vitamin D intake and inadequate sun exposure, or multiple myeloma can all mimic or contribute to low bone mass among patients on glucocorticoids. In particular, a 25-OH vitamin D measurement is helpful in identifying patients with low or low normal vitamin D stores who might benefit from supplementation. Although not indicated in all glucocorticoid users with low BMD, laboratory evaluation for these and other conditions should be undertaken based on clinical suspicion (Saag, 2003).

1.1. Treatment

Based on data showing an increased risk for bone loss among RA patients, particularly on steroid, there is a need to identify effective strategies aimed at mitigating possible toxicity. The American College of Rheumatology and other specialty groups have released recommendations advocating an increasingly aggressive approach to this serious problem based on accumulating literature demonstrating good efficacy of several antiosteoporosis compounds, particularly the bisphosphonates (ACR, 2001).

The most effective intervention for the prevention of bone loss and fractures among glucocorticoid users is glucocorticoid discontinuation or dose reduction (Pocock et al., 1987). This is not always possible because of the severity of many chronic inflammatory diseases. Suppression of the pituitary–adrenal axis occurs rapidly with exogenous glucocorticoid therapy. A single dose can be associated with a blunted response to a major stressor, such as surgery, and when glucocorticoid therapy is continued for several days, the hypothalamic–pituitary–adrenal axis response is impaired. Streck and Lockwood (1979) showed that 50 mg of prednisone per day for 5 days has been associated with decreased responsiveness to insulin-induced hypoglycemia and adrenocorticotropin (ACTH) stimulation. Generally, after 1 month of high-dose glucocorticoid therapy, steroid-withdrawal syndromes should be considered, and doses should be tapered. Longer-acting steroids such as dexamethasone result in more axis suppression than shorter-acting steroids such as prednisone or prednisolone (Byyny, 1976). Symptoms of steroid withdrawal are adrenal insufficiency with lethargy, malaise, nausea, arthralgias, myalgias, headache, and fever. Postural hypotension may occur. Protocols for steroid taper should include small, graduated dose decreases over increments of 1–2 weeks for those who have been on long-term therapy to prevent precipitating an exacerbation of the underlying disease process treated with glucocorticoid. When a dose of 5 mg of prednisone or its equivalent is reached, an assessment of adrenal reserve is indicated (Trence, 2003).

A number of therapeutic agents used in postmenopausal osteoporosis have particular relevance for GIOP. Vitamin D and calcium increase gastrointestinal calcium intake and limit renal losses; thiazide diuretics decrease urinary calcium excretion; estrogens and testosterone supplements help offset gonadal deficiency; bisphosphonates and calcitonin help prevent bone resorption; and PTH stimulates osteoblastic bone formation (Saag, 2003).

The prevention and treatment of glucocorticoid-induced bone loss include nonpharmacologic and pharmacologic approaches (Table 1). The lowest dose for the shortest interval of therapy should be used. Weight-bearing exercise, fall prevention, smoking cessation, and alcohol intake limitation should all be recommended. Calcium and vitamin D supplementation recommendations include 400 IU/day of vitamin D and approximately 1500 mg of calcium. Thiazide diuretics with sodium restriction can improve intestinal absorption of calcium and further decrease urinary calcium loss (Adams et al., 1981).

The mainstays of glucocorticoid-induced bone loss prevention and treatment are the bisphosphonates. Adachi et al. (1994, 1997) showed that cyclic etidronate, 400 mg/day for 2 weeks every 3 months, prevents bone loss at initiation of glucocorticoid therapy, increases bone density over time, and decreases fracture incidence. Alendronate, 10 mg daily, increases BMD, decreases fracture rate (Saag et al., 1998), and is well tolerated. If gastrointestinal side effects make oral bisphosphonates difficult to use, intravenous infusion of pamidronate increases lumbar and, to a lesser extent, hip BMD (Bentsen et al., 2001), and has the additional advantage of being given only every 3 months. Zoledronic acid is also used this way. Calcitonin, given subcutaneously or nasally, can protect against glucocorticoid-induced bone loss but bone mass does not increase and does not decrease fracture risk (Healey et al., 1996). Despite accumulating data on the effectiveness of anti-osteoporotic therapies in GIOP, only 5–35% of patients on glucocorticoids in the US, Canada, and Great Britain receive therapies to prevent or treat GIOP (ACR, 2001).

Table 1
Recommendations for the prevention and treatment of glucocorticoid-induced osteoporosis

Patient begining therapy with glucocorticoid (prednisone equivalent of ⩾5 mg/day) with plans for treatment duration of ⩾3 months:
Modify lifestyle risk factors for osteoporosis
Smoking cessation or avoidance
Reduction of alcohol consumption if excessive
Instruct in weight-bearing physical exercise
Initiate calcium supplementation
Initiate supplementation with vitamin D (plain or activated form)
Prescribe bisphosphonate (use with caution in premenopausal women)
Patient receiving long-term glucocorticoid therapy (prednisone equivalent of ⩾5 mg/day):
Modify lifestyle risk factors for osteoporosis
Smoking cessation or avoidance
Reduction of alcohol consumption if excessive
Instruct in weight-bearing physical exercise
Initiate calcium supplementation
Initiate supplementation with vitamin D (plain or activated form)
Prescribe treatment to replace gonadal sex hormones if deficient or otherwise clinically indicated
Measure bone mineral density (BMD) at lumbar spine and/or hip.
If BMD is not normal (i.e., T-score <-1), then
Prescribe bisphosphonate (use with caution in premenopausal women)
Consider calcitonin as second-line agent if patient has contraindication to or does not tolerate bisphosphonate therapy
If BMD is normal, follow up and repeat BMD measurement either annually or biannually

Adapted from: Recommendations for the prevention and treatment of glucocorticoid-induced osteoporosis: 2001 update. American College of Rheumatology, Ad Hoc Committee on Glucocorticoid-Induced Osteoporosis.

1.1.1. Calcium and vitamin D

Calcium decreases bone resorption as measured by urinary hydroxyproline. However, calcium alone may not prevent bone loss, especially those prone to poor absorption. Elemental calcium at 1200–1500 mg/day is necessary but not sufficient as a sole therapy for patients on glucocorticoids. Vitamin D can be administered in a variety of formulations (Sambrook et al., 2003). In a prevention study, calcium, calcitriol, and calcitonin used in varying combinations were given to patients for 1 year. Patients were followed for an additional second year off therapy. At the lumbar spine, subjects randomized to receive a combination containing calcitriol experienced significantly less bone loss than those receiving calcium alone. In year 2, a slight lumbar spine BMD increase was seen among subjects who received calcitonin. No differential effects between the three treatment arms were observed at the femoral neck, where bone loss occurred in all three treatment groups (Sambrook et al., 1993).

Inactivated vitamin D preparations may also have merit in GIOP. In a 2-year randomized controlled trial of RA patients on chronic low doses of glucocorticoids (mean prednisone dosage 5.6 mg/day) 1000 mg of calcium carbonate and 500 IU of vitamin D prevented bone loss in the lumbar spine and trochanter (Buckley et al., 1996). An earlier study of smaller doses of vitamin D and calcium did not demonstrate a different effect than that of calcium alone, although a small increase in BMD was noted in both groups (Bijlsma et al., 1988). Due to the impairment in calcium absorption mediated by glucocorticoids and the common occurrence of vitamin D deficiency among housebound patients suffering with chronic inflammatory conditions, vitamin D should be supplemented in all glucocorticoid users.

1.1.2. Thiazide diuretics

Adams (1981), specifically examined the efficacy of thiazide agents in glucocorticoid-treated patients. In combination with dietary sodium restriction, hydrochlorothiazide 50 mg twice a day improved the total body calcium balance. Despite the scarcity of evidence, use of thiazides during the early phase of glucocorticoid use when there is profound hypercalciuria, may be useful, while carefully monitoring for side effects.

1.1.3. Calcitonin

Calcitonin is weakly effective at preventing and treating GIOP when bone mass is measured at the lumbar spine. Adachi et al. (1997) found that spinal bone density declined on placebo (5%), whereas the calcitonin-treated group had a nonsignificant decline of 1.3% over 1 year. Although less lumbar bone was lost in an observational study of sarcoid patients who received calcitonin for GIOP prevention, a randomized controlled prevention study in polymyalgia rheumatica patients did not show greater bone preservation with injectable calcitonin (Healey et al., 1996). In one of the three treatment studies, placebo patients lost 7.8% BMD over 2 years, whereas the nasal calcitonin-treated group had an increase of 2.8% (Luengo et al., 1994). For GIOP, calcitonin is a relatively weak antiresorptive agent. It potentially maintains bone mass, but in most studies calcitonin does not lead to a marked increase in BMD. There has not been a documented benefit of its effects on fracture reduction.

1.1.4. Estrogen

In the only published randomized controlled trial of estrogen replacement therapy (ERT) in GIOP, postmenopausal women with RA received transdermal estradiol, 50 μg/day, or calcium supplementation (400 IU/day) (Hall et al., 1994). At the end of 2 years, women on ERT had higher bone density in the spine than those receiving calcium alone. There were no significant differences at the femur. Two small observational studies of ERT by Lukert et al. (1992) and Sambrook et al. (1992) demonstrated reduced bone loss in the spine among chronic glucocorticoid users. Selective estrogen modulators (SERMs) may offer a therapeutic option in the treatment of GIOP but have an increased risk of thrombosis and menopausal symptoms.

1.1.5. Bisphosphonates

When administered over 1 or 2 years to patients on glucocorticoids for a variety of chronic inflammatory disorders, etidronate, pamidronate, alendronate, and risedronate are efficacious in preventing or treating bone loss at the spine and in regions of the hip (Table 2). Randomized controlled clinical trials looking at effects of etidronate on GIOP revealed increased or preserved lumbar BMD compared with placebo, which often included calcium. In the largest prevention trial, cyclical etidronate was instituted within 100 days of prednisone initiation in 141 men and women, beginning prednisone therapy for a variety of conditions (Adachi et al., 1997). The placebo group had a decrease in lumbar BMD of 3.2%, whereas the treatment group had an increase of 0.6% at 1 year. Similar effects were seen at the trochanter. Bone density at the femoral neck did not differ significantly between groups. A trend toward a significant fracture reduction was seen in the postmenopausal women in this study. The largest treatment study with etidronate also confirmed that etidronate, when administered with calcium and vitamin D, resulted in a significant 4.5% increase in lumbar BMD (Pitt et al., 1998).

Alendronate has proven efficacy in preventing and treating bone loss associated with glucocorticoid use and in preventing vertebral fractures. In the combined report from two multinational studies, 477 new and chronic glucocorticoid users were studied, including postmenopausal women. At the spine, there was a significant increase in BMD of 2.9% on 10 mg of alendronate and a loss of 0.4% on placebo. Similar effects were seen at the trochanter, and smaller but significant gains in BMD were noted at the femoral neck (Saag et al., 1998). A second year extension to this study among 208 (37%) of the original subjects who continued to take >7.5 mg of prednisone documented similar beneficial effects at the spine, trochanter, and femoral neck. A significant 90% reduction in an overall small number of incident vertebral fractures was observed. Alendronate (5 mg) was statistically equivalent to 10 mg except among postmenopausal women not receiving estrogen, where 10 mg resulted in significantly greater increases in lumbar BMD (Adachi et al., 2001).

Risedronate at 2.5 and 5.0 mg/day maintained or increased bone mass at the lumbar spine, trochanter, and femoral neck in patients beginning

Table 2

Comparison of five large randomized controlled trials assessing bisphosphonates in the treatment and prevention of glucocorticoid-induced osteoporosis[a]

Characteristic or outcome measure	Adachi et al. [25] ($n = 141$)	Roux et al. [38] ($n = 117$)	Saag et al. [20] ($n = 477$)	Cohen et al. [26] ($n = 228$)	Reid et al. [21] ($n = 290$)
Drug studied	Etidronate	Etidronate	Alendronate	Risedronate	Risedronate
Sex and menopausal status (%)					
Postmenopausal women	50	49	49	46	53
Premenopausal women	12	15	22	20	9
Men	38	36	29	34	38
Baseline vertebral fractures (%)					
Treatment group	45	3.4	15	30	33
Placebo group	49	1.7	17	29	37
Baseline osteoporosis defined by BMD criteria (%)	NA	24.5	32	NA	23
Mean daily prednisone dosage (mg)					
Baseline	22	NA	18	21	15
End of study	11	11	9	11	13
Supplements provided during study					
Calcium (mg/day)	500	500	800–1000	500	1000
Vitamin D (IU/day)	None	None	250–500	None	400
BMD increase (%)[b]					
Lumbar spine					
From baseline	0.6	0.3	2.9[c]	0.6[c]	2.9[c]
From placebo	3.7	3.1	3.3[c]	3.4[c]	2.5[c]
Trochanter					
From baseline	1.5	NA	2.7[c]	1.4[c]	2.4[c]
From placebo	4.1	NA	3.4[c]	4.4[c]	1.4[c]
Femoral neck					
From baseline	0.2	NA	1.0[c]	0.8[c]	1.8[c]
From placebo	1.9	NA	2.2[c]	3.8[c]	2.1[c]
Vertebral fracture reduction (%)					
Overall	40 (*P* NS)	NA	38 (*P* NS)[d]	67 (*P* NS)[c]	67[c]
Postmenopausal women	85 ($P = 0.05$)	NA	51 (*P* NS)[d]	60 (*P* NS)[c]	NA

Adapted from: Recommendations for the prevention and treatment of glucocorticoid-induced osteoporosis: 2001 update. American College of Rheumatology, Ad Hoc Committee on Glucocorticoid-Induced Osteoporosis.

[a] NA = information not available; BMD = bone mineral density; NS = non significance.

[b] Only 1-year values that were significant at the $P < 0.05$ level are shown.

[c] For alendronate at 10 mg/day and risedronate at 5 mg/day.

[d] Results shown are for the primary fracture outcome measured using vertebral morphometry among pooled alendronate users (both 5 and 10 mg/day dosages).

glucocorticoids (Cohen et al., 1999). At the lumbar spine, bone mass was maintained with an increase of 0.6% in the group receiving 5 mg of risedronate compared with a loss of 2.8% in the control group. Similar effects were seen at the trochanter. At the femoral neck, bone mass increased 0.8% in those given 5 mg of risedronate with a loss of 3.1% in the control group. In patients already on long-term glucocorticoids, 2.5 and 5.0 mg of risedronate maintained or increased bone mass at the lumbar spine, trochanter, and femoral neck. (Reid et al., 2000). Pooled data from the two risedronate studies demonstrated a 58–70% reduction in vertebral fracture rate (Wallach et al., 2000).

Intravenous pamidronate may afford another effective therapeutic alternative for highly selected individuals who are not candidates for oral bisphosphonate therapy. As measured by QCT, a >19% increase in lumbar BMD at 1 year was seen in a randomized controlled study (Reid et al., 1988).

In all large randomized controlled trials of bisphosphonates, bone mass was maintained or increased with bisphosphonate therapy, whereas a decline was generally seen in the control group of the prevention studies. In the treatment studies, a bisphosphonate was always more effective than control therapy, although the control groups did not always lose bone at a significant rate. A Cochrane review further concluded that bisphosphonates are effective in preventing and treating glucocorticoid-associated bone loss at the lumbar spine and the femoral neck (Homik et al., 1999).

Zoledronic acid is the most potent bisphosphonate that has been studied in clinical trials to-date (Body et al., 1999). It is superior to pamidronate in the treatment of cancer-related hypercalcemia (Major et al., 2001). It has high potency; therefore only small doses are required for the inhibition of bone resorption, and long dosing intervals may be used. Intermittent intravenous administration of zoledronic acid results in changes in biochemical markers of bone turnover and in BMD that are similar to those observed with daily oral bisphosphonate therapy. The reductions in markers at 1 year (Reid et al., 2002) are similar to those seen with 5 mg of risedronate per day and 10 mg of alendronate per day. Zoledronic acid increases spinal BMD at 12 months to 5% above values found in patients receiving placebo; an increase similar to that achieved with a daily 10 mg dose of alendronate (5%) (Liberman et al., 1995), a daily 5 mg dose of risedronate (3%) (Harris et al., 1999), or a daily 150 mg dose of pamidronate (5%) (Reid et al., 1994). Intravenous zoledronic acid also produced results similar to those of the oral regimens at the femoral neck (alendronate, 3% increase in bone density; risedronate, 2%; pamidronate, 3%) and in the total body (alendronate, 1.5% increase; pamidronate, 1%). An annual infusion of zoledronic acid might be an effective treatment for postmenopausal osteoporosis for patients who cannot tolerate conventional oral bisphosphonates.

1.1.6. Parathyroid hormone and growth factors

Most therapies for osteoporosis, including the bisphosphonates, hormone replacement therapy (HRT), SERMs, and calcitonin, act by reducing bone turnover. Inhibition of bone resorption is usually associated with an increase in BMD during the first 1–3 year of treatment by an amount that varies from 4–8% for bisphosphonates and raloxifene to only 1–2% for calcitonin. This reduction in bone turnover and increase in BMD are associated with a 30–50% lower risk of subsequent fracture. Patients with osteoporosis have already lost skeletal mass of more than 25% below the young adult mean. Even with treatment, many patients continue to have a BMD that remains within the osteoporotic range, and many continue to fracture (Hodsman et al., 2003).

Anabolic agents that directly stimulate bone formation have the potential to increase skeletal mass to levels at least equal to those seen in age- and sex-matched normal patients. These agents can potentially restore bone mass to young adult levels. Sodium fluoride, the first anabolic agent studied, increased BMD to a greater extent than antiresorptive agents (Riggs et al., 1982). However, bone containing fluoride is weaker than naturally mineralized bone, and the antifracture efficacy of fluoride is inconsistent.

The anabolic activity of PTH and the N-terminal fragment analogs of PTH have been investigated for many years. Although these agents increase both resorption and formation of bone, animal models have demonstrated that their primary effects when given by daily injection reflect their role as potent anabolic agents capable of inducing large and rapid increases in bone mass and strength. A large randomized, placebo-controlled trial of PTH analog human PTH-(1–34) (teriparatide) reported dose-related increases in lumbar spine BMD of 9.7–13.7% after a median treatment period of 21 months (Neer et al., 2001). Significant gains of 2.8–5.1% also occurred at the femoral neck, but a decrease in BMD of 2.1–3.2% was seen at the radial shaft, which is primarily a cortical bone site. Neer showed a significant reduction in both incident vertebral fractures (65–69%) and nonvertebral fractures (53%).The ideal treatment of osteoporosis should preferably prevent fractures through normalization of bone mass and bone micro-architecture. Biosynthetic human PTH 1–34 (teriparatide) was recently approved as the first anabolic treatment of osteoporosis. The effects of teriparatide are mediated by the G-protein-dependent, PTH receptor-1 in the cell membrane. The binding of the ligand to the receptor activates adenylate cyclase and a number of phospholipases (A, C, and D), and increases intracellular levels of cAMP and calcium. Intermittent teriparatide increases the number of osteoblasts and bone formation of pre-existing osteoblasts, increased differentiation of lining cells, and reduced osteoblast apoptosis. The anabolic effects of teriparatide on bone have been demonstrated in several species. It increases bone mass, structural integrity, bone diameter, and bone strength. Clinical efficacy was demonstrated in a randomized study comprising of 1637 postmenopausal women with osteoporosis showing a 65 and 35% reduction of the relative risk of vertebral and appendicular fractures, respectively, during 18 months of treatment. Moreover, BMD in the lumbar spine and hip increased by 9.7 and 2.6%, respectively. Similar effects on BMD have been reported in glucocorticoid osteoporosis; however, fracture data are limited in these groups (Brixen, 2004).

Teriparatide should be used in combination with calcium plus vitamin D, and may be combined with HRT. In contrast, alendronate attenuates the effect of teriparatide. The efficacy of other combinations remains uncertain. After termination of teriparatide, BMD of the lumbar spine is reduced by approximately 2–3% after 2.5 years. This decrease may be prevented by treatment with bisphosphonates. Reduced dosage or termination of therapy due to hypercalcemia was necessary in 3% of the patients studied. In a rat toxicology study, in which teriparatide was administered in high dosages for an extended period of time, osteosarcoma was seen in a significant number of animals. None of the patients followed in clinical trials has developed osteosarcoma (Brixen, 2004).

2. Rheumatoid arthritis

Rheumatoid arthritis affects approximately 1% of the US population, imposing enormous societal costs. In addition to causing significant morbidity and posing a substantial economic burden, an increasing number of population-based studies have shown that RA leads to premature mortality. Great strides have been made in the treatment of RA in the last 15–20 years, but several major comorbidities have been identified. They include CVD and osteoporosis leading to fracture (Mikuls and Saag, 2001).

The association of diseases with systemic inflammation, such as RA or SLE and CVD has gained much attention because increasing evidence has showed that inflammation is a direct risk factor for atherosclerosis. Solomon et al. (2003) in a prospective cohort study involving 114,342 women, showed that women with RA had a greater than two-fold higher risk of myocardial infarction (MI) and that this association remained after adjusting for known and potential cardiovascular risk factors.

CVD is generally considered to be the leading contributor to mortality in RA, accounting for one-half of all deaths. Although the overall incidence of CVD in RA does not seem to be disproportionately increased, it does seem to result in death at earlier ages in RA compared to controls (Mikuls and Saag, 2001). Wolfe et al. (1994) observed 361 deaths attributable to CVD in the RA cohorts, which was over twice the number expected deaths (161 expected deaths). In an investigation of the United Kingdom National Health Service Central Register, Symmons et al. (1998) reported a standardized mortality ratio of 2.2 (95% CI: 1.8–2.6) for CVD in RA patients. CVD accounted for 34% of excess deaths observed in this large RA cohort. In another longitudinal study, RA was an independent risk factor for the development of congestive heart failure (CHF), with a trend toward increased incidence of MI (Gabriel et al., 1999).

The pathogenesis of CVD in the setting of RA is multifactorial. There is increasing evidence that inflammatory mediators intrinsic to the disease represent major culprits in the development of

CVD and that agents used to ameliorate inflammation may paradoxically promote the development of accelerated atherogenesis, thrombosis, and CHF (Mikuls and Saag, 2001).

Inflammation, characteristic of active RA, likely plays a primary role in CVD. It has been suggested that subclinical vasculitis, common in RA, leads to endothelial injury and accelerated atherosclerosis. Inflammatory mediators, such as C-reactive protein (CRP), are an independent risk factor for CVD. In a retrospective case-control trial of 211 patients with seropositive RA, baseline erythrocyte sedimentation rates were predictive of first cardiovascular events. CRP may have a direct role in the development of CVD. CRP activates components of the complement cascade (implicated in early atherogenesis) and along with complement, has been localized in human atheromatous lesions (Wallberg-Jonsson et al., 1999). RA patients have a three-fold risk of atheroma compared to normal and hypertensive controls; the risk is directly related to duration and severity of disease (Roman et al., 2005 submitted for publication).

The relationship between RA and CVD has become a major focus of attention since many of the cells comprising the inflammatory infiltrate in the joint lining are also found in atherosclerotic plaques. Although inflammation in RA centers on the synovium, inflammatory mediators spill into the systemic circulation, where they interact with endothelial cells (Solomon et al., 2003). Interleukin 1 (IL-1) and tumor necrosis factor alpha (TNF-alpha), found in high concentrations in the blood of RA patients, have profound effects on endothelial cells, up-regulating them to express adhesion molecules, increasing their permeability, and facilitating migration of inflammatory cells into vessel walls. It has long been known that T-cells play a critical role in the pathogenesis of RA. Recent data also suggest that T-cell abnormalities may play a role in acute coronary syndromes and atherosclerotic plaque instability. In addition, several different investigators have found that cytokines, CRP, and other inflammatory markers, known to be elevated in RA, are also elevated before and at the time of ischemic injuries. CRP stimulates macrophages to produce tissue factor, an important procoagulant (del Rincon et al., 2001). However, single time evaluation of inflammatory cytokines does not distinguish RA patients with atherosclerotic plaque from those without (Roman et al., 2005 submitted for publication).

Other possible links between RA and CVD include the reduced physical activity often associated with RA, medications taken for RA, and differential use of cardiovascular protection for patients with RA. The therapies used to treat RA, such as glucocorticoids, methotrexate (MTX), hydroxychloroquine, and cyclooxygenase inhibitors may induce or protect from thrombotic events or atherogenesis. Corticosteroids have a recognized atherogenic effect, mediated through their effects on plasma lipids. However, these agents are used in about half of all RA patients and usually in low dosage. Some studies even suggest that they have not been able to demonstrate an association between CV mortality and steroid use in RA. MTX, known to down regulate T-cell activity, has been associated with reduced cardiovascular mortality in patients with RA. Conversely, MTX may cause atherosclerosis by inducing hyperhomocysteinemia. This effect may be counterbalanced by the concomitant use of folic acid in MTX-treated RA (Solomon et al., 2003).

2.1. Treatment

It is paramount that those physicians caring for RA patients recognize patients at highest risk and implement primary and secondary preventative measures to reduce the effects of CVD in this population. Cigarette smoking cessation is of added value, because smoking increases the risk of atherosclerosis and CVD-associated mortality, but also increases RA severity. In the absence of contradictory evidence, it is appropriate to attempt to minimize the exposure of at-risk patients to glucocorticoids. Folic acid supplementation, used to prevent dose-related toxicity of MTX, also lowers serum homocysteine levels and may be preventative in patients receiving MTX. Given the frequency of dyslipidemia in RA, lipid measurements should be part of routine health care screening, with abnormal lipid values treated appropriately. Of interest, hydroxychloroquine, a commonly used disease modifying antirheumatic drug (DMARD), has a favorable effect on serum lipids, implying this may be a preferred therapy for patients at risk (Mikuls and Saag, 2001).

The cardioprotective role of HRT in postmenopausal women remains controversial based on results from recent studies. Compared with placebo, HRT is associated with a significant increase in CRP levels and a decline in serum homocysteine. In contrast, raloxifene, a SERM used for osteoporosis, does not adversely effect CRP levels, and, similar to estrogen, lowers serum homocysteine, raising speculation that this agent may have a preferential role in the primary and secondary prevention in RA patients (Walsh et al., 2000). This small increase in thromboembolic events suspected with estrogens and SERMs require carefully balancing the risk safety profile for many patients.

It seems imperative that aggressive cardiac preventive measures in patients with RA need to be considered to address established coronary heart disease (CHD) risk factors. In addition, it seems that early aggressive treatment of RA with disease-modifying antirheumatic drugs may reduce the future risk of MI.

3. Systemic lupus erythematosus

In spite of considerable improvements in treatment, morbidity and mortality in patients with systemic lupus erythematosus (SLE) are substantial, with mortality rates of 5–10% at 5 years and 15–30% at 10 years. Patients with SLE have a nearly five-fold increased risk of death compared with the general population. The standardized mortality ratio is high, 9.16, in patients aged less than 55 years. A bimodal pattern of mortality has been described, with early deaths predominately due to active SLE and intercurrent infection and late deaths due to atherosclerotic disease. CVD currently accounts for a proportionately greater percentage of deaths in late disease. With the increased life expectancy of SLE patients due to improved therapy, CVD has emerged as a significant threat to the health of these women (Manzi et al., 1997). Having improved therapy for active SLE disease, the challenges that face physicians today include how to understand and prevent the long-term complications of the disease and accumulation of chronic damage (Bessant et al., 2004).

Jonsson et al. (1989) showed that MI rate in Swedish patients with SLE was increased nine-fold. While clinical evidence of coronary disease is found in 6.7–8.3% of patients with SLE, subclinical atherosclerosis is more common. Petri and Civelek (1998) and Manzi et al. (1999) showed atheromatous carotid plaques have been demonstrated by ultrasonography in 25–40% of patients with SLE. Studies have suggested that not all of the increased risk of CVD seen in SLE patients is attributable to traditional risk factors such as hypertension, diabetes, smoking, and hypercholesterolemia (Doria et al., 2003). Esdaile et al. (2001) showed that after removing the effect of these known risk factors, there is still a 7.9-fold increase in the risk of stroke and a 10.1-fold increase in the risk of nonfatal MI in patients with SLE. Bruce et al. (2000) found that the mean age at a first coronary event was 49 years in patients with SLE compared with 65–74 years in the general population. Manzi et al. (1997) investigated CVD in 498 women with SLE, and found the risk of MI relative to age-matched controls was highest, at 52.4, in those aged 35–44 years. Two-thirds of all cardiovascular events in this cohort occurred in patients aged less than 55 years.

The hypothesis that premature atherosclerosis in SLE is solely attributable to an increased frequency of conventional risk factors, such as hypertension, dyslipidemia, and diabetes, all of which may be provoked or exacerbated by corticosteroid therapy does not hold true (Roman et al., 2001). Current knowledge indicates that atherosclerosis is an active inflammatory and immune-mediated process (Fischer et al., 2004). The chronic inflammation and immune dysregulation characteristic of SLE likely contributes to the accelerated vascular disease in these patients. Esdaile et al. (2001) suggested that SLE itself may be atherogenic through chronic activation of the immune system. Roman et al. (2003) confirmed that the prevalence of atherosclerosis is significantly increased among patients with SLE and that the prevalence is not attributable to traditional risk factors for CVD, but that chronic inflammation is atherogenic in this population, an effect that is additive to that of aging in promoting atherosclerosis. Kao et al. (2003) reveals the striking similarities between processes inherent to SLE and atherogenesis and speculates that treatment strategies directed toward specific immune dysregulation in SLE will be beneficial in preventing premature vascular disease in this population.

Parallels between the inflammatory and immune-mediated mechanisms of both atherogenesis and SLE may provide clues to understanding premature vascular disease in these patients (Gordon, 2002). SLE-related factors are likely involved in all stages of atherogenesis from the formation of the atherosclerotic lesion to its rupture, as well as in the thrombotic event itself. Processes critical to the pathogenesis of SLE, such as immune complex formation and complement activation, are involved in endothelial injury and local inflammation, influence LDL uptake by regulating cholesterol metabolism, and affect the functional integrity (compliance) of the vessel, thereby promoting an atherogenic milieu. The upregulated CD40–CD40L interactions in SLE potentially influence many processes, ranging from promoting inflammatory processes to contributing to thrombus formation.

Other links between SLE and atherosclerosis involve sources of injury to the endothelium, such as homocysteine, and contributions to local inflammation and plaque vulnerability by the effects of chronic viral infections. CRP, an acute-phase reactant commonly measured in inflammatory autoimmune diseases such as RA and SLE, is now known not to be an innocent bystander but an active participant. CRP activates complement, increases the inflammatory response, enhances uptake of LDL into macrophages, and induces monocyte production of tissue factor, leading to plaque formation and thrombosis. The enhancement of macrophage uptake of ox-LDL by antiphospholipid antibodies recognizing ox-LDL–beta2-glycoprotein-I complexes illustrates how the propensity of autoantibodies in SLE may influence various atherogenic processes. Furthermore, macrophage uptake of LDL may be modulated by hyperlipidemia as well as genetic factors related to SLE (Kao et al., 2003).

4. Hormone replacement therapy

Hormone replacement therapy (HRT) is treatment with estrogen alone or in combination with progestin to compensate for the decrease in natural hormones that occurs at menopause. HRT has been shown to increase BMD, but data supporting reduction of vertebral and nonvertebral osteoporotic fractures with HRT are inconsistent. After the publication of the Heart Estrogen/Progestin Replacement Study (HERS) results in 1998 (Hulley et al., 1998), recommendations for HRT use changed dramatically. Experts advocated HRT only in women with menopausal symptoms or in women with documented osteoporosis or osteopenia who were at relatively low risk for breast cancer (Kim and Kwok, 2003). In July 2002, the Women's Health Initiative (WHI) study was halted early when the study demonstrated that combination estrogen/progestin increased the risk of CHD and breast cancer in women with and without known CHD. In March 2004, the study also halted the estrogen-alone portion of the trial when data revealed significantly increased risk of stroke and deep vein thrombosis in postmenopausal women (Humphries and Gill, 2003).

Almost all autoimmune diseases are more common in women, but the female predominance in SLE is particularly strong. At least 85% of patients with SLE are women. Reduced androgen levels, increased 16 alpha-hydroxylation of estradiol, and increased prolactin levels have been reported in SLE patients. Additional evidence that hormonal differences may contribute to the increased risk of SLE experienced by women comes from experimental studies in mouse models of SLE demonstrating disease exacerbation by estrogen and prolactin and amelioration by androgens. In the NZB/NZW F1 murine model of SLE, females have earlier onset of more severe disease and greater antibody formation, as well as earlier mortality compared with their male counterparts. Furthermore, castration of male NZB/NZW F1 in mice accelerates disease and estrogen treatment further potentiates this effect (Roubinian et al., 1977, 1978; Elbourne et al., 1998).

IL-1 is produced predominantly by monocytes and macrophages. In addition to being a mediator of innate immunity, it is also a stimulator of bone resorption. Acceleration of bone resorption is the principal contributing factor to osteoporosis in postmenopausal women. Treatment with estrogen and progesterone for 1 month caused a decrease in IL-1 activity in nonosteoporotic and osteoporotic postmenopausal women (Pacifici et al., 1989). Alterations in IL-1 production may underlie the postmenopausal acceleration in bone loss and its inhibition by HRT. TNF-alpha also is produced by cells of monocyte and macrophage lineage and has biologic functions similar to those of IL-1. TNF-alpha is present in the local bone environment and is a potent stimulator of bone resorption. Estradiol inhibits TNF-alpha release and may be a part of the mechanism by which it exerts a protective effect on the skeletons of postmenopausal women.

The safety of hormone therapy in SLE remains an area of controversy except for lupus patients with antiphospholipid antibodies, in which estrogens are contraindicated.

There are concerns that estrogen administration to SLE patients may trigger an increase in disease activity, including the exacerbation of lupus-like disease in animal models and epidemiologic data in humans. Epidemiologic data include the strong female predominance observed in lupus, with onset occurring during the childbearing years, and the association between postmenopausal hormone therapy and an increased risk for subsequent development of SLE (Sanchez-Guerrero et al., 1995). The prospective Nurses' Health Cohort Study reported an increased relative risk for the development of SLE in a cohort of nurses exposed to HRT. The calculated age-adjusted relative risk of development of SLE on patients who received HRT was 2.1 (95% CI: 1.1–4.0). A proportional increase in the risk of SLE related to the duration of HRT was also observed. Although this study suggested a linkage between HRT and SLE onset, it did not give information on whether HRT exacerbates the disease in patients with preexisting SLE (Mok et al., 1998).

Given the improved prognosis for SLE, more women with SLE survive to undergo menopause. Few studies have explored SLE activity in postmenopausal women. Investigators have reported a decrease in the number or severity of disease flares in female patients after menopause (Mok et al., 1999a). If the risk of developing SLE is related to estrogen exposure, disease risk would be expected to be reduced in women with early menarche. These associations have been observed in numerous epidemiologic studies of breast cancer. Cooper et al. (2002) observed earlier natural menopause among women who subsequently developed SLE compared with population-based controls, and early menarche was not related to SLE risk.

In women with SLE, the reduction of estradiol to testosterone ratio by the administration of cyproterone acetate reduces the episodes of exacerbation. Mok et al. (1999b) reported significantly fewer flares ($p = 0.03$) and severe flares ($p = 0.01$) among patients with cyclophosphamide-induced ovarian failure when compared with patients who were still menstruating and concluded that ovarian failure with hypoestrogenemia was protective against lupus flares. In a small cohort of 30 women, Sanchez-Guerrero et al. (2001) concluded that disease activity is mild during the premenopausal and postmenopausal periods in women with SLE. A modest decrease, especially in the maximum disease activity is seen after natural menopause.

A case-control study of 16 postmenopausal patients on HRT compared with 32 controls not receiving HRT showed no difference in the rate of flares over a follow-up period of 1 year. Although no significant flares could be demonstrated in the HRT users over 12 months, patients who received HRT had more serological but less clinical relapses (Kreidstein et al., 1997). In another small study of 34 patients, the rate of flare was equivalent in a group of patients given HRT ($N = 11$) to that in patients ($N = 23$) not receiving replacement. The magnitude of the observed flares was also not significantly different between the two groups (Mok et al., 1998). A preliminary report of HRT given to a larger group of postmenopausal lupus patients ($N = 106$) also showed no exacerbation of disease activity in the 52 patients randomized to receive therapy compared to patients receiving placebo

(Sanchez-Guerrero et al., 2001), however an increased number of thrombotic events was seen. SELENA (Safety of Estrogen in Lupus Erythematosus-National Assessment) was an equivalence trial that showed that the rate of severe or mild/moderate flares in SLE was not increased by oral contraception and is thus far the only prospective trial to-date to support the safe use of oral contraceptives in SLE (Petri and Buyon et al., 2004). The use of HRT was also studied in SELENA with results not yet published.

Early menopause is often a manifestation of autoimmune conditions involving the ovary or the adrenal or thyroid glands (Hoek et al., 1997). Antiovarian autoantibodies have been detected in women with SLE (Moncayo-Naveda et al., 1989) and in women with premature ovarian failure (Luborsky et al., 1990). Cyclophosphamide treatment is often the main etiological factor of premature menopause in patients with SLE (Mok et al., 1998).

Before the conclusion of the estrogen plus progestin portion of the WHI, approximately 8 million women in the United States were taking estrogen alone, and approximately 6 million women were taking the combined hormone regimen. The use of HRT for primary and secondary prevention of CHD is no longer recommended. Although HRT is effective for the prevention of postmenopausal osteoporosis, therapy should be considered for women at significant risk of osteoporosis and who cannot take nonestrogen medications. The FDA recommends that estrogens and progestins should be used at the lowest doses for the shortest duration required to achieve treatment goals. As overall prognosis and survival for persons with autoimmune diseases especially SLE and RA has improved, attention is now being focused on complications leading to late mortality and progressive morbidity in these women.

References

Adachi, J., Benson, W.G., Brown, J., et al. 1997. Intermittent etidronate therapy to prevent corticosteroid-induced osteoporosis. New Eng. J. Med. 337, 382–387.

Adachi, J., Cranney, A., Goldsmith, C.H., et al. 1994. Intermittent cyclical therapy with etidronate in the prevention of corticosteroid-induced bone loss. J. Rheumatol. 21, 1922–1926.

Adachi, J.D., Bensen, W.G., Bell, M.J., et al. 1997. Salmon calcitonin nasal spray in the prevention of corticosteroid-induced osteoporosis. Br. J. Rheumatol. 36, 255–257.

Adachi, J.D., Bensen, W.G., Hodsman, A.B. 1993. Corticosteroid-induced osteoporosis. Semin. Arthritis Rheum. 22, 375–384.

Adachi, R., Saag, K., Emkey, R., et al. 2001. Effects of alendronate for two years on BMD and fractures in patients receiving glucocorticoids. Arthritis Rheum. 44, 202–211.

Adami, S., Fossaluzza, V., Rossini, M., et al. 1991. The prevention of corticosteroid induced osteoporosis with nandrolone decanoate. J. Bone Miner. Res. 15, 72–81.

Adams, J.S., Wahl, T.O., Lukert, B.P. 1981. Effects of hydrochlorothiazide and dietary sodium restriction on calcium metabolism in corticosteroid treated patients. Metabolism 30, 217–221.

Bentsen, Y., Jamart, J., Esselinkx, W., et al. 2001. Primary prevention of glucocorticoid-induced osteoporosis with intavenous pamidronate and calcium: a prospective controlled 1-year study comparing single infusion given once every three 3 months, and calcium. J. Bone Miner. Res. 16, 104–112.

Bessant, R., Hingorani, A., et al. 2004. Risk of coronary heart disease and stroke in a large British cohort of patients with systemic lupus erythematosus. Rheumatology 43, 924–929.

Bijlsma, J.W.J., Raymakers, J.A., Mosch, C., et al. 1988. Effect of oral calcium and vitamin D on glucocorticoid-induced osteopenia. Clin. Exp. Rheumatol. 6, 113–119.

Body, J.J., Lortholary, A., Romieu, G., Vigneron, A.M., Ford, J. 1999. A dose-finding study of zoledronate in hypercalcemic cancer patients. J. Bone Miner. Res. 14, 1557–1561.

Brixen, K.T. 2004. Teriparatide (biosynthetic human parathyroid hormone 1–34): a new paradigm in the treatment of osteoporosis. Basic Clin. Pharmacol. Toxicol. 94, 260–270.

Bruce, I.N., Gladman, D.D., Urowitz, M.B. 2000. Premature atherosclerosis in systemic lupus erythematosus. Rheum. Dis. Clin. North Am. 26, 257–278.

Buckley, L.M., Leib, E.S., Cartularo, K.S., Vacek, P.M., Cooper, S.M. 1996. Calcium and vitamin D supplementation prevents bone loss in the spine secondary to low dose corticosteroids in patients with rheumatoid arthritis: a randomized, double-blind, placebo controlled trial. Ann. Intern. Med. 125, 961–986.

Byyny, R.L. 1976. Withdrawal from glucocorticoid therapy. New Eng. J. Med. 295, 30–32.

Cohen, S., Levy, R.M., Keller, M., et al. 1999. Risedronate therapy prevents corticosteroid-induced bone loss: a twelve-month, multicenter, randomized, double-blind, placebo-controlled, parallel-group study. Arthritis Rheum. 42, 2309–2318.

Cooper, C., Coupland, C., Mitchell, M. 1995. Rheumatoid arthritis, corticosteroid therapy and hip fracture. Ann. Rheum. Dis. 54, 49–52.

Cooper, G.S., Dooley, M.A., Treadwell, E.L., StClair, E.W., Gilkeson, G.S. 2002. Hormonal and reproductive risk factors for development of systemic lupus erythematosus. Arthritis Rheum. 46, 1830–1839.

d'Elia, F.H., Larsen, A., et al. 2003. Radiographic joint destruction in postmenopausal rheumatoid arthritis is strongly associated with generalized osteoporosis. Ann. Rheum. Dis. 62, 617–623.

Del Rincon, I., Williams, K., Stern, M.P., Freeman, G.L., Escalante, A. 2001. High Incidence of cardiovascular events in a rheumatoid arthritis cohort not explained by traditional cardiac risk factors. Arthritis Rheum. 44, 2737–2745.

Dempster, D.W., Arlot, M.A., Meunier, P.J. 1983. Mean wall thickness and formation periods of trabecular bone packets in corticoid-induced osteoporosis. Calcif. Tissue Int. 35, 401–407.

Dequecker, J., Westhovens, R. 1995. Low dose corticosteroid associated osteoporosis in rheumatoid arthritis and its prophylaxis and treatment: bones of contention. J. Rheumatol. 22, 1013–1019.

Doria, A., Sheffield, Y., Wu, R., Gambari, P.F., Puato, M., Ghirardello, A., Gilburd, B., Corbanese, S., Patnaik, M., Zampieri, S., Peter, J.B., Favaretto, E., Iaccarino, L., Sherer, Y., Todesco, S., Pauletto, P. 2003. Risk factors for sub clinical atherosclerosis in a prospective cohort of patients with systemic lupus erythematosus. Ann. Rheum. Dis. 62, 1071–1077.

Elbourne, K.B., Keisler, D., McMurray, R.W. 1998. Differential effects of estrogen and prolactin on autoimmune disease in the NZB/NZW F1 mouse model of systemic lupus erythematosus. Lupus 7, 420–427.

Esdaile, J., Abrahamowicz, M., Grodzicky, T., Li, Y., Panaritis, C., du Berger, R., Cote, R., Grover, S.A., Fortin, P.R., Clarke, A.E., Senecal, J.L. 2001. Traditional Framingham risk factors fail to fully account for accelerated atherosclerosis in systemic lupus erythematosus. Arthritis Rheum. 44, 2331–2337.

Fischer, L., Schlienger, R., Matter, C., et al. 2004. Effect of rheumatoid arthritis or systemic lupus erythematosus on the risk of first-time acute myocardial infarction. Am. J. Cardiol. 93 (2), 198–200.

Gabriel, S., Crowson, C., O'Fallon, M. 1999. Comorbidity in arthritis. J. Rheumatol. 26, 2475–2479.

Gluck, O.S., Murphy, W.A., Hahn, T.J., et al. 1981. Bone loss in adults receiving alternate day glucocorticoid therapy: a comparison with daily therapy. Arthritis Rheum. 24, 892–898.

Gordon, C. 2002. Long-term complications of systemic lupus erythematosus. Rheumatology 41, 1095–1100.

Hall, G.M., Daniels, M., Doyle, D.V., Spector, T.D. 1994. Effect of hormone replacement therapy on bone mass in rheumatoid arthritis patients treated with and without steroids. Arthritis Rheum. 37, 1499–1505.

Hall, G.M., Spector, T.D., Griffin, J.A., et al. 1993. The effect of rheumatoid arthritis and steroid therapy on bone density in postmenopausal women. Arthritis Rheum. 36, 1510–1516.

Hansen, M., Podenphant, J., Florescu, A., et al. 1999. A randomised trial of differentiated prednisolone treatment in active rheumatoid arthritis: clinical benefits and skeletal side effects. Ann. Rheum. Dis. 58, 713–718.

Harris, S.T., Watts, N.B., Genant, H.K., et al. 1999. Effects of risedronate treatment on vertebral and nonvertebral fractures in women with postmenopausal osteoporosis: a randomized controlled trial. JAMA 282, 1344–1352.

Healey, J.H., Paget, S.A., Williams-Russo, P., et al. 1996. A randomized controlled trial of salmon calcitonin to prevent bone loss in corticosteroid-treated temporal arteritis and polymyalgia rheumatica. Calcif. Tissue Int. 58, 73–80.

Hodsman, A.B., Hanley, D.A., Ettinger, M.P., Bolognese, M.A., Fox, J., Metcalfe, A.J., Lindsay, R. 2003. Efficacy and safety of human parathyroid hormone (1–84) in increasing bone mineral density in postmenopausal osteoporosis. J. Clin. Endocrinol. Metab 88, 5212–5220.

Hoek, A., Schoemaker, J., Drexhage, H.A. 1997. Premature ovarian failure and ovarian autoimmunity. Endocr. Rev. 18, 107–134.

Homik, J., Suarez-Almazor, M., Shea, B., et al. 1999. Calcium and Vitamin D for Corticosteroid-Induced Osteoporosis (Cochrane review). Update Software, Oxford.

Hulley, S., Grady, D., Bush, T., et al. 1998. Randomized trial of estrogen plus progestin for secondary prevention of coronary heart disease in postmenopausal women. Heart and Estrogen/Progestin Replacement Study (HERS) Research Group. J. Am. Med. Assoc. 280, 605–613.

Humphries, K., Gill, S. 2003. Risks and benefits of hormone replacement therapy: the evidence speaks. Can. Med. Assoc. J 168 (8), 1001–1010.

Jee, W.S., Park, H.Z., Roberts, W.E., et al. 1977. Corticosteroid and bone. Am. J. Anat. 129, 477–480.

Jonsson, J., Nived, O., Sturfelt, G. 1989. Outcome in systemic lupus erythematosus: a prospective study of patients from a defined population. Medicine 68, 141–150.

Kao, A., Sabatine, J., Manzi, S. 2003. Update on vascular disease in systemic lupus erythematosus. Curr. Opin. Rheumatol. 15, 519–527.

Kim, C., Kwok, Y. 2003. Decision analysis of hormone replacement therapy after the Women's Health Initiative. Am. J. Obstet. Gynecol. 189, 5.

Kipen, Y., Buchbinder, R., Forbes, A., et al. 1997. Prevalence of reduced bone mineral density in systemic lupus erythematosus and the role of steroids. J. Rheumatol. 24, 1922–1929.

Kreidstein, S., Urowitz, M., Gladman, D., Gough, J. 1997. Hormone replacement therapy in systemic lupus erythematosus. J. Rheumatol. 24, 2149–2152.

Lane, N.E., Lukert, B. 1998. The science and therapy of glucocorticoid induced bone loss. Endocrinol. Metab. Clin. North Am. 27, 465–483.

Liberman, U.A., Weiss, S.R., Bröll, J., et al. 1995. Effect of oral alendronate on bone mineral density and the incidence of fractures in postmenopausal osteoporosis. New Eng. J. Med. 333, 1437–1443.

LoCascio, V., Bonucci, E., Imbimbo, B., et al. 1984. Bone loss after glucocorticoid therapy. Calcif. Tissue Int. 36, 435–438.

Luborsky, J.L., Visintin, I., Boyers, S., Asari, T., Caldwell, B., DeCherney, A. 1990. Ovarian antibodies detected by immobilized antigen immunoassay in patients with premature ovarian failure. J. Clin. Endocrinol. Metab. 70, 69–75.

Luengo, M., Pons, F., Martinez de Osaba, M.J., et al. 1994. Prevention of further bone mass loss by nasal calcitonin in patients on long term glucocorticoid therapy for asthma: a two year follow up study. Thorax 49, 1099.

Lukert, B.P., Johnson, B.E., Robinson, R.G. 1992. Estrogen and progesterone replacement therapy reduces glucocorticoid-induced bone loss. J. Bone Miner. Res. 7, 1063–1069.

Lukert, B.P., Raisz, L.G. 1990. Glucocorticoid-induced osteoporosis: pathogenesis and management. Ann. Intern. Med. 112, 352–364.

Lukert, B.P., Raisz, L.G. 1994. Glucocorticoid therapy induced osteoporosis. Rheum. Dis. Clin. North Am. 20, 629–651.

Major, P., Lortholary, A., Hon, J., et al. 2001. Zoledronic acid is superior to pamidronate in the treatment of hypercalcemia of malignancy: a pooled analysis of two randomized, controlled clinical trials. J. Clin. Oncol. 19, 558–567.

Manolagas, S.C., Weinstein, R.S. 1999. New developments in the pathogenesis and treatment of steroid-induced osteoporosis. J. Bone Miner. Res. 14, 1061–1066.

Manzi, S., Meilahn, E., et al. 1997. Age-specific incidence rates of myocardial infarction and angina in women with systemic lupus erythematosus: comparison with the Framingham study. Am. J. Epidemiol. 145, 408–415.

Manzi, S., Selzer, F., Sutton-Tyrell, K., et al. 1999. Prevalence and risk factors of carotid plaque in women with systemic lupus erythematosus. Arthritis Rheum. 42, 51–60.

Michel, B.A., Bloch, D.A., Wolfe, F., Fries, J.F. 1993. Fractures in rheumatoid arthritis: an evaluation of associated risk factors. J. Rheumatol. 20, 1666–1669.

Mikuls, T., Saag, K. 2001. Co morbidity in rheumatoid arthritis. Rheum. Dis. Clin. North Am. 27 (2), 283–303.

Mok, C., Lau, C., et al. 1998. Safety of hormonal replacement therapy in postmenopausal patients with syatemic lupus erythematosus. Scand. J. Rheumatol. 27, 342–346.

Mok, C.C., Lau, C.S., Ho, C.T.K., Wong, R.W.S. 1999a. Do flares of systemic lupus erythematosus decline after menopause? Scand. J. Rheumatol. 28, 357–362.

Mok, C.C., Wong, R.W.S., Lau, C.S. 1999b. Ovarian failure and flares of systemic lupus erythematosus. Arthritis Rheum. 42, 1274–1280.

Moncayo-Naveda, H., Moncayo, R., Benz, R., Wolf, A., Lauritzen, C.H. 1989. Organ-specific antibodies against ovary in patients with systemic lupus erythematosus. Am. J. Obstet. Gynecol. 160, 1227–1229.

Neer, R., Sanchez, S., et al. 2001. Effect of parathyroid hormone (1–34) on fractures and bone mineral density in postmenopausal women with osteoporosis. New Eng. J. Med. 344, 1434–1441.

Pacifici, R., Rifas, L., McCracken, R., et al. 1989. Ovarian steroid treatment blocks a postmenopausal increase in blood monocyte interleukin 1 release. Proc. Natl. Acad. Sci. USA 86, 2398–2402.

Peel, N.F.A., Moore, D.J., Barrington, N.A., et al. 1995. Risk of vertebral fracture and relationship to bone mineral density in steroid treated rheumatoid arthritis. Ann. Rheum. Dis. 54, 801–806.

Petri, M., Buyon, J. et al. 2004. Combined oral contraceptives are not associated with an increased rate of flare in SLE patients in SELENA. Presented at ACR Annual Scientific Meeting October 18, San Antonio, TX.

Petri, M., Civelek, C. 1998. Discordance of myocardial SPECT and carotid duplex in systemic lupus erythematosus (abstract). Arthritis Rheum. 41 (S), 218.

Pitt, P., Todd, P., Webber, D., et al. 1998. A double blind placebo controlled study to determine the effects of intermittent cyclical etidronate on bone mineral density in patients on long term oral corticosteroid treatment. Thorax 53, 351–356.

Pocock, N.A., Eisman, J.A., Dunstan, C.R., et al. 1987. Recovery from steroid-induced osteoporosis. Ann. Intern. Med. 107, 319.

Ramsey-Goldman, R., Dunn, J.E., Huang, C., et al. 1999. Frequency of fractures in women with systemic lupus erythematosus. Arthritis Rheum. 42, 882–890.

Ramsey-Goldman, R., Manzi, S. 2001. Association of osteoporosis and cardiovascular disease in women with systemic lupus erythematosus. Arthritis Rheum. 44, 2338–2341.

Reid, I.R., Brown, J.P., Burckhardt, P. 2002. Intravenous zoledronic acid in postmenopausal women with low bone mineral density. New Eng. J. Med. 346, 653–661.

Reid, I.R., Evans, M.C., Stapleton, J. 1992. Lateral spine densitometry is a more sensitive indicator of glucocorticoid induced bone loss. J. Bone Miner. Res. 7, 1221–1225.

Reid, I.R., Evans, M.C., Wattie, D.J., et al. 1992. Bone mineral density of the proximal femur and lumbar spine in glucocorticoid-treated asthmatic patients. Osteoporos. Int. 2, 103–105.

Reid, D.M., Hughes, R., Laan, R.F. 2000. Efficacy and safety of daily risedronate in the treatment of corticosteroid-induced osteoporosis in men and women: a randomized trial. J. Bone Miner. Res. 15, 1006–1013.

Reid, I.R., King, A.R., Alexander, C.J., et al. 1988. Prevention of steroid-induced osteoporosis with (3-amino-1-hydroxypropylidene)-1,1-bisphosphonate (APD). Lancet 1, 143–146.

Reid, I.R., Wattie, D.J., Evans, M.C., Gamble, G.D., Stapleton, J.P., Cornish, J. 1994. Continuous therapy with pamidronate, a potent bisphosphonate, in postmenopausal osteoporosis. J. Clin. Endocrinol. Metab. 79, 1595–1599.

Repa-Eschen, L. 2000. The necessity of a managed care approach for osteoporosis. In: L.V. Avioli (Ed.), The Osteoporotic Syndrome, 4th ed, Academic Press, San Diego, pp. 2–23.

Riggs, B., Seeman, E., et al. 1982. Effects of the fluoride/calcium regimen on vertebral fracture occurrence in postmenopausal osteoporosis. New Eng. J. Med. 306, 446–450.

Roman, M.J., Moeller, E., Davis, A. 2005. Early onset atherosclerosis in rheumatoid arthritis. Ann. Int. Med., submitted for publication.

Roman, J., Salmon, J., Sobel, R., Lockshin, M., et al. 2001. Prevalence and relation to risk factors of carotid atherosclerosis and left ventricular hypertrophy in systemic lupus erythematosus and antiphospholipid antibody syndrome. Am. J. Cardiol. 87, 663–666.

Roman, M.J., Shanker, B.A., Davis, A., Lockshin, M.D., Sammaritano, L., Simantov, R., Crow, M.K., Schwartz, J.E., Paget, S.A., Devereux, R.B., Salmon, J.E. 2003. Prevalence and correlates of accelerated atherosclerosis in systemic lupus erythematosus. New Eng. J. Med. 349, 2399–2406.

Roubinian, J.R., Papoian, R., Talal, N. 1977. Androgenic hormones modulate autoantibody responses and improve survival in murine lupus. J. Clin. Invest. 59, 1066–1070.

Roubinian, J.R., Talal, N., Greenspan, J.S., Goodman, J.R., Siiteri, P.K. 1978. Effect of castration and sex hormone treatment on survival, anti-nucleic acid antibodies and glomerulonephritis in NZB/NZW F1 mice. J. Exp. Med. 147, 1568–1583.

Saag, K. 2003. Glucocorticoid-induced osteoporosis. Endocrinol. Metab. Clin. 32 (1), 135–157.

Saag, K.G. 1997. Low-dose corticosteroid therapy in rheumatoid arthritis: balancing the evidence. Am. J. Med. 103 (Suppl. 6A), 31S–39S.

Saag, K.G., Emkey, R., Schnitzer, T.J., et al. 1998. Alendronate for the prevention and treatment of glucocorticoid induced osteoporosis. New Eng. J. Med. 339, 292–299.

Saag, K.G., Koehnke, R., Caldwell, J.R., et al. 1994. Low dose long-term corticosteroid therapy in rheumatoid arthritis: an analysis of serious adverse events. Am. J. Med. 96, 115–123.

Sambrook, P., Birmingham, J., Champion, D., et al. 1992. Postmenopausal bone loss in rheumatoid arthritis: effect of estrogens and androgens. J. Rheumatol. 19, 357–361.

Sambrook, P., Birmingham, J., Kelly, P., et al. 1993. Pre vention of corticosteroid osteoporosis: a comparison of calcium, calcitriol, and calcitonin. New Eng. J. Med. 328, 1747–1752.

Sambrook, P., Kotowicz, M., Nash, P., et al. 2003. Prevention and treatment of glucocorticoid-induced osteoporosis: a comparison of calcitriol, vitamin D plus calcium, and alendronate plus calcium. J. Bone Miner. Res. 18, 919–924.

Sambrook, P. 2004. Glucocorticoid-induced osteoporosis, Chapter 16, Rheumatology. 3rd ed., Elsevier, Toronto, pp. 2109–2114.

Sanchez-Guerrero, J., Gonzalez-Perez, M., et al. 2001. Effect of hormone replacement therapy on disease activity in postmenopausal patients with SLE. Arthritis Rheum. 44 (suppl.), S263.

Sanchez-Guerrero, J., Liang, M.H., Karlson, E.W., Hunter, D.J., Colditz, G.A. 1995. Postmenopausal estrogen therapy and the risk for developing systemic lupus erythematosus. Ann. Intern. Med. 122, 430–433.

Sanchez-Guerrero, J., Villegas, A., Mendoza-Fuentes, A., et al. 2001. Disease activity during the premenopausal and postmenopausal periods in women with systemic lupus erythematosus. Am. J. Med. 111, 464–468.

Sasaki, N., Kusano, E., Ando, Y., et al. 2001. Glucocorticoid decreases circulating osteoprotegerin (OPG): possible mechanism for glucocorticoid induced osteoporosis. Nephrol. Dial Transplant 16, 479–482.

Solomon, D., Karlson, E., et al. 2003. Cardiovascular morbidity and mortality in women diagnosed with rheumatoid arthritis. Circulation 107, 1303–1307.

Steinweg, K. 2002. Menopause, bone physiology, and osteoporosis prevention. Clin. Fam. Prac. 4 (1), 89.

Streck, W.F., Lockwood, D.H. 1979. Pituitary adrenal recovery following short term suppression with corticosteroids. Am. J. Med. 66, 910–914.

Symmons, P., Jones, M., Scott, D., et al. 1998. Long term mortality outcome in patients with rheumatoid arthritis: early presenters continue to do well. J. Rheumatol. 25, 1072–1077.

The American College of Rheumatology ACR 2001. Recommendations for the prevention and treatment of glucocorticoid-induced osteoporosis: 2001 update. American College of Rheumatology Ad Hoc Committee on Glucocorticoid-Induced Osteoporosis. Arthritis Rheum. 44, 1496–1503.

Thompson, J.T., Modin, G., Arnaud, C., et al. 1997. Not all postmenopausal women on chronic steroids and estrogen are osteoporotic: risk factors for osteoporosis. Calcif. Tissue Int. 61, 377–381.

Trence, D. 2003. Management of patients on chronic glucocorticoid therapy: an endocrine perspective. Primary Care; Clin. Office Practice 30 (3), 593–605.

van Staa, T., Leufkens, H., Abenhaim, L., et al. 2000. Use of oral corticosteroids and risk of fractures. J. Bone Miner. Res. 15, 993–1000.

Walsh, B., Paul, S., Wild, R., et al. 2000. The effects of hormone replacement therapy and raloxifene on C-reactive protein and homocysteine in healthy postmenopausal women: a randomized, controlled trial. J. Clin. Endocrinol. Metab. 85, 214–218.

Wallach, S., Cohen, S., Reid, D.M., et al. 2000. Effects of risedronate treatment on bone density and vertebral fracture in patients on corticosteroid therapy. Calcif. Tissue Int. 67, 277–285.

Wallberg-Jonsson, S., Johansson, H., Ohman, M., et al. 1999. Extent of inflammation predicts cardiovascular disease and overall mortality in seropositive rheumatoid arthritis. A retrospective cohort study from disease onset. J. Rheumatol. 26, 2562–2571.

Wolfe, F., Mitchell, D., Sibley, J., et al. 1994. The mortality of rheumatoid arthritis. Arthritis Rheum. 37, 481–494.

Further Reading

Roux, C., Oriente, P., Laan, R., Hughes, R.A., et al. 1998. Randomized trial of effect of cyclical etidronate in the prevention of corticosteroid-induced bone loss. J. Clin. Endocrinol. Metab. 83, 1128–1133.

Index

A

ACE-inhibitor 53
adverse effects of hormonal contraceptives 126
alpha-fetal protein (AFP) 50
anti beta 2 Glycotroptein I antibodies 111–116, 118
anti-dsDNA antibodies 49, 52
anti-La/SSB antibodies 45, 49
antinuclear antibodies 117
anti-phospholipid antibodies 45–46
anti-phospholipid antibody 44, 49
anti-rheumatic drugs 101, 103, 105, 107, 109
anti-Ro/SSA 45, 49, 50
anti-Ro/SSA antibodies 96–98
anti-U1RNP antibody 85
antimalarials 116
antiphospholipid 59, 61–63, 65, 67, 69–75
antiphospholipid antibodies 118–121
antiphospholipid antibody 129
antiphospholipid antibody and hormonal contraceptives 44, 126–130
anti platelet antibodies 114
arterial thrombosis and hormonal contraceptives 128
autoantibodies 112–115, 117–119
autoimmune disease 29–31, 33, 35, 37, 39–41, 111, 113–117, 119–121, 142, 145, 147–148, 150
autoimmune diseases 141, 143, 145, 147, 149, 151, 153, 155, 157, 159
autoimmunity 3–4, 6, 8–9, 29–30, 33–35, 40–42
azathioprine cyclosposrin-A 53–54, 115, 118

B

barrier contraception 124
Behçet disease 89
benefits of hormonal contraceptives 126

C

cardiovascular disease 161, 178–179
cervical dysplasia 147–149, 159
cesarean section 44
Churg–Strauss syndrome 88
combination oral contraceptive 123–124, 126–130
complement 45, 49–52, 54
congenital complete heart block 83
congenital heart block 20, 25–28, 45, 95
connective tissue diseases and hormonal contraceptives 129, 134–135
contraception 123, 126–127, 129, 132–136
corticosteroid 45
corticosteroids 115–116, 118, 120
cyclophosphamide 43, 53–54

D

depo-medroxyprogesterone acetate (DMPA) (Depo-provera) 123
dermatomyositis 84
diabetes 43
disorders 141–142, 144, 147, 150–151, 153–155, 157–158

E

eclampsia 52
effects of hormonal contraceptives on hemostasis 127
environmental influences 4–6, 8–9

F

female sexual 151, 157
female sexual dysfunction 150, 155, 159
fertility 29–33, 35–37, 39–43
fetal echocardiogram 45
fetal growth restriction 62, 67
fetal lung maturity 49
fetal ultrasound 48
flurinated corticosteroids 115–116

G

genetic background 116–117
gestational 43

H

HELLP syndrome 44, 51–52, 54
heparin 66–75
HLA 11–13, 18–24
hormonal contraception 123–125

hormonal contraceptives 126–130
hormone replacement therapy 170, 174, 177, 179
human chorionic gonadotropin (hCG) 50
hydroxychloroquine 47, 53, 101, 105–107
hypertension 43–45, 49, 52–53

I

immune system 118–119
imprinting 6, 8
infertility 29–37, 39–42
influences 8
intrauterine devices 123

L

lactation 101, 106
learning disabilities 115, 118–120
leflunomide 43
long term outcome of children born to patients with autoimmune disease 117
low birth weight 45
lupus anticoagulant 59, 61–62, 64–65, 67, 71, 73–74
lupus flare 47, 50–51
lupus nephritis 46, 54
lupus-prone mice 117

M

maternal mortality 43
medications 135–136
medication interactions with hormonal contraceptives 135
menopause 161–163, 174–176, 178–179
method and use effectiveness (of contraception) 123, 126
β-methasone
methotrexate 43, 53–54
(-methasone) 45
microchimerism 12–13, 21
microscopic polyangiitis 89
mixed connective tissue disease 85
mycophenolate mofetil 43, 53–54

N

necrotizing vasculitis 87
neonatal lupus 20, 24, 28, 45, 49, 95, 99, 111, 113–114, 117–121
neonatal thromboses 114
non-reversible contraception 123
non-steroidal anti inflammatory drug (NSAID) 53

O

orgasmic disorders 151, 155, 158
osteoporosis 161–167, 169–171, 173–179

P

placenta 45–46
polyarteritis nodosa 88
polymyositis 84
pre-eclampsia 43–44, 50–52
prednisone 101, 104–106
preeclampsia 62–63, 67, 69, 71, 111–112
pregnancy 43–50, 52–54, 101–109
pregnancy complication 118
pregnancy loss 45
premature delivery 112
preterm birth 45
preterm births 44, 46
progestin-only contraception 136
progestin-only contraceptives 125
progestins, generations of 125
proteinuria 48

R

Raynaud's phenomenon and estrogen 134
reversible contraception 123
rheumatoid 154
rheumatoid arthritis: effects of estrogen on 133, 162, 171, 176–179

S

secondary female sexual disorders 144–145, 148–149, 153–154, 156–157
sex differences 3–6, 8–9
small for gestational age infants 112, 114
systemic lupus erythematosus: effects of estrogen on 43, 129, 131, 134, 162, 173, 176–179
systemic lupus erythematosus and hormonal contraceptives 43, 126–131, 134, 162, 173, 176–179
systemic sclerosis 111, 120–121, 134
systemic sclerosis and estrogen 125–131, 134–136
systemic vasculitis 87, 89

T

Takayasu arteritis 86
thalidomide 43, 54

U

undifferentiated connective tissue diseases 77, 82

V

vaginitis 144–147
vasculitides 86
vasculitis 86–89
venous thrombosis and hormonal contraceptives 127
vulvar disorders 141, 144

W

Wegener's granulomatosis 87

X

X and Y chromosome 6–8
X-inactivation 6, 8